NANOPARTICLE BASED THERAPEUTICS

Volume – I

Dr. Wei Chen, Ph. D.

Copyright © 2023

All rights reserved. No part of this publication may be reproduced, distributed, or transmitted in any form or by any means, including photocopying, recording, or other electronic or mechanical methods, without the prior written permission of the AUTHOR, except in the case of brief quotations embodied in critical reviews and certain other non-commercial uses permitted by copyright law. For permission requests, write to the author, addressed "Attention: Permissions Coordinator," at the address below.

Index of Sciences Ltd.

Kemp House,

160 City Road, London.

www.indexofsciences.com

Ordering Information:

Quantity sales. Special discounts are available on quantity purchases by corporations, associations, and others. For details, contact the publisher at the address above.

Printed in the United Kingdom

ISBN: 9-798-86050793-7

Preface

The straightforward format of this book makes it an easy read. It is written in a straightforward and clear style, making it accessible to a broad audience of students and academics. The areas covered in this book include the Photodynamic therapy, as well as Microwave induced photodynamic therapy. This book provides an overview of Cancer and discusses the use of the Cancer Resistance and Therapy.

In this book, different phases and management of X-ray induced photodynamic therapies are described and also studied the Chemodynamic therapy. Sonodynamic therapy is also explained in detail in this book.

This is a fairly unique book in terms of the depth and complexity with which the subject is discussed. Tables, equations, and approximately one hundred illustrations are used to illustrate the data.

About the Author

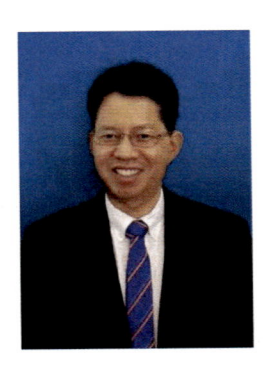

Professor Chen, Wei

Wei Chen, Ph.D., graduated from the School of Earth Sciences, Jilin University, received a master's degree from Central South University and a Ph.D. degree from the School of Chemistry, Peking University. After postdoctoral research at The University of Science and Technology at Beijing, he worked at the Institute of Semiconductors of the Chinese Academy of Sciences as a senior scientist and became a deputy director of the Materials Key Laboratory.

He won the president of the Academy of Sciences Outstanding Fund and the Academy of Sciences Young Scientist Award. From August 1998 to May 1999, he was a senior visiting scholar in the Department of Materials Chemistry, Lund University, Sweden; from June 1999 to March 2000, he was a senior researcher at the Center for Chemical Physics, University of Western Ontario, Canada. From 2000 to 2006, he worked at Nomadics Inc. and was the leader of the nanotechnology research group. He joined the University of Texas at Arlington as an assistant professor in 2006 and is now a full professor in the Department of Physics, the University of Texas at Arlington. He has been engaged in cutting-edge nanotechnology research for many years and is an internationally renowned expert in nanomedicine and cancer nanotechnology. He is well known for his inventions in cancer nano-targeted therapy and deep cancer photodynamic therapy.

Currently, he has published 340 papers in famous academic journals such as PNAS, Nano Letters, Signal Transduction and Targeted Therapy, Advanced Materials, Advanced Functional Materials, Bioactive Materials, Materials Today Physics, presided over the compilation of 1 monograph (three volumes), and participated in the compilation of 18 monographs. With an h-index is 63, Dr. Chen's articles have been cited more than 15900 times, including one paper with 740 citations. He has 22 US patents granted and has been funded with more than 45 scientific research projects with a total funding of more than 11 million U.S. dollars. His early pioneering work on thermoluminescence of nanoparticles was adopted by Charles P. Poole Jr. and Frank J. Owens in their first Textbook 'Introduction to Nanotechnology' published in 2003. Dr. Chen's scientific research work has attracted wide attention and has been reported by the American TV program CBS.

Dr. Chen received the University distinguished record of research and creative activity award in 2020. He is one of the 35 scientists from the USA to be included in the National Academy of Inventors 2020 class of Senior Members. He was elected to be a Fellow of the International Association of Advanced Materials and a Vebleo Fellow in 2020 and a Sigma Xi full member and the fellow of Royal Society of Chemistry in 2021. Dr. Chen received the Pencis award for International Research Awards on Oncology and Cancer Research in 2021 and the scientist award from IAAM in 2022 for outstanding contribution in Nanotechnology and was elected as a fellow of National Academy of Inventors in 2022 and a fellow for the University Academy of Distinguished Scholars in 2023. Dr. Chen serves as an associate editor for Cancer Nanotechnology, Journal of Biomedical Nanotechnology and Nano Translational Medicine and as an editorial members for 20 international scientific journals.

His major contributions are summarized as below:

(1) The first to propose the concept of "nanoparticle self-lighting photodynamic therapy" for the treatment of deep cancer. Two representative papers: JNN (2006) has been cited 656 times so far and won the Best Paper Award from the American Science and Technology Press in 2017. Advanced Drug Delivery Reviews (2008) became a popular article in 2008 and 2009 and has been cited more than 741 times.

(2) Invented the fourth-generation photosensitizer copper-cysteamine. This new type of photosensitizer can generate active oxygen species in ultraviolet light, X-rays, microwaves, and ultrasound for the treatment of cancer and infectious diseases: 8 US, European, and Asian patents.

(3) The new research direction of copper sulfide (CuS) used in cancer nanotherapy technology has become a hot spot in the field of photothermal therapy. The representative paper 'Copper Sulfide Nanoparticles for Photothermal Ablation of Tumor Cells' (Nanomedicine, 2010, 5:1161) ranked 384 among 123573 articles in the category of 'Biotechnology Applied Microbiology' from 2010 to 2014 (Web of Science). It has been cited 618 times so far.

(4) The invention of a new type of cancer treatment, Microwave Induced Photodynamic Therapy (MIPDT), which won a US patent, has also become an important research hotspot.

Contents

Preface 3
About the Author 4
Chapter -1 8
Introduction to Cancer 8
Chapter-2 20
Photodynamic Therapy 20
Chapter 3 94
X-ray induced photodynamic therapy 94
Chapter 4 132
Microwave induced photodynamic therapy 132
Chapter 5 182
Sonodynamic Therapy 182
Chapter 6 199
Chemo dynamic Therapy 199
Chapter 7 236
Photothermal Therapy 236
Chapter 8 261
Hypoxia and Therapy 261
Chapter 9 290
Cancer Resistance and Therapeutic Strategies 290
Chapter 10 316
Targeting and delivery 316

Chapter -1

Introduction to Cancer

Cancer is a set of diseases with more than 100 cancer types that involve the uncontrolled growth of cells, as well as the ability to invade or spread to other parts of the body. The symptoms and signs can include lumping, abnormal bleeding, prolonged cough, unexplained weight loss, and changes in bowel movements. Although these symptoms may show cancer, they may also have other causes. Although epidemiology, incidence rates, and the study of who gets cancer and why are not covered in this class, they are critical. Old age is a condition that makes people susceptible to cancer. More people today have cancer and die of it than have in the past.

Cancer mortality
- lung cancer, 31%
- prostate cancer, 10%
- colorectal cancer, 8%
- pancreatic cancer, 6%
- liver & intrahepatic bile duct, 4%
- leukemia, 4%
- esophageal cancer, 4%
- bladder cancer, 3%
- non-Hodgkin lymphoma, 3%
- kidney cancer, 3%
- other, 24%

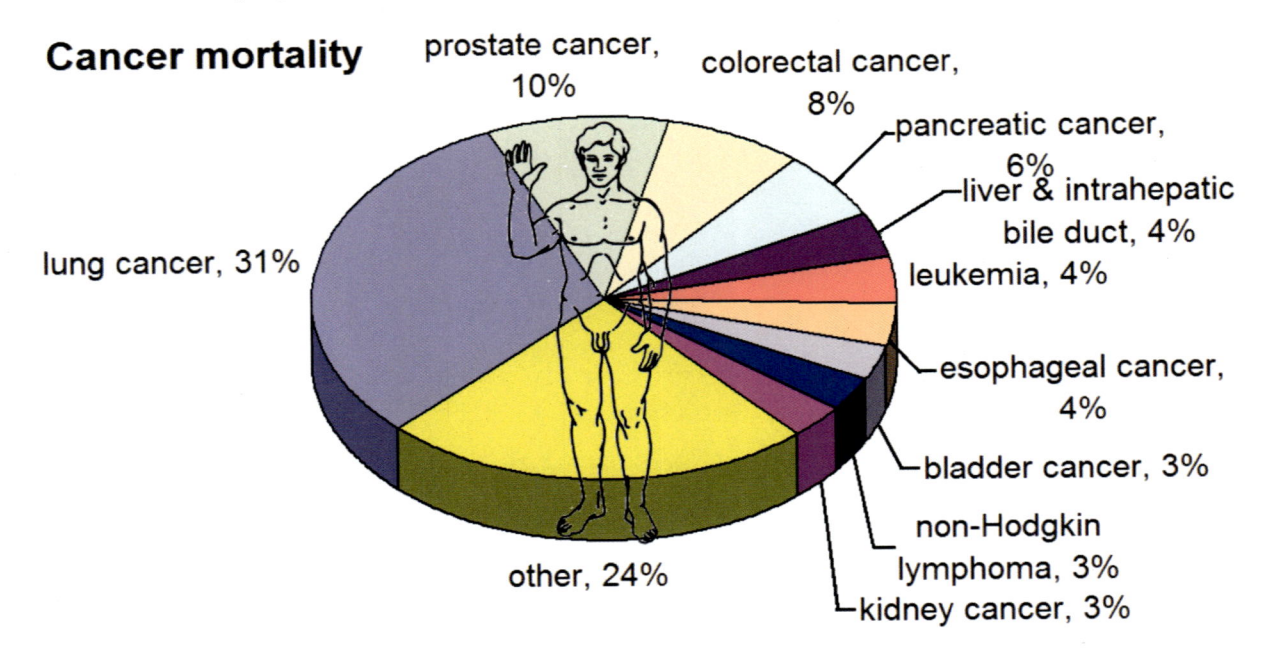

Figure 1-1 Cancer Classification and Mortality Image from Kleinsmith, Principles of Cancer Biology, (adopted with permission from ref. 1)

Figure 1-1 shows the Cancer Classification and Mortality. The following is a list of the most frequently diagnosed cancers in the United States, excluding nonmelanoma skin cancers:

- Bladder Cancer
- Breast Cancer
- Colon and Rectal Cancer
- Endometrial Cancer
- Kidney Cancer
- Leukemia
- Liver
- Lung Cancer
- Melanoma
- Non-Hodgkin Lymphoma
- Pancreatic Cancer
- Prostate Cancer
- Thyroid Cancer

This list was compiled using cancer incidence and mortality statistics from the National Cancer Institute and other sources. The estimated annual incidence in 2021 had to be at least 40,000 cases to be included on the list of common cancers.

Breast cancer is the most prevalent type of cancer on the list, with 284,200 new cases expected in the United States in 2021. Prostate and lung cancers are the next most common types of cancer.

Because colon and rectal cancers are frequently referred to collectively as "colorectal cancers," the list includes both cancer types. Colon and rectal cancers are expected to increase by 104,270 and 45,230 new cases, respectively, for a total of 149,500 new cases of colorectal cancer in 2021.

Types of Cancer

Cancer is classified into over a hundred distinct diseases based on a variety of criteria. In this section, we categorize cancers into four broad categories based on a few key characteristics.

Carcinomas

Carcinomas are tumours that are found on the epithelial cell layers that line various organs. About 80% of cancer-related deaths are caused by carcinomas. A tumour that originates in sheets of cells lining a cavity, like the lining of the skin or the esophagus, is referred to as a squamous cell carcinoma. Secretory cell tumours that originate in a glandular duct and secrete substances into the cavity they line are known as adenocarcinomas.

Although carcinomas can occur anywhere on the body, you may frequently hear people discuss the following common types of carcinoma:

- Basal cell carcinoma
- Squamous cell carcinoma
- Renal cell carcinoma
- Ductal carcinoma in situ (DCIS)
- Invasive ductal carcinoma
- Adenocarcinoma

Basal cell carcinoma: This is the most prevalent type of cancer. It is found in the cells that line the deepest part of the outer layer of the skin. You should seek treatment for basal cell carcinoma as soon as possible to avoid scarring. However, this type of carcinoma rarely spreads to other parts of the body.

Basal cell carcinomas frequently resemble the following:

- Sores that are still open
- Patches of red
- Pink enlargements
- Bumpy or scarred areas

Squamous cell carcinoma: The second most common type of skin cancer is squamous cell carcinoma. Cancerous cells develop from the flat, squamous cells that make up the epidermis, the skin's outermost layer. Squamous cell carcinomas typically grow slowly and rarely spread, but they are more likely than basal cell carcinomas to invade fatty tissue beneath the skin or to spread further.

Renal cell carcinoma: The most common type of kidney cancer is renal cell carcinoma. Cancerous cells typically develop in the lining of the kidney's very small tubes, called tubules. These cells may aggregate and form an obstruction over time. Cancer can develop in one or both kidneys.

Ductal carcinoma in situ (DCIS): The most common type of breast cancer is ductal carcinoma in situ.

Cancerous cells are contained within the milk duct lining and have not spread through the duct walls into surrounding breast tissue.

Invasive ductal carcinoma: This type of breast cancer begins in a milk duct and spreads to the breast's fatty tissue. It has the potential to spread to other parts of the body via the lymphatic and bloodstream systems.

Sarcomas

Tumours formed in connective tissue cells form sarcomas. Only 1% of human clinical tumours are sarcomas. The tumours originate from mesenchymal (muscle, fat, bone, cartilage, and nerve) cells such as bone, muscle, fat, cartilage, and nerve cells.

Sarcomas are classified into more than 70 subtypes. Sarcoma treatment varies according to the type, location, and other factors of the sarcoma.

Leukemias

Leukemias and lymphomas are cancers that arise as a result of abnormal blood cell growth. Malignancies of the blood, including erythrocytes, plasma cells, and lymphocytes, comprise hematopoietic malignancies. Leukemia, which can be either a blood or bone marrow disease, is a liquid tumor that consists of uncontrolled growth of white blood cells throughout the bloodstream. Lymphomas are solid masses made of lymphoid cell clusters that are formed in lymph nodes.

Leukemia, in general, refers to cancers of the white blood cells. WBCs are critical components of the immune system. They defend your body against bacteria, viruses, and fungi, as well as abnormal cells and foreign substances. WBCs in leukaemia do not function normally. Additionally, they can divide too rapidly, eventually crowding out normal cells.

Although the majority of WBCs are produced in the bone marrow, certain types are also produced in the lymph nodes, spleen, and thymus gland. WBCs are formed in the bone marrow and circulate throughout the body in the blood and lymph (fluid that circulates through the lymphatic system), concentrating in the lymph nodes and spleen.

Lymphomas

Lymphoma is a type of cancer that begins in the immune system's infection-fighting cells called lymphocytes. These cells are found throughout the body, including the lymph nodes, spleen, thymus, and bone marrow. When a person has lymphoma, lymphocytes undergo mutations and grow out of control.

Lymphoma is classified into two subtypes:

1. Non-Hodgkin: This is the most common type of lymphoma.
2. Hodgkin

Types of Cancer Treatment

Figure 1-2 Five Year Survival rates by cancer type reported in 2009 and the rates are mainly the same as today. There are numerous cancer treatment options. The type of treatment you receive will be determined by the type of cancer and its stage. Certain cancer patients will receive only one treatment. However, the majority of patients receive a combination of treatments, such as surgery in conjunction with chemotherapy and/or radiation therapy. When you require cancer treatment, there is a great deal to learn and consider. It is perfectly natural to feel overwhelmed and perplexed. However, speaking with your doctor and becoming informed about the various treatment options available to you can help you feel more in control.

Cancer is treated with surgery (by removing cancerous cells), radiation (by damaging cancer cells and causing them to die), and medicine (slowing down or killing cancer cells). As we discuss oncogenic processes, it is inevitable that we will discuss the expected effects of radiation and chemotherapy on cancer cells. Additionally, as we discuss metastasis, we will inevitably discuss when surgery will be effective.

In addition, we will introduce new therapeutics that are under development, such as photodynamic therapy, photothermal therapy, and Chemodynamic therapy.

Tumour level: dysplasia, invasion, and metastasis

Tumours develop from healthy tissues as illustrated in Figure 1-3. The primary tumour is the tumour from which the cancer develops, and cancer types are classified according to the tissue in which the primary tumour was discovered. Thus, liver cancer refers to cancer that began in the liver, even if the cancer spreads to other parts of the body. Cancer is highly variable in a variety of ways, including the host tissue's nature, and cancers derived from distinct primary tissue sources behave differently. Tumour is a term that refers to an abnormal cell mass. This mass is caused by abnormal cell growth, which is described in a variety of ways.

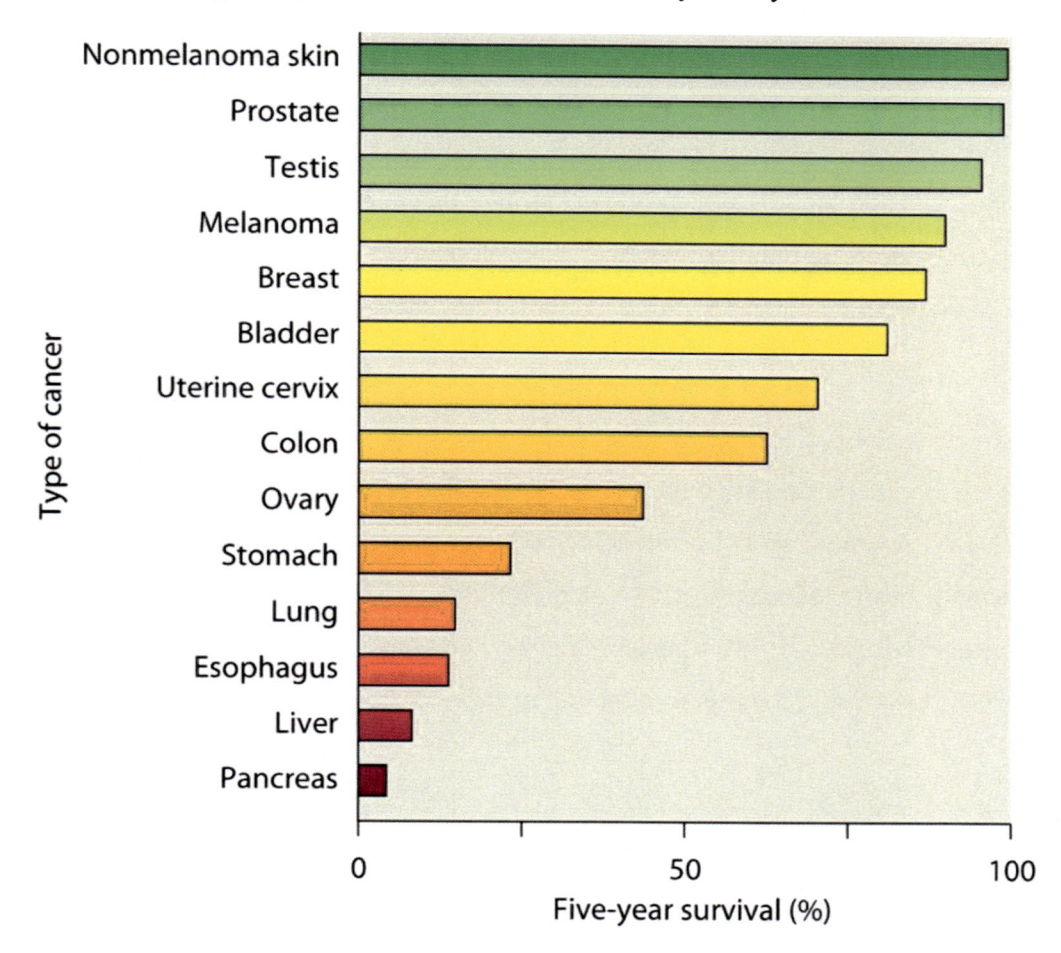

Figure 1-2 Five-year survival rates 1995–2000 by organ of origin.

Image from Kleinsmith, Principles of Cancer Biology, **(adopted with permission from rfe.2)**

Hyperplasia

Hyperplasia is an increase in the number of cells in a given area caused by uncontrolled proliferation. However, hyperplasia implies that the cells appear normal. Hyperplasia is frequently the initial stage of tumor growth. Hyperplasia results in an increase in the number of cells.

Dysplasia

Dysplasia is the next stage of tumour development. Typically, this indicates that cells appear abnormal and/or are located abnormally microscopically. Dysplasia is characterized by abnormal cell organization and proliferation.

Neoplasia

Neoplasia is the uncontrolled growth of cells that is not regulated by the body's physiological processes. A "tumour" or "mass lesion" is merely a "growth" or "enlargement" that is not necessarily malignant (such as a granuloma). While the term "cancer" implies malignancy, benign and malignant neoplasms exist. A neoplasm does not develop in a single way. Neoplasms are caused by a variety of different mechanisms, which complicate diagnosis and treatment.

Invasiveness

Cancer cells are characterized by their invasiveness—their proclivity to spread locally. A tumour is an uncontrolled growth of cells. A benign tumour is distinct from a malignant tumour, which is synonymous with cancer. It is not capable of invading adjacent tissue or spreading to other parts of the body, as cancer is. In the majority of cases, benign tumours have a favourable prognosis. However, benign tumours can become life-threatening if they press against vital structures such as blood vessels or nerves. As a result, they require treatment at times and do not at others.

Metastases

Cancer cells spread from the site of their formation to another part of the body. Metastasis occurs when cancer cells disperse from the primary tumour, travel through the blood or lymph system, and form a new tumour in other organs or tissues of the body. The new, metastatic tumour is identical to the primary tumour in terms of cancer type. If breast cancer spreads to the lung, for instance, the cancer cells in the lung are breast cancer cells, not lung cancer cells.

Staging

The stage of your cancer indicates the extent of the disease, such as the size of the tumour and whether it has spread. Knowing the stage of your cancer assists your doctor in the following ways:

- Recognize the severity of your cancer and your chances of survival
- Determine the most effective course of treatment for you.
- Identify clinical trials that may offer you a treatment option.

Even if cancer progresses or spreads, it is always referred to by the stage assigned at diagnosis.

The original stage is updated with new information about how cancer has progressed over time.

As a result, the stage does not change, even if cancer does.

Metastasis

Metastatic cancer occurs when cancer spreads from the site of origin to a distant part of the body. It is also referred to as stage IV (4) cancer in many types of cancer. Metastasis is the process by which cancer cells spread to other parts of the body.

When viewed under a microscope and tested in other ways, metastatic cancer cells exhibit characteristics similar to those of primary cancer, rather than those of the cells in the location of metastatic cancer. This is how physicians determine whether cancer has spread from another part of the body.

Cancer that has spread to other organs is referred to as metastatic cancer. Breast cancer that has spread to the lung, for example, is referred to as metastatic breast cancer, not lung cancer. It is treated as breast cancer at stage IV, not as lung cancer.

Drug delivery

The two most common methods of drug delivery (IV injection and oral dosing) require the drug to travel from the bloodstream to the tumour (in both cases) and from the digestive system to the bloodstream (in the case of oral drugs). Thus, understanding the interaction of tumours and the circulatory system is critical for predicting the effect of medical intervention on cancer.

Cell level

Multicellular organisms that are healthy maintain tight control over each individual cell in the body. Cancer is a disease in which cells escape this control and proliferate uncontrollably, and the majority of cancer research in the last few decades has been conducted at the cellular level.

Engineers and physicists, in particular, have the potential to have a significant impact on cancer research by expanding it to the tissue and body level. Hypertrophy, hyperplasia, dysplasia, and neoplasia are all examples of new tissue growth. Each of these growth types is related to (or can be related to) a different type of aberrant cell behaviour in a unique way. Hypertrophy refers to an increase in the size of cells, while hyperplasia refers to an increase in the number of cells.

These could be considered normal behaviour (for example muscle growth is hypertrophy while healing is hyperplasia). Dysplasia is a term that refers to abnormal, disorganized growth. Neoplasia is a term that refers to an unorganized growth pattern characterized by an increase in the number of dividing cells. Neoplasia implies the presence of a tumour. Neoplasia occurs when the balance between cell growth and death is disturbed.

Growth Factors

Normal cells proliferate and divide only in response to growth factors (e.g., EGF and PDGF from their environment). This ensures that normal cells grow only in response to instructions.

Growth factor signals are transmitted to the interior of the cell via growth factor receptors (for example, EGFR and PDGFR). Cancer cells become aberrant when their growth becomes independent of external signals, either due to erroneous growth factor receptor responses or because the cell produces its own growth factors.

When cancer cells are supposed to self-destruct, they do not.

Healthy cells have a tightly controlled programme for when to die, and the majority of cell death in humans occurs as a result of programmed, purposeful death. Necrosis, or uncontrolled death, is a relatively uncommon occurrence that typically occurs in response to injury. By contrast, apoptosis occurs continuously throughout the body and is a necessary component of both development and normal function. When cells are no longer required or are defective, they self-destruct. When cells are infected with pathogens or when their DNA is found to be defective, they self-destruct. Cells that are somehow misplaced (unable to bind in the expected manner, not receiving paracrine or endocrine signals in the expected manner) self-destruct.

On the contrary, cancer cells typically have a disrupted apoptotic programme and do not initiate apoptosis. This has a significant effect, particularly on the cellular DNA. Due to the fact that cells with DNA mutations self-destruct, the genetic integrity of the cells is maintained. Cancer cells, on the other hand, frequently have mutations in the proteins that monitor DNA integrity and induce apoptosis when that integrity is compromised. As a result, cancer cells do not self-destruct when they should, and cancer cells can develop significant DNA disruptions.

Many of the cancer cells have damaged or destroyed genetic information.

Mutations in DNA spontaneously arise during DNA replication because it is not always perfect.

Additionally, mutagens cause mutations to occur at a higher frequency.

When large-scale mutations are included, cancer cells display gross chromosomal abnormalities that are different from healthy cells. In addition, cancer cells exhibit gross chromosomal abnormalities, unlike healthy cells, which are diploid. Large-scale mutations make cancer cells different from healthy cells in addition to altering the gross chromosomal structure. In some cases, this leads to incorrect repairs of DNA, which is referred to as chromosomal translocation.

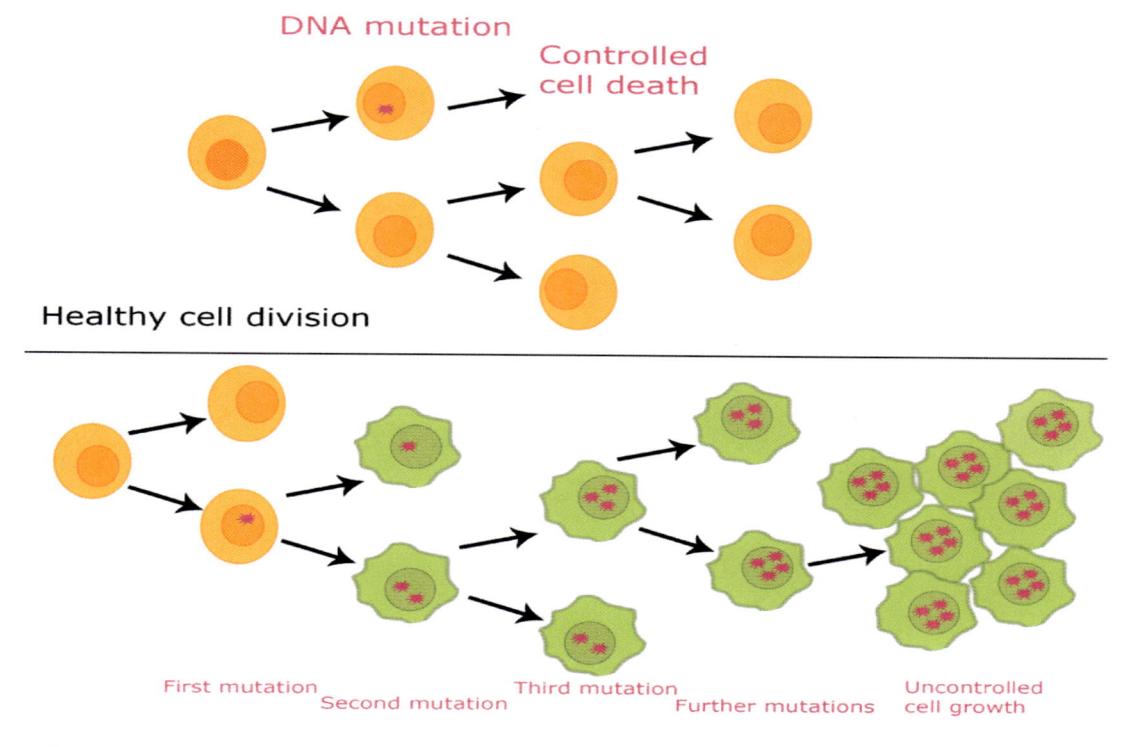

Figure 1-3 Heathy cell and cancer cell division and development, adopted from ref. 3 with permission

With sporadic cancers, many mutations build up in cells over time, eventually leading to cancer.

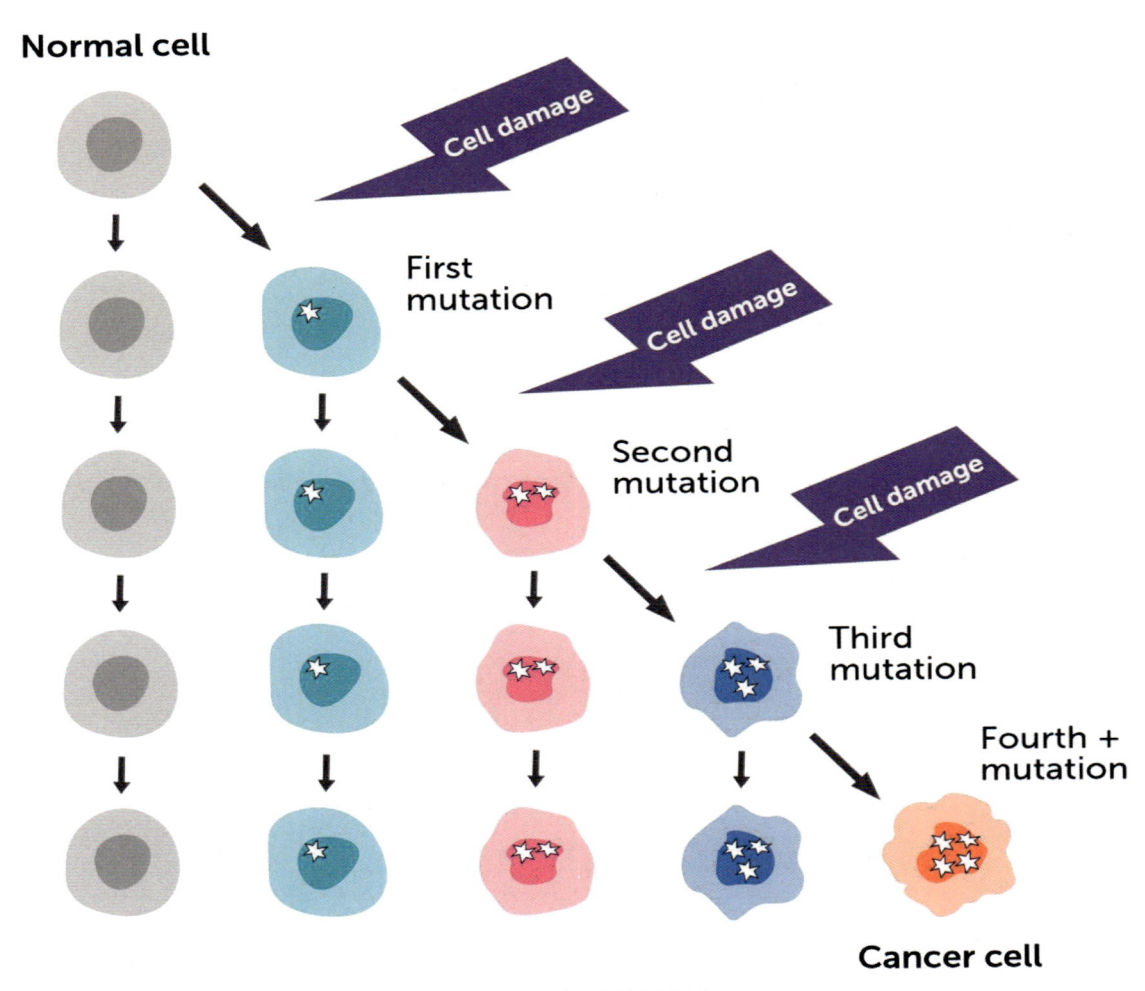

Adapted from "Understanding Gene Testing" - NIH 1995

Figure 1-4 Cell Mutation and Cancer Development

Changes in molecular adhesiveness, paracrine signaling, and angiogenesis are frequently observed in cancer cells.

New molecular changes are observed in cancer cells. Gap junction proteins are decreased, while cell adhesion proteins are reduced. These play a role in making cancer cells less adhesive. Cancer cells secrete factors that help promote angiogenesis, while at the same time, secreting proteases that help degrade their surroundings. Cancer is a complex system with a multitude of causes, but it is limited by the observable symptom of uncontrolled and invasive growth that occurs at the cellular level. It is possible that many of the phenomena that lead to cancer may also lead to other system failures – such as the loss of a person's life during development or death during infancy. The process is referred to as cancer when something in an organism is working correctly, but then localized uncontrolled growth results in disease.

Cancer is a disease characterized by abnormal cell growth and unrestricted cell replication. Cancerous cells form tumours, and as these tumours metastasize, they support angiogenesis, resulting in greater hypoxia in the area. This means that identifying cancer based on the properties of cancer cells and tumours can be used for diagnostic and therapeutic purposes.

References for this chapter

1. Epidemiology of cancer https://en.wikipedia.org/wiki/Epidemiology_of_cancer
2. **Lewis J. Kleinsmith,** Principles of Cancer Biology, 1st edition Published by Pearson (November 1, 2005) © 2006
3. Cancer Management through Genomics Study, https://stayrelevant.globant.com/en/technology/healthcare-life-sciences/cancer-management-through-genomics-study/

Chapter-2

Photodynamic Therapy

2.1 Photodynamic therapy – General Introduction

A treatment that combines light energy with a photosensitizer is called photodynamic therapy (PDT). Photochemicals are activated by light of a specific wavelength, such as from a laser. The photosensitizers themselves are nontoxic, however, as the photosensitizers become toxic after light activation.

Photocarcinogenesis and multiple other photodynamic diseases are commonly treated with medications that use a variety of photosensitizers, including those for acne, psoriasis, age-related macular degeneration, and multiple cancers, such as skin, lung, brain, bladder, pancreas, bile duct, esophagus, head and neck.

Additionally, PDT helps to treat infections caused by bacteria, fungi, and viruses. Studies show that this light-based therapy has the potential to engage the body's immune system, thereby increasing the number of cancerous and precancerous cells the body is capable of destroying.

Photodynamic therapy is used to diagnose and treat a variety of conditions, including the following:

- Pancreatic Cancer
- Cancer of the bile ducts (cholangiocarcinoma)
- Esophagus Cancer
- Certain skin conditions, such as precancerous changes of the skin (actinic keratosis) and nonmelanoma skin cancer
- Lung Cancer

Photodynamic therapy (PDT) was discovered over a century ago (in 1900) by chance observation of microorganisms (Paramecia) being killed when exposed to both a photosensitizing dye (acridine) and sunlight simultaneously. However, for the majority of that time period, PDT was studied and developed as an anticancer therapy, not an antimicrobial therapy. Although the mechanism of action has been studied in detail, it is still not fully understood. It is a process that begins with the absorption of a photon of light (with a wavelength matching the dye's absorption band) and ends with the dye (also called a photosensitizer, PS) being excited to its short-lived (nanoseconds) excited singlet electronic state.

This singlet-state PS can undergo an electronic transition (spin-flip) to a much more stable triplet state with a much longer lifetime (microseconds). Due to the triplet PS's longer lifetime, it can react with ambient (ground state) oxygen via one of two distinct photochemical pathways, Type I or Type II. The type I involves electron transfer to generate superoxide radicals ($•O_2^-$) and then hydroxyl radicals (HO•), whereas the second type involves energy transfer to generate excited state singlet oxygen ($^1O_2$). Both HO• and $^1O_2$ are extremely reactive oxygen species (ROS) capable of causing significant damage to nearly all types of biomolecules (proteins, lipids, and nucleic acids) and cell death. The Jablonski diagram (Figure 2-1) illustrates the photochemical generation of various ROS during PDT and their broad-spectrum antimicrobial activity. The Jablonski diagram illustrates the PS energy levels in their ground state, excited singlet state, and triplet state configurations (top of Figure 2-1).

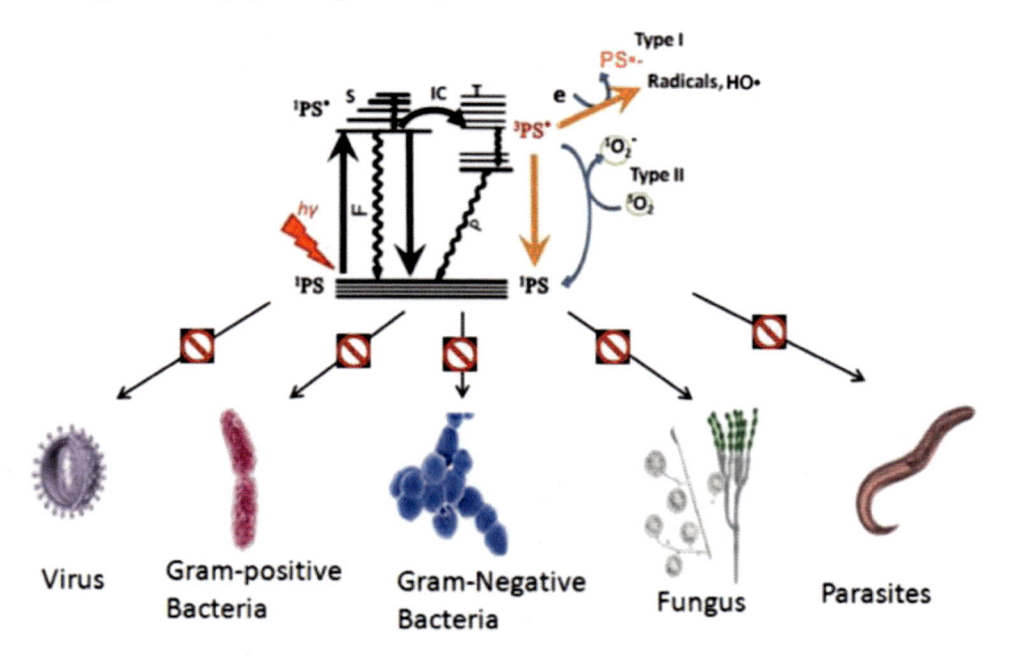

Figure 2-1 **Jablonski diagram showing photochemical pathways in aPDI**

The ground state 1PS absorbs a photon to form excited singlet state 1PS* that can undergo intersystem crossing (IC) to form the triplet state 3PS*. This long-lived species can undergo energy transfer (Type II) to form singlet oxygen $^1O_2$ or electron transfer (Type I) to form hydroxyl radicals HO•. Both these ROS are capable of killing a broad spectrum of pathogens. (adopted from ref. 1 Curr Opin Microbiol. 2016, 33: 67–73 with permission)

As previously stated, PDT was investigated as a cancer therapy for many years by developing PS that could be administered systemically (via intravenous injection) or topically (e.g. aminolaevulinic acid), and then the tumour would be irradiated with light (either as a surface spot or by insertion of interstitial fibre optics). However, beginning in the 1990s, it was recognized that PDT could also exert a potent antimicrobial effect if PS could be engineered to bind selectively to microbial cells while remaining non-toxic to host mammalian cells.

The best way to accomplish this goal of antimicrobial photodynamic inactivation (aPDI) was to ensure that the PS had a strong cationic charge, as microbial cells in general have a higher negative charge than mammalian cells, and cationic PS will bind selectively to them. Additionally, PS binding to microbial cells is rapid, whereas cationic PS uptake by mammalian cells is slow, resulting in high selectivity when a short drug-light interval (a few minutes) is used.

The advantages of aPDI as a potential clinical antimicrobial therapy were bolstered when it was discovered that it works equally well regardless of the microbial cells' antibiotic resistance status and, additionally, that aPDI has not been shown to produce resistance in bacteria even after 20 consecutive cycles of partial killing followed by regrowth. Additionally, aPDI has the advantage of being applied topically or locally to the infected area. Numerous chronic infections are caused by the formation of microbial biofilms, which systemically administered antibiotics cannot penetrate. However, it has been demonstrated that aPDI can kill biofilm-grown cells *in vitro* and *in vivo*.

This anti-biofilm technique has been found to be particularly effective against dental infections such as periodontitis and peri-implantitis. Additionally, infections in burns or damaged tissue have a compromised blood supply, which means that antibiotics administered systemically do not reach the infection site in sufficient concentrations. aPDI kills microbial cells rapidly (seconds), whereas antibiotics take hours or days to act, providing a potential advantage against rapidly spreading infections such as necrotizing fasciitis. Additionally, the broad-spectrum nature of aPDI enables treatment to be initiated prior to the identification of infectious agents.

Although many infections occur deep within the body, it is now possible to deliver PS and light to virtually any anatomical region via endoscopes, narrow-diameter interstitial needles, and fibre optics.

The optimal molecular design of an antimicrobial PS (aPS) should incorporate a number of distinct characteristics. First, the aPS must be non-toxic in the dark, particularly to mammalian cells. Second, they should have a high quantum yield of reactive oxygen species production and a high molar absorption coefficient at a wavelength that allows for good tissue penetration (red and near-infrared).

Thirdly, aPS should exhibit selectivity for microbial cells over mammalian host cells, particularly when incubation times are short (short drug-light interval). Fourthly, and perhaps most importantly, an aPS should contain cationic charges, which are best provided by quaternary nitrogen atoms or basic amino groups.

Polycationic conjugates

It was previously established that an overall cationic charge was required for an antimicrobial PS to be effective (especially for one that is required to kill many logs of Gram-negative bacteria).

As a result, attaching a photochemically efficient PS to a polycationic polymer with a large number of them made sense.

Fullerenes

Fullerenes are allotropes of closed-cage carbon with a roughly spherical shape and a diameter of about 1 nm. Due to their highly conjugated double bonds, they absorb visible light well and generate a high quantum yield of the triplet state and reactive oxygen species (ROS) when illuminated.

Although fullerenes in their natural state are extremely hydrophobic, insoluble in water, and prone to aggregation, when functionalized with cationic groups, they become water-soluble and rather specific for binding to microbial cells.

A variety of cationic fullerenes were evaluated *in vitro* and *in vivo* in animal models of localized infection. The advantages of fullerenes as antimicrobial PS are their high photostability and ability to generate highly toxic hydroxyl radicals, while the disadvantage is that the excitation light is of a relatively short wavelength and thus does not penetrate very well into tissue. This limitation may not be significant for topical applications to infected areas.

Bacteriochlorins

Bacteriochlorins (BCs) are tetrapyrroles with two double bonds reduced (1 in each of two opposing pyrrole rings), making them tetrahydroporphyrins. When a porphyrin's double bond is reduced to form a chlorin, the long-wavelength band is redshifted and enlarged, and when a second double bond is reduced to form a BC, the effects on the absorption are even more pronounced. For effective light penetration into living tissue, strong long-wavelength absorption bands are required.

The only remaining requirement is for the BC to contain quaternary cationic groups that facilitate the binding and penetration of bacterial cells. Interestingly, we discovered that an asymmetric di-cationic BC was significantly more active against Gram-positive bacteria and fungi than a symmetrically substituted tetra cationic BC (which was only effective against Gram-negative bacteria), presumably because the molecular asymmetry allowed for greater penetration into the bacterial cells. This difference was most noticeable in eukaryotic fungal cells.

Without a doubt, the most frequently used antimicrobial PS are the phenothiazinium dyes, such as methylene blue and toluidine blue. Both of these compounds have received regulatory approval for aPDI in a variety of countries worldwide. Nonetheless, these compounds are not carcinogenic and highly active, and numerous laboratories have attempted to introduce compounds with significantly higher activity, or alternatively, naturally occurring dyes that are supposed to be easier to pass regulatory hurdles.

The cationic zinc phthalocyanine RLP068, the cationic phenalenone derivative SAPYR, and the porphyrin Sylsens B are notable examples of synthetic high activity compounds. A cationic hypericin compound derived from St John's Wort, a cationic riboflavin compound derived from vitamin B2, and a cationic derivative of curcumin (a yellow spice found in turmeric) known as SACUR-3 are all examples of compounds derived from natural products.

Potentiation by inorganic salts

Azide

To quench the singlet oxygen produced during PDT, sodium azide has been used widely. Contrary to expectations, we discovered that adding azide to methylene blue (MB), aPDT did not inhibit but rather enhanced bacterial killing. The addition of azide enhanced the killing of other phenothiazinium dyes and cationic fullerenes. Although azide's ability to enhance microbial photo-killing is intriguing from a mechanistic standpoint, azide's toxicity precludes clinical application.

Iodide

Given that the azide ion-mediated potentiation involves the photochemical production of azidyl radicals via an electron transfer mechanism, we investigated the possibility that the non-toxic salt potassium iodide could be used to enhance antimicrobial PDI mediated by MB. Photoproduction of reactive iodine radicals was demonstrated to be the mechanism. Potentiation with iodide is also used to enhance the activity of aPDI mediated by cationic fullerenes such as LC16.

Bromide

Neither phenothiazinium dyes nor cationic fullerenes demonstrated any enhancement of microbial killing when bromide anion was added. However, antimicrobial photocatalysis mediated by UVA excited titanium dioxide nanoparticles (a semiconductor with a large bandgap) can be enhanced by the addition of bromide, resulting in the production of hypobromite as a byproduct.

F. PDT of infections in animal models

Bioluminescent microbial imaging

Contag and colleagues pioneered the use of genetically engineered bioluminescent microbial cells (that glow in the dark) in combination with a low-light imaging camera to enable real-time, non-invasive monitoring of the progression and response to treatment of localized infections.

This technology laid the groundwork for the now widely used bioluminescence imaging protocols, which enable real-time, non-invasive, longitudinal imaging of a variety of disease states in a variety of fields of biomedical research.

PDT of infections

We used this bioluminescence imaging technique to demonstrate aPDT's efficacy in a variety of different animal models of localized infections. When the bacterial strain is particularly virulent and invasive (as is the case with Pseudomonas aeruginosa), timely administration of aPDT may prevent mice from dying of systemic sepsis.

In 2015, the O'Neill's report issued dire predictions that by 2050, antibiotic resistance acceleration could result in 300 million additional deaths and cost an additional US$100 trillion. Given that the antibiotic era is widely believed to be nearing an end and the likelihood of discovering novel classes of antibiotics is considered to be rather remote, it is critical to develop alternative antimicrobial technologies to which bacteria cannot develop resistance and that work equally well regardless of current resistance status.

aPDT will play a significant role in the development of this new armamentarium that is unavoidably occurring in the twenty-first century. This grand endeavor will benefit from novel PS, novel photochemical potentiation strategies, and useful animal models for testing.

2.2 A Comprehensive Review of Photodynamic Therapy

Since antiquity, light has been recognized as having healing properties, with phototherapy dating all the way back to 3000 B.C. Historically, sunlight exposure was used to treat a variety of ailments, ranging from mood and mental health problems to locomotor abnormalities and skin diseases. The infrared spectrum, ultraviolet radiation, and electromagnetic induction discoveries, together with the advent of artificial light sources, all contributed considerably to the development of modern phototherapy.

Oscar Raab, a medical student working with Professor Hermann von Tappeiner, created photodynamic treatment (PDT) more than a century ago. He discovered that paramecia that had been cultured with a fluorescent dye and exposed to light died, whilst those kept in the dark were unaffected. The phrase "photodynamic response" was coined by Von Tappeiner for the first time.

Despite being recognized since early 1900, PDT's clinical application dates from the 1970s. Thus, PDT is a non-invasive, cutting-edge technology for identifying and treating a variety of disorders. PDT is a promising treatment method for a wide variety of malignancies and non-oncological disorders because to its spatiotemporal selectivity, and its antibacterial impact makes it useful for non-clinical applications as well.

PDT has acquired popularity as a result of the positive interplay between light, photosensitive chemicals (referred to as photosensitizers), and oxygen. The primary advantages of PDT over conventional treatment options such as chemotherapy, radiation, and surgery include improved cosmetic outcomes, minimal functional disruptions, good patient tolerance, fertility preservation, and minimum systemic toxicity.

However, significant disadvantages persist, primarily due to the use of classic organic photosensitizers. Nanotechnology can be used to improve PS's solubility, optical absorption, and tumour targeting capacity. In this regard, nanoplatforms have been developed to enhance the efficiency of existing photosensitizers.

This article will discuss the biophysical mechanics underlying PDT, the evolution of photosensitizers, and the role of nanomaterials in achieving exceptional PDT therapy performance. Additionally, an in-depth examination of present and emerging PDT applications was conducted.

The Photodynamic Therapy Principle of Action

PDT is a type of light treatment that is unique in that it utilizes three primary components: a photosensitizer (PS), a light source, and molecular oxygen. The three primary types of light sources used in PDT are lasers, light-emitting diodes, and lamps, with the type selected based on the target location, absorption spectrum of the photosensitizer utilized and required light dose. When exposed to sufficient light, the non-toxic photosensitizing substance deposited at the target spot becomes activated, absorbing and transferring electrons, while the in situ discovered oxygen molecules operate as electron acceptors. Thus, harmful reactive oxygen species (ROS) are created, causing irreversible damage to microbes and target tissues by membrane rupturing and cell death via necrosis or apoptosis.

ROS are classified into two broad categories, each of which corresponds to a separate PDT mechanism (Figure 2-2). Oxygen radicals are formed via electron transfer (e.g., superoxide anion $O_2^{·-}$, hydroxyl radical $HO^·$, hydroperoxyl radical $HOO·$), whereas singlet oxygen is formed via energy transfer ($^1O_2$). The transition of PS molecules from the ground state to the singlet excited state and then to the triplet excited state is referred to as the type I mechanism. The excited PS molecules then interact with the substrate via electron transfer to create free radicals. In contrast, in the photodynamic reaction of type II, excited PS molecules combine with molecular oxygen to form highly active singlet oxygen, which then interacts with lipids, proteins, and nucleic acids, ultimately inducing cell death by necrosis or apoptosis.

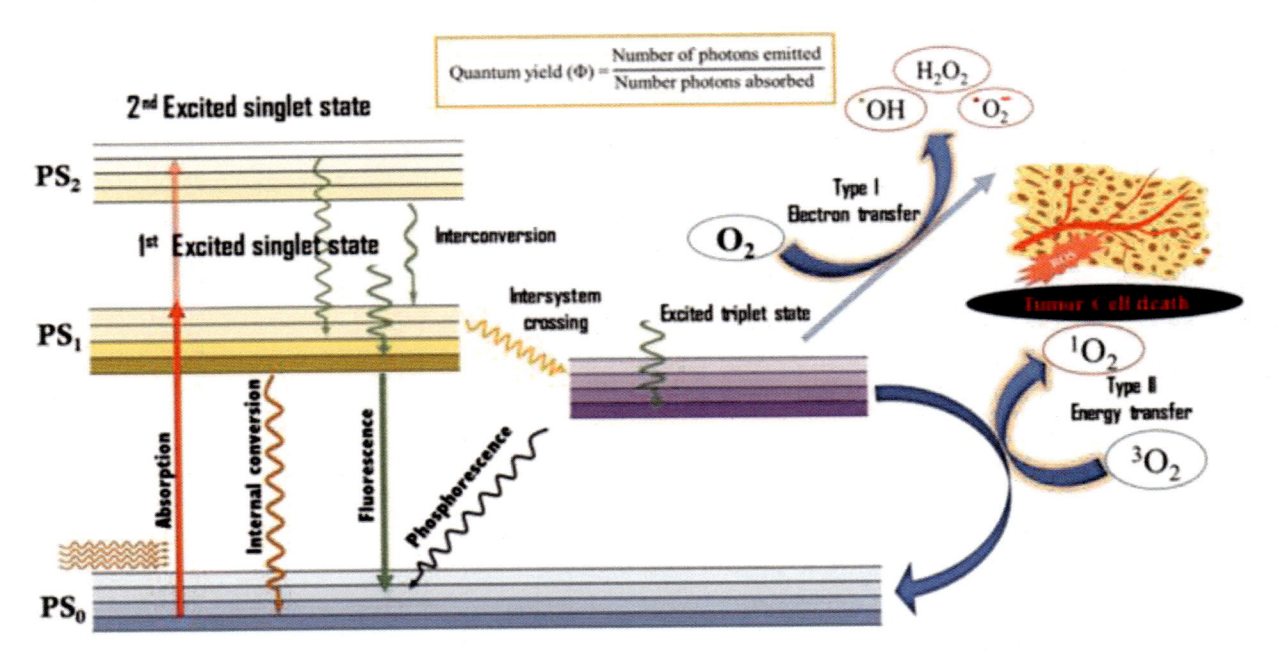

Figure 2-2. Schematic illustration of the mechanism of photodynamic treatment (PDT), adopted with permission from ref. 2

Photosensitizers

Apart from light and oxygen, one of the critical components of PDT is the presence of photosensitizers. The intrinsic features of these chemicals dictate their therapeutic efficacy, as PSs can absorb light of a certain wavelength and initiate photochemical or photophysical reactions. A perfect PS should be chemically pure and uniform in composition, be an efficient ROS generator, accumulate selectively in target tissue in the absence of radiation, absorb light in the long-wave part of the spectrum (600–850 nm, referred to as the "phototherapeutic window"), be stable in solution, serum, or plasma, and be easily eliminated from the organism.

Photosensitizers, in the form of water-soluble mixtures of hematoporphyrin derivative (HpD), were first tested for their utility in commercial photodynamic treatment in the 1970s. More than 1000 naturally and synthetically produced PSs have been identified. The creation of PSs has seen centuries of iteration, where each generation strives to find optimum optical and biological qualities.

The first generation of PSs is based on several versions of HpDs that have been utilized in clinical studies on thousands of patients for over 30 years. Photofrin (Axcan Pharma, Mont-Saint-Hilaire, QC, Canada) was the first clinically licensed PS and has been used to treat numerous forms of cancer, including non-small cell lung, bladder, esophagus, and brain cancer. Despite their widespread use, first-generation PSs have a number of drawbacks. Due to their low chemical purity, these PSs can be activated efficiently only at wavelengths below 640 nm, limiting tissue penetration. Additionally, the prolonged half-life of PSs causes the skin to become hypersensitive to light for several weeks, necessitating that patients treated with them remain in a dark room for up to six weeks. To address these constraints, it became critical to build a new generation of PSs.

As a result, research on the next generation of photosensitizers began in the late 1980s. PSs of the second generation are composed entirely of pure synthetic chemicals that contain an aromatic macrocycle (e.g., porphyrins, benzoporphyrins, chlorins, bacteriochlorins, and phthalocyanines). Temoporfin (Foscan®, Biolitec, Gina, Germany), motexafin lutetium (Lutex®, Pharmacyclics, Sunnyvale, CA, USA), palladium bacteriopheophorbide (Tookad® soluble, Negma-Lerads, Elancourt, France), tin ethyl etiopurpurin (Purlytin®, Miravant, in comparison to first-generation PSs, these porphyrinoid compounds exhibit increased tumour selectivity and penetration into deep-lying tissues, owing to their absorption spectra in the 650–800 nm range. Additionally, they are excreted from the body more rapidly, resulting in fewer side effects and less time (less than two weeks) spent in a dark room by the patient. However, their primary disadvantage is their low water solubility. Under physiological settings, this feature causes second-generation PSs to congregate, lowering the yield of ROS production. Additionally, the hydrophobic nature precludes intravenous administration, necessitating the development of novel drug delivery systems. As a result, it was necessary to develop a new generation of photosensitizers to simplify transport and cell absorption, thereby improving treatment effects.

The third-generation PSs are being developed with the primary goal of synthesizing structures having a better affinity for the target cells. Typically, these PSs contain a second-generation PS or a photoactivatable medication coupled to or encapsulated in biodegradable/biocompatible NPs. As a result, the stability and hydrophilicity of PSs are raised, the pharmacokinetics, pharmacodynamics, and biodistribution of PSs are improved *in vivo*, undesirable side effects are decreased, and dark toxicity is controlled. Despite significant advancements over the last decade, third-generation PSs are still in development. Difficulties in administering PSs to children limit the general clinical application of PDT, and new drug delivery systems are an important demand for boosting the photodynamic method's bioavailability.

Photodynamic Therapy Using Nanomaterials

Integrating PSs with nanotechnology was identified as a highly promising strategy for increasing therapeutic effectiveness while researching novel techniques to improve PDT. Nanomaterials have lately emerged as a critical component of PDT, enabling enhanced results in terms of selective targeting, high drug loading, multifunctional integration, increased solubility of hydrophobic PSs, preservation of a steady PS delivery rate, and decreased toxicity to healthy cells.

The high surface-to-volume ratio of NPs is one of their enticing properties. This feature enhances loading capacity, which results in increased concentration delivery and uptake by target cells. NPs' small size also enables them to imitate biological molecules, which enables these nanocarriers to easily pass-through immune system barriers. Additionally, their surface can be functionalized with specific ligands that are recognized exclusively by specific receptors, with this unique match serving as the trigger for drug release.

In this regard, PSs may be encapsulated in or immobilized on nanoplatforms and given to the tumour selectively. A number of nanostructures can be used for this purpose, including dendrimers, micelles, liposomes, quantum dots, nanoparticles, and antibody–drug conjugates.

A promising strategy is represented by metal-based NPs capable of transporting and delivering hydrophobic PSs to tumoral tissues via the increased permeability and retention (EPR) effect. In comparison to conventional photosensitizers, metal-based NPs have a long cycle time, a moderate rate of degradation, and a focused and regulated release, making them ideal candidates for PDT.

Gold is a suitable material for metallic NPs due to its low toxicity, inertness, and outstanding biocompatibility. Additionally, its affinity for thiol and amine groups makes surface functionalization with ligands such as antibodies, proteins, nucleic acids, and polysaccharides simple. Gold nanocages, nanorods, and nanoshells are regarded as dazzling photo response structures because they are capable of sensitizing singlet oxygen production and creating reactive oxygen species (ROS) that can kill cancer cells [69]. Gold nanoclusters have been shown to be an excellent carrier for the administration of clinically authorized PSs, allowing for spatiotemporal control and minimizing undesired side effects.

Silver is another element of interest in PDT because it possesses antibacterial characteristics in addition to its capacity to create singlet oxygen. The huge specific area of silver NPs increases the surface area of this substance in contact with bacteria or viruses, improving its bactericidal impact. Additionally, when utilized as nanocontainers for PSs, these particles exhibit a bimodal effect, enhancing the efficacy of fault detection and pathogen isolation.

Copper sulphide NPs are commonly utilized in PDT because they are inexpensive, simple to produce, and easily functionalized on the surface. CuS NPs also exhibit photothermal and photodynamic capabilities, which, when combined with their low cytotoxicity, make them ideal for eradicating germs from infected wounds. CuS nanodots can also be used as a template for nanotheranostics due to their high biocompatibility.

Titanium dioxide can also operate as a photosensitive agent, generating singlet oxygen when exposed to light. These NPs attracted attention due to their changeable bandgap, band location, outstanding photostability, low toxicity, strong catalytic activity, abundance, and low cost. TiO_2 NPs, either alone or in combination with other chemicals, have been successfully used in PDT to treat malignant tumours and inactivate antibiotic-resistant bacteria.

Manganese oxide-based nanoplatforms for drug delivery have also been demonstrated to be successful in PDT. MnO_2 nanosheets can renew oxygen in the tumour microenvironment via a reaction with H_2O_2, while also consuming glutathione to boost anticancer activity. Additionally, these materials exhibit high PS absorption capacity and biocompatibility, which are desirable characteristics for PS carriers.

Additionally, molybdenum oxide, zinc oxide, and tungsten oxide NPs, yttrium oxide NPs, ruthenium nanomaterial complexes, transition metal dichalcogenide nanosheets, and transition metal carbides nanosheets and NPs are purportedly employed in PDT.

Another appealing alternative to conventional PDT is the encapsulation of PSs in silica NPs. Despite the fact that silica is not active, it has several properties that make it a good candidate for this light-based therapy, including nontoxicity, chemical inertness, and optical transparency. Mesoporous silica NPs have been extensively employed as nanocarriers for hydrophobic PSs, most notably zinc phthalocyanine, in this regard.

Carbon-based nanomaterials have also generated substantial interest in the realm of PDT research. Their unique optical and mechanical qualities, superior biocompatibility, low toxicity, variable chemical functionalization, improved permeability effect, and capacity to generate ROS make them ideal for cancer PDT and antimicrobial photodynamic inactivation. Carbon nanotubes, fullerenes, and graphene-based nanomaterials are the most widely used allotropic forms of carbon.

Carbon nanotubes have generated interest for PDT applications due to their unusual structure and properties. Single-walled carbon nanotubes, in particular, have been investigated as potential sensitizers in cancer therapy due to their efficiency as delivery vehicles for hydrophobic PSs.

Fullerenes can also be utilized as PSs due to their beneficial qualities, which include their capacity to perform photochemistry, their ability to self-assemble into supramolecular fullerosomes, and their strong resistance to photobleaching. Additionally, fullerene derivatives can be used to deliver medications specifically to the nuclear pore complex and tumour vasculature.

Nanomaterials based on graphene, such as graphene quantum dots, graphene oxide, and reduced graphene oxide, have also been used in cancer therapy, either for anticancer drug delivery or for PDT. The capacity of graphene quantum dots to generate singlet oxygen in particular can be used to eliminate harmful germs and cancer cells. Polymeric NPs' adaptability and diversity have garnered attention in PDT. Their capacity to shield pharmaceuticals from initial degradation, boost drug permeability into targeted tissue, and reduce systemic toxicity increased the attractiveness of polymer-based nanosystems over free medications. The chosen class of such materials is biodegradable polymers, as they release the PS cargo when destroyed by the biological environment. Numerous topologies have been developed as delivery systems for photo-based cancer treatment, ranging from linear and branching to crosslinked polymers.

Polyacrylamide is an example of a suitable polymer for PDT use (PAA). PAA NPs can be functionalized with amine or carboxyl groups, a targeting moiety, and/or polyethylene glycol, as well as loaded with actuating molecules, making them ideal for tumor-selective PDT. PAA NPs are very soluble in water, making them ideal vehicles for the delivery of PSs such as methylene blue, Photofrin, 5,10,15,20-tetrakis(1-methyl-4-pyridinio) porphyrin tetra(p-toluenesulfonate) (TMPyP), and Temoporfin (m-THPC).

Due to its biodegradability and ease of formulation, poly (D,L-lactide-co-glycolide) (PLGA) has also garnered interest for PSs encapsulation. The photoactivity of PLGA NPs loaded with PSs was found to be greater than that of free PDT medicines against breast tumour and ovarian cancer cells.

Dendrimers have been used in PDT for PS delivery due to their highly branched structure and monodispersity. Additionally, dendrimer-based delivery vehicles benefit from increased permeability, sustained drug release, high solubility, high loading capacity, and enhanced colloidal, biological, and shelf stability. Dendrimers were specifically used as carriers for 5-aminolevulinic acid (ALA), an FDA-approved precursor of a PS used in topical PDT.

Natural polymers, like as proteins and polysaccharides, can be converted into NPs that are effective for PDT. Human serum albumin, bovine serum albumin, xanthan gum, alginate, chitosan, and gelatin are only a few of the materials that have been studied for PDT.

Additionally, lipid-based nanostructures can be useful in PDT. Liposomes may be a promising targeted delivery nanosystem since they can contain and assist the penetration of unstable PSs to and through the cell membrane. PS administration through liposomes was found to be effective against metastatic melanoma, breast cancer, skin cancer, and tumor-derived angiogenic vascular endothelial cells.

Another possibility is to mix PSs with low-density lipoproteins (LDL), particularly given the high number of LDL receptors on the surface of tumour cells. Studies have demonstrated that covalently bonding PS to LDL prior to injection results in increased PDT efficiency as compared to free PS delivery.

Organic–inorganic hybrid materials, such as nanoscale metal–organic frameworks (MOFs), have also been identified as promising PDT delivery platforms. Their versatility is a result of their chemical composition, well-defined crystalline structures, high surface-to-volume ratio, high porosity, low density, regular channel, changeable aperture, and various architecture and tailoring. MOFs have been successfully used to treat a variety of cancers.

Applications of Photodynamic Therapy

PDT has attracted significant interest in treating both malignant and non-malignant disorders due to its non-invasive nature. PDT has been used in a variety of medical sectors for the last 40 years, from oncology to dermatology, urology, ophthalmology, and dentistry, and has been shown to be effective in treating a wide variety of disorders.

Cancerous Diseases

PDT was developed as a promising alternative to the invasive nature of prior anticancer therapeutic techniques (e.g., radiotherapy, chemotherapy, and surgery). The primary advantage of PDT is its selectivity for tumoral tissues, with minimal harm to non-malignant cells. PDT can kill cancer cells in three ways: directly by raising ROS production, indirectly by shutting down tumour blood arteries, and indirectly by stimulating the patient's immune system by increasing cancer cell-derived antigen presentation to T cells.

PDT was initially tested on humans in 1976, when it was used to treat patients with bladder cancer. Following that, encouraging responses were observed in early-stage patients with lung, esophagus, and gastric carcinomas. PDT was then used to treat a variety of different cancers and cancer types, including brain tumours, intraocular cancer, breast cancer, head and neck cancer, pancreatic cancer, and gynecological tumours.

PDT can be used to treat both melanoma and non-melanoma skin cancers, the latter of which are classified into two subgroups: basal cell carcinoma (BCC) and squamous cell carcinoma (SCC) (SCC). Melanoma develops from pigment-producing cells (melanocytes) and is the most aggressive kind of skin cancer, prone to grow and spread if left untreated. As a result, it is critical to recognize this disease early and to provide therapy immediately. PDT is a therapy option for melanoma. However, certain obstacles remain, including improved tumour targeting and the requirement for near-infrared absorbent PSs.

Non-melanoma skin cancers, on the other hand, are most frequently found in areas exposed to the sun. BCC begins in the epidermis's lowest layer (which is composed of basal cells) and grows slowly, with a low potential for metastasis. SCCs, on the other hand, are more prone to enter deeper layers of the skin and spread to other parts of the body, but this is quite uncommon. Nonetheless, these tumours should not be left untreated in order to avoid spreading to neighboring sites and causing multicentric, synchronic, and metachronic lesions. PDT has been shown to give the best optimal cosmetic and functional outcomes in this regard. However, individuals treated in this manner should be closely followed because an incomplete response and relapse are still possible.

Breast cancer is the most prevalent type of carcinoma in females, accounting for the majority of cancer-related deaths in women globally. Breast cancer treatment begins with a mix of chemotherapy medicines, radiation therapy, and surgical intervention. Nonetheless, medications do not enter tumour tissue sufficiently, resulting in systemic adverse effects. Once these disadvantages are overcome, PDT is viewed as a promising, safe, and minimally intrusive therapy. Additionally, if only a portion of a tumour with a known and limited extent is visible on an MRI scan, PDT treatment is significantly easier to repeat than traditional therapies.

Lung cancer is one of the top three malignancies in the United States in terms of diagnosed cases and deaths. While chemotherapy is the most often used therapeutic technique, cancer cells develop drug resistance and eventually cease to respond to therapy. Consequently, a new treatment approach must be implemented, either as a backup to chemotherapy or as the primary treatment modality. PDT has a lengthy track record of clinical effectiveness in this regard, having been licensed by the FDA for the ablation of microinvasive endobronchial non-small cell lung cancer (NSCLC) that is not amenable to other treatments, as well as totally or partially obstructive endobronchial NSCLC.

Cervical cancer is the fourth most frequent malignancy in women worldwide, both in terms of incidence and fatality rate. Conventional therapy options for this condition create adverse effects such as pain and bleeding, and can even impair individuals' reproductive capacity, which do not occur when PDT is used.

Prostate cancer, on the other hand, is one of the most common types of cancer among males globally. Unfortunately, the majority of prostate tumours are detected in advanced stages, when the prognosis is poor due to pathophysiological alterations and an insufficient response to treatment. To address these limitations, PDT was developed as a substitute, and several PSs have been evaluated in the clinic for focused prostate tumour ablation.

PDT was found to be helpful in the treatment of gastrointestinal tract tumours, with esophageal, gastric, liver, pancreatic, and colorectal cancers being treated. The primary benefits of PDT for various forms of cancer are that it is less intrusive than surgery and has a broader indication than endoscopic resection. Additionally, it can be utilized as a supplementary treatment following the failure of chemoradiotherapy on a local level.

Additionally, there has been increasing interest in the use of PDT to treat several types of brain cancers. Brain malignancies can be extremely aggressive and infiltrative, with a poor overall prognosis for patients. Tumor excision is a time-consuming and non-curative procedure that requires following chemotherapy and fractionated radiotherapy. A potential solution to these problems would be to combine fluorescence-guided surgery and PDT, which would allow for synergic tumour cell visualization and selective annihilation.

Non-Cancerous Diseases

Despite its widespread use in cancer treatment, PDT is not restricted to the destruction of tumour cells. The photodynamic effect was first proven against bacteria at the turn of the twentieth century. With the current issues of antibiotic resistance and the emergence of novel infections, it is unsurprising that PDT has garnered interest for its ability to combat bacteria, fungus, viruses, and protozoa.

Antimicrobial photodynamic treatment (also known as "photodynamic inactivation" in the literature) is a safe and cost-effective way for treating a variety of infectious infections. This is critical because skin and soft tissue lesions can readily get infected with multidrug-resistant bacteria, hence preventing appropriate healing. Additionally, traditional local treatments for infected wounds caused by burns, trauma, surgery, or disease are costly and frequently ineffective. PDT has been recommended as a therapy option for localized bacterial infections. PDT has demonstrated superior wound healing effects, increasing tissue repair by eliminating germs while simultaneously encouraging the proliferation of fibroblasts.

Dental infections are one of the fastest growing areas of antibacterial PDT in clinical practise. Photodynamic treatment has been shown to successfully eradicate pathogens found in subgingival periodontal plaques (e.g., Porphyromonas gingivalis, Fusobacterium nucleatum, and Staphylococcus spp.), both in aqueous suspension and as a biofilm.

PDT is also used to treat fungal infections. These infections are becoming more prevalent globally, in part because there are only three primary classes of antifungal medicines available for invasive infections, and treatment efficacy is dependent on the patient's immune response. Onychomycosis, one of the most common and serious nail fungal infections, is a case in point. PDT is deemed promising for treating this illness when used in conjunction with a PS and keratolytic medicines that improve the permeability of the nail plates to active agents.

PDT has been shown to be effective at inactivating mammalian viruses such as HIV, human papillomavirus (HPV), hepatitis A, B, and C viruses, herpes viruses, human parvovirus B19, human cytomegalovirus, enteroviruses, and adenoviruses. PDT became a focus of intense investigation during the pandemic as an alternate or complementary therapy option for SARS-CoV-2 infection. The photodynamic effect has the potential to disrupt the viral envelope, proteins, and RNA membrane structures. As a result, PDT is proving to be an extremely effective method of inactivating infectious pathogens.

Apart from pathogen-related disorders, PDT can also be used to treat central serous chorioretinopathy (CSC). This disorder is characterized by serous retinal detachment and retinal pigment epithelial detachment at the macula, resulting in vision impairment in low light. Numerous therapies for CSC have been offered (e.g., laser photocoagulation, carbonic anhydrase inhibitors), but they are insufficiently targeted in addressing this core choroidal vascular problem. Fortunately, PDT appears to be useful in treating CSC, as it alters the structure and permeability of the choroidal vasculature.

Additional Applications

PDT's usefulness extends beyond clinical uses. This method is advantageous for a variety of additional applications. One example is the decontamination of medical devices from biofilms. This is critical, all the more so because infected equipment can represent a major hazard to human health via nosocomial diseases. PDT can be used to repel biofilm infections from implants, such as prosthetic joint infections and infections produced by biofilms associated with ventilator-associated pneumonia.

PDT can also be used to create photoactive fabrics by integrating PSs that are activated by sunshine. Masks, suits, and gloves can be created in this manner to ensure that healthcare professionals are dressed in a sterile, safe, and decontaminated environment. Similarly, antimicrobial surfaces can be obtained to help healthcare institutions avoid infectious illness outbreaks.

PDT's targeted pathogen inactivation is advantageous for environmental water treatment. Without establishing resistance, microorganisms such as Gram-positive and Gram-negative bacteria, viruses, fungi, and parasites can be eradicated from the surface, ground, drinking water, and wastewaters.

Biotechnology is another intriguing subject in which to apply PDT ideas. For example, inactivating bacteria on the surfaces of fruits extends their shelf life, with PDT being a high-efficiency, non-thermal sterilizing method. Another advantageous application is to substitute PDT for antibiotic treatment of milk in order to eliminate microorganisms in dairy products.

The food sector can be enhanced with PDT, not just by eliminating germs within the product but also by developing better packaging. This sterilization procedure was purportedly used to produce packaging materials that limit bacterial development.

The Benefits and Drawbacks of Photodynamic Therapy

Due to its widespread use, it is obvious that PDT has a number of advantages over more traditional forms of therapy. One of the most significant is spatiotemporal selectivity, which is a result of spatial and temporal irradiation control. This property enables low invasiveness, low systemic toxicity, and minimum functional disruption.

PDT is well tolerated by patients, may be repeated at the same site, and causes little or minimal harm to target tissues inside the body when used to treat them. In addition, unlike other therapies, PDT retains fertility and has no adverse effect on pregnancy or delivery. Additionally, because ROS can cause damage to a wide variety of cells, PDT is suited for a wide variety of clinical and non-clinical applications.

While PDT is a promising and useful therapy method for a variety of illnesses, its implementation is hampered by conventional PSs. Traditional PDT's most frequently cited disadvantages include its low water solubility, limited light penetration depth, and ineffective tumour targeting. Additionally, complex scheduling, the necessity of multiple surgeries, patient supervision following treatment, and photosensitivity issues during the first few weeks following therapy are negatives. As a result, establishing a new generation of PSs is critical for the advancement and standardization of PDT in clinical practice.

Combinatorial techniques with different therapy modalities represent another way to overcome PDT's limitations (Figure 2-3). This way, the benefits of each treatment can be maximized while the drawbacks are mitigated. For example, PDT may increase the immune response to tumours, and when combined with immunotherapy, "abscopal" responses can be produced from lesions that are too deep to be effectively treated with PDT.

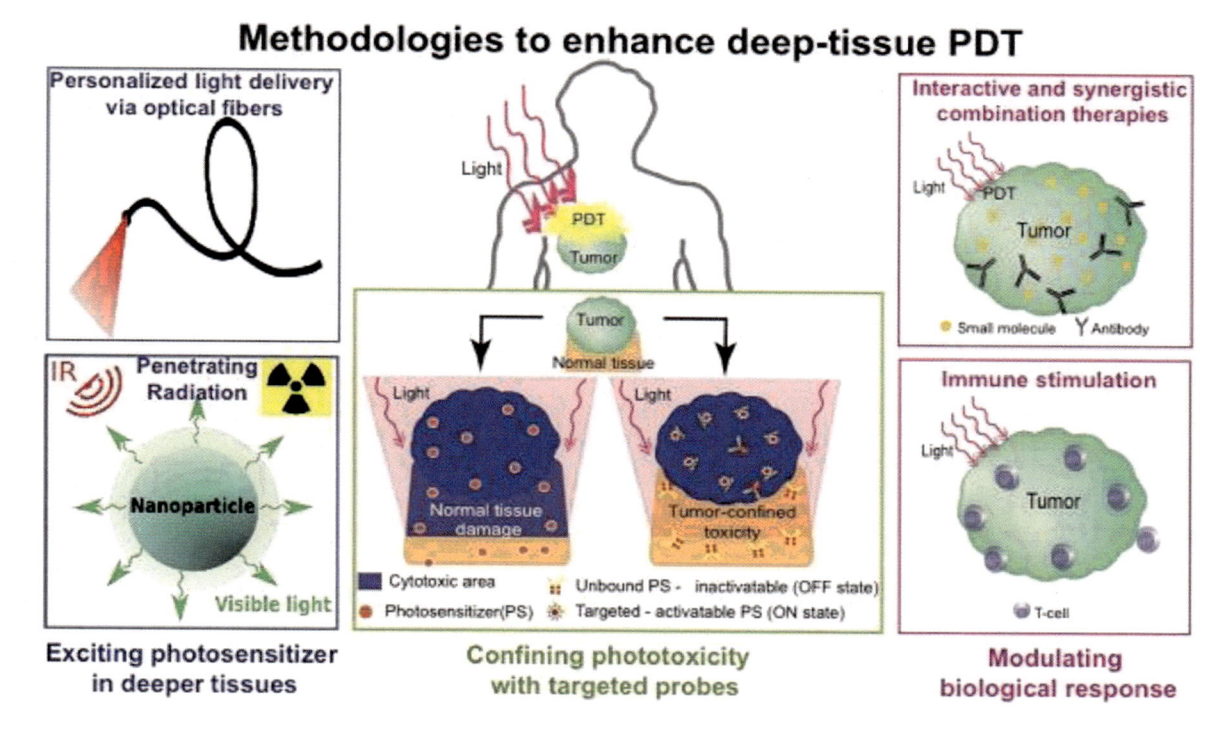

Fig. 2-3 Combinations of PDT with various treatment methods to enhance efficiency. Adopted from ref. 3 with permission

The Bottom Line

To summarize, photodynamic treatment has grown in popularity over the previous few decades, with a variety of practical applications. PDT has proven interesting for eliminating tumoral tissues, bacteria, fungi, and viruses due to its technique of creating ROS via the combined interaction of light, oxygen, and photosensitizing chemicals. Due to the non-invasive and non-toxic nature of this therapy, it has become popular for treating a variety of tumours and infections.

PDT, on the other hand, has not yet reached its full potential since conventional photosensitizers have restrictions on light absorbance, penetration depth, and cellular uptake. In this regard, research into nanotechnology-enhanced PDT has begun. Numerous materials with nanoscale dimensions were evaluated as PSs or PSs carriers, with encouraging results. Nonetheless, the majority of investigations are still in the *in vitro* testing stage, with only a few progressing to clinical trials.

Despite its ease of use, PDT has not yet reached the magnitude of conventional chemotherapy and radiotherapy. With breakthroughs in material testing and integrated multimodal platforms, recent focused research is projected to modify this aspect in the near future.

2.3 An updated evaluation of photodynamic therapy in cancer treatment

Cancer continues to be a major public health issue on a global scale. Breast cancer, in particular, is the disease with the greatest worldwide health impact. Despite recent technical advances, recurrence and metastasis remain the leading causes of death. Indeed, the significant mortality rate associated with distant metastasis in patients continues to be a barrier to effective therapy in clinic. Metastasis is a progressive and complex process in which cancer cells invade and spread to specific organs such as the lung, liver, brain, and bone. Metastatic lesions are frequently many and resistant to standard therapies, endangering the outcome of surgical resection, chemotherapy, and radiation therapy.

For thousands of years, light has been recognized as having medicinal potential. Since the Ancient, Indian, and Chinese civilizations over 3000 years ago, it has been used to cure a variety of disorders, primarily in combination with reactive chemicals, for example, to treat vitiligo, psoriasis, and skin cancer. Following the discovery of phototherapy in 1895, which earned Niels Ryberg Finsen the 1903 Nobel Prize in Physiology/Medicine for his work on the treatment of diseases, particularly lupus vulgaris, using concentrated light beams, several studies involving the use of light and chemicals arose.

Photodynamic therapy (PDT) is currently being investigated as a potential alternative treatment for malignant disorders. It is based on the uptake of a photosensitizer (PS) molecule that, when stimulated by light of a specific wavelength, combines with oxygen in target tissues, generating oxidant species (radicals, singlet oxygen, and triplet species) that cause cell death. The cytotoxic effects of PDT have been demonstrated to be caused by the oxidation of a wide variety of biomolecules in cells, including nucleic acids, lipids, and proteins, resulting in severe disruption of cell signalling cascades or gene expression regulation. As with other newly proposed treatments, there is still room for improvement, and significant resources have been devoted recently to this subject. We set out in this study to provide a comprehensive update on PDT and its implications for cancer research and treatment. We have discussed everything from the photochemical mechanisms at work to the various cell death pathways caused by a variety of photosensitizers, all the way up to the most recent preclinical studies and ongoing clinical trials.

PDT's photochemical principles and constituents

As previously stated, PDT is characterized by the photosensitized oxidation of biomolecules via two distinct pathways. In Type I reactions, light energy is transferred from excited molecules to biomolecules via electron/hydrogen transfer (radical mechanism) and results in particular damage to biomolecules and the commencement of radical chain reactions [Figure 2-4]. In contrast, the Type II mechanism transfers the excitation energy to molecular oxygen ($^3O_2$), resulting in the creation of singlet oxygen ($^1O_2$), which is exceedingly electrophilic and capable of damaging membranes, proteins, and DNA [Figure 2-4]. While direct contact reactions generally result in more severe damage to biomolecules, they also result in photodegradation of the PS, whereas diffusive species are necessary for PS replenishment. In any case, the generation of triplet excited species is critical to the PS's performance. Both tricyclic phenothiazinium salts and macrocyclic polypyrroles (porphyrins and derivatives) yield a significant number of triplets upon electronic excitation and are thus frequently utilized as PSs in PDT. Without a doubt, the outcome of PDT is highly dependent on the PS's intrinsic efficiency. Even if the quest for novel PS is primarily focused on the synthesis of chemicals that create singlet oxygen more efficiently, several aspects such as aggregation and photodegradation must be studied.

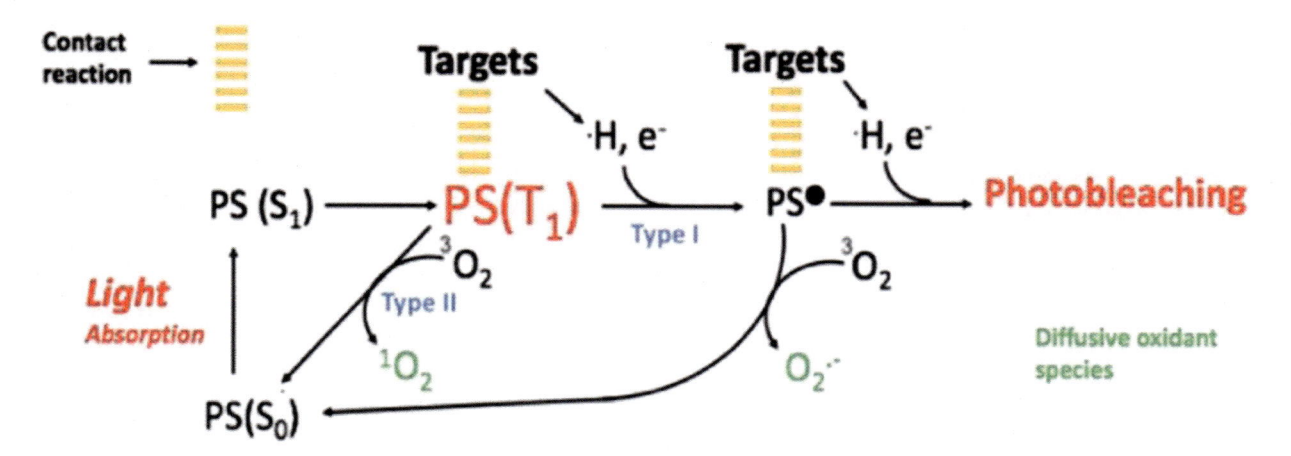

Figure 2-4. Mechanisms of photosensitization. The photosensitizer (PS), is a molecule capable to absorb energy from light in a specific wavelength. Once excited, the PS transits from its ground

state PS(S$_0$), to its singlet excited PS(S$_1$) and triplet excited PS(T$_1$) states. At this point PS(T$_1$) can react directly with biomolecules, like proteins or lipids (targets), via Type I photochemical reaction, resulting in formation of radicals, like PS•, capable to initiate radical chain reactions. Otherwise, PS (T$_1$) can react with molecular oxygen ^{3}O$_2$, via the Type II photochemical reaction. Both generates diffusive oxidant species like radical superoxide, O$_2^-$, and singlet oxygen, ^{1}O$_2$, via type I and II respectively, capable to extend the damage. Adopted from ref. 5 with permission

Protein and membrane damage is critical for optimizing the cytotoxic efficacy of PDT. Indeed, PSs with a higher degree of accumulation in the membranes of cells and/or organelles are typically more cytotoxic. Recently, the process by which photosensitized oxidation of lipids results in membrane leakage was identified. In broad terms, phospholipid alterations occur as a result of lipid peroxidation, which are reactions initiated by the generation of free radicals and singlet oxygen. After this stage, the reaction becomes autocatalytic, producing hydroperoxides and other byproducts. The essential steps in photo-induced membrane degradation are summarized in Figure 2-5. Typically, the first one includes the "ene" reaction between the lipid (LH) and singlet oxygen (produced by a type II photochemical reaction between the PS triplet PS(T$_1$) and molecular oxygen), resulting in the synthesis of hydroperoxide (LOOH). The remaining steps include direct photochemical interactions with the PS(T$_1$). Irreversible damage occurs when a hydrogen atom is extracted from an unsaturated fatty acid (LH), forming a lipid radical (L•). This one is affected by the addition of an oxygen molecule, resulting in the development of the peroxyl radical (LOO•), which is capable of reacting with another LH fatty acid, commencing a new oxidation cycle and resulting in the formation of lipid hydroperoxide (LOOH) and another L•. The propagation phase involves the peroxyl radical (LOO•) initiating a new oxidation chain and the breakdown of the lipid hydroperoxides into various intermediate radicals. The synthesis of alkoxides is catalyzed in light-induced reactions by direct contact interactions between the triplet photosensitizer, the lipid double bond, and the lipid hydroperoxide, which results in chain breakage by -scission. This reaction produces lipid truncated aldehydes and other products, which are the chemicals that initiate the leaking process. This explains the success of the experiments and offers up new options for cellular targeting tactics, which will be addressed in greater detail below.

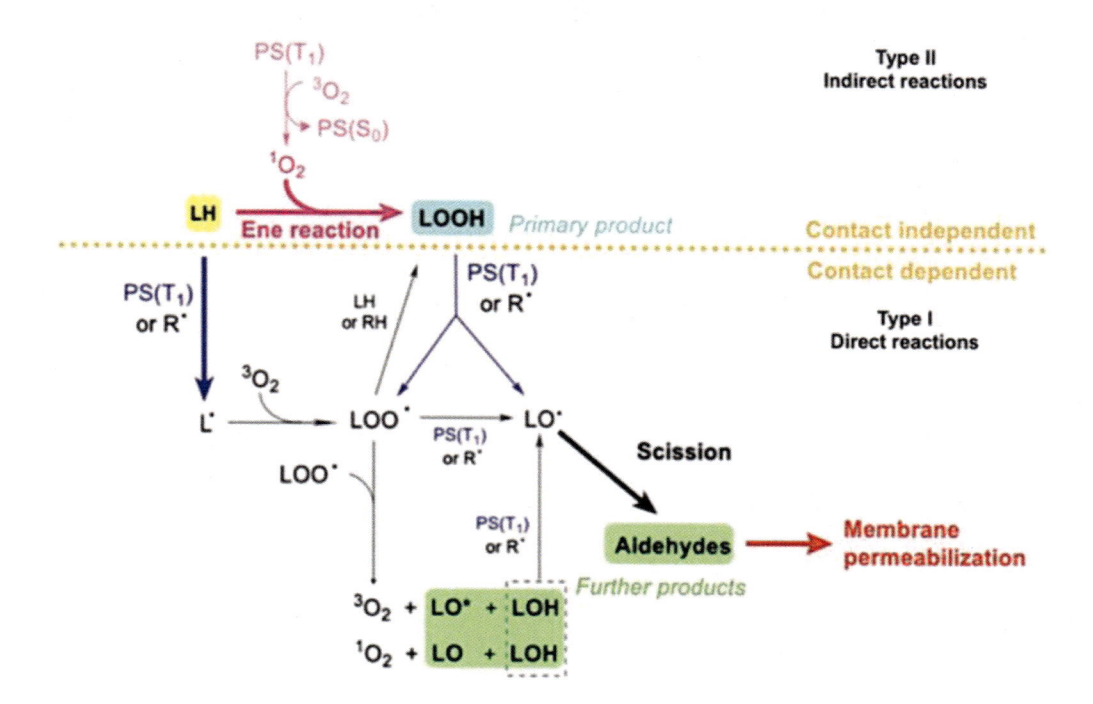

Figure 2-5. Photo-induced membrane damage mechanisms. **This diagram illustrates how photochemical reactions of Type I and Type II contribute to membrane leakage via lipid degradation. Type I reactions alter membrane fluidity as a result of direct interaction between the PS triplet [PS (T1)] and either the LH or LOOH lipid double bond. Type II reactions [PS (T1) and molecular oxygen ($^3O_2$)] produce singlet oxygen ($^1O_2$), which is converted to hydroperoxide (LOOH) as the principal product. From. R•, LOO•, LO•: lipid carbon-centered, peroxyl, and alkoxyl radicals; LOOH, LOH, LO, LO*: lipid hydroperoxide, alcohol, ketone, and excited state ketone.** Adopted from ref. 5 with permission

PDT research

Photosensitizers and mechanisms of photocytotoxicity

Apart from light and oxygen, the PS is one of the three critical components of PDT. Due to their photochemistry features and uptake efficiency, only a few PSs are now approved and utilized clinically on a global scale. Porfimer sodium (Photofrin), mTHPC (Foscan), NPe6 (Laserphyrin), SnEt2 (Purlytin), Visudyne (Veteporfin), and Motexafin lutetium (LuTex) are all being studied therapeutically or preclinically in the treatment of breast cancer. These photosensitizers exhibit a high degree of selectivity for tumour cells and are therefore suited for cellular and vascular-targeted photodynamic therapy. Additionally, their interference with cytoprotective molecular responses is a rising field of investigation. Additionally, other chemicals such as porphyrin precursors [e.g., aminolevulinic acid (ALA), phenothiazines (e.g., methylene blue), cyanines (e.g., merocyanine, indocyanine green), hypericin, and xanthenes (e.g., Rose Bengal) have been investigated as potential PS for PDT.

Significant research has been conducted over the previous decades to define the efficacy and selectivity of PS. Several of them have concentrated on the development of agents with longer absorption wavelengths, which allow for greater penetration of illuminating sources and hence increase the depths to which tumour cells can be targeted, dubbed second-generation PDT agents. Third-generation PSs, such as antibody-directed PS and PS-loaded nanocarriers, have recently appeared. These techniques were developed to enhance the potency and efficacy of PDT and to expand the sorts of sick tissues that may be treated.

Apart from the photoactive ability of PSs, which enables them to serve as a therapeutic agent when activated by light, their autofluorescence is also a significant property. Indeed, the fluorescence of PS enables them to be used as imaging agents for the detection of precancerous lesions and early malignancies, as well as tumour margins. Additionally, this feature can be exploited to identify residual dysplastic tissue following surgical tumour resections and to evaluate the PDT treatment's progress. As a result, their combination of imaging, detection, and therapeutic properties endows them with theranostic properties. PS 5-ALA, which is a prodrug that is enzymatically transformed to the active PS agent protoporphyrin IX during heme production, exhibits theranostic qualities and has contributed significantly to the field of PDT research and treatment. Additionally, 5-ALA has demonstrated clinical efficacy in a variety of tumour types in clinical trials.

PDT is thought to contribute to at least three distinct processes of tissue damage. The first is the capability of PS excitation to directly destroy cells via the action of harmful reactive chemical species. Cell described above, the direct phototoxic action of PDT results in irreversible photodamage to specific targets such as membranes and organelles. The level of damage and the processes of cell death are depending on the PS type, concentration, subcellular location, applied energy, and also on the intrinsic resistance features of each tumour type. When the intracellular and/or extracellular milieu is perturbed to an excessive degree, cells can either perish as a result of a total breakdown of the plasma membrane (necrosis morphology) or by specialized cell death processes. Additionally, PDT tumour elimination may result in damage to the tumour vasculature, impairing the provision of oxygen and vital nutrients, as well as activation of the immune system, through the induction of an inflammatory and immunological response against tumour cells.

Subroutines of cell death are substantially associated with good therapeutic outcomes. Even if a full explanation of cell death pathways is beyond the scope of this study, we highlight some of their most salient characteristics, as characterizing one or more of them that contribute to cell toxicity is a critical area of research in the field of PDT.

PDT has been demonstrated to activate numerous cell death subroutines, which may be unintentional or deliberate [Figure 2-6]. Accidental cell death is an uncontrollable type of cell death produced by the physical breakdown of the plasma membrane in response to strong physical, chemical, or mechanical stimuli. On the other hand, controlled cell death (RCD) occurs as a result of the activation of one or more signal transduction modules, and hence can be modified pharmacologically or genetically to a degree. Apoptosis and various processes of controlled necrosis are already associated with RCD subroutines (such as necroptosis and lysosome-dependent cell death). Apoptosis is a type of RCD that is triggered by perturbations in the extracellular or intracellular microenvironment. It is classified as extrinsic (when signals are detected by plasma membrane receptors, propagated by caspase-8, and precipitated by executioner caspases, primarily caspase-3), or intrinsic (when signals are detected by mitochondrial membrane permeabilization (MOMP), unbalance of pro and anti-apoptotic proteins, and precipitated by execution Necroptosis is a type of RCD that is triggered by perturbations in extracellular or intracellular homeostasis and is critically dependent on the phosphorylation, oligomerization, and migration of MLKL (mixed lineage kinase domain-like protein) to the plasma membrane, as well as the kinase activities of RIPK3 and (in some settings) RIPK1 (receptor interacting protein kinases-1 and -3, respectively). Finally, lysosome-dependent cell death (LDCD) occurs as a result of the permeabilization of the lysosomal membrane and the release of cathepsins, with or without the participation of MOMP and caspases. Indeed, one of the advantages of PDT is that it has been shown to be capable of dealing with malignant cells' well-documented ability to evade many resistance mechanisms.

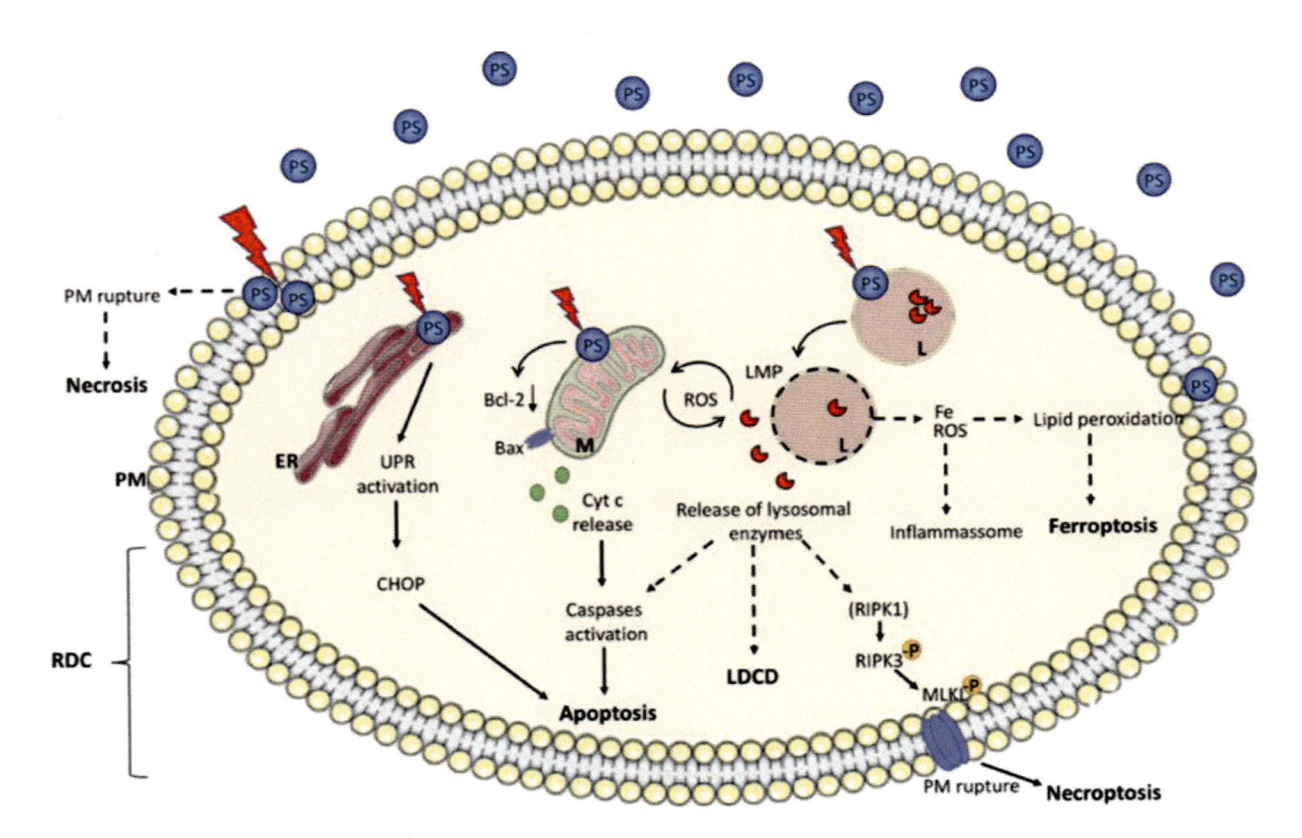

Figure 2-6. Overview of cell death subroutines that can be elicited by Photodynamic therapy. The most described locations of different photosensitizers (PS) are the plasma membrane (PM), endoplasmic reticulum (ER), mitochondria (M) or the lysosome (L). Depending on its localization, after activation by light (red light bolt) it can directly damage the PM causing unregulated necrosis or culminate in one or more regulated cell death (RCD) mechanisms. UPR: unfolded protein response; LMP: lysosome membrane permeabilization; Fe: iron; ROS: reactive oxygen species; -P: phosphate group presented in the active forms of RIPK3 and MLKL on necroptosis pathway; LDCD: lysosomal dependent cell death. Adopted from ref. 5 with permission

PS location within or on the cell surface is crucial for determining the mechanism by which cells die and consequently the cellular response to photodamage. As a result, it is critical to have a detailed understanding of the preferred subcellular location of PS accumulation in order to identify its cytotoxic potential when used in PDT. PS absorption by tumorigenic cells, as well as its preferred intracellular location, is determined by the chemical properties of each substance. While hydrophobic compounds can diffuse rapidly through plasmatic membranes, more polar medicines are often absorbed by endocytosis or facilitated transport by serum lipids and proteins. Due to their same chemical core, the majority of PSs are localized in organelle membranes during internalization. PS's cellular location is variable and has been found to include the endoplasmic reticulum (ER), mitochondria, Golgi complex, lysosomes, and plasma membrane. PS should not accumulate in the nuclei of cells to avoid DNA damage and the creation of genetically resistant cells. Accidental necrosis occurs more frequently when the PS action site is in the plasma membrane and/or when it is stimulated with high energy doses. To avoid causing unintended injury to normal tissues, this impact should be avoided in general. Autophagy is induced in an organelle-specific photodamage situation as a coordinated intracellular response aimed at reestablishing homeostasis. When inadequate or insufficient autophagy is induced, cell death is the most frequently reported outcome. PDT's most well-documented organelle-specific cytotoxicity is associated with photodamage to mitochondria, lysosomes, and endosomes.

Porphyrins can exhibit a wide range of localization patterns, but are most frequently found in plasma membranes and mitochondria. PSs localized in the mitochondria can permeabilize the inner mitochondrial membrane and selectively damage antiapoptotic BCL-2 family proteins located on the outer mitochondrial membrane, while leaving proapoptotic proteins intact, resulting in an imbalance of pro- and antiapoptotic players and caspase activation. On the other hand, as previously demonstrated in 5-ALA-PDT), certain mitochondria-associated porphyrins can also induce necroptosis. Using negatively charged porphyrins, NPe6, and phenothiazinium methylene blue, a lysosome localization pattern was identified. A possible advantage of lysosome-targeted PDT is that lysosomal damage may readily bypass autophagic defense, which can be activated concurrently with cell damage. PDT that causes lysosome damage results in LDCD. Following PDT, the release of cathepsins can result in the cleavage of the pro-apoptotic protein Bid to a truncated version called tBid. As previously demonstrated in NPe6-PDT, this product can interact with mitochondria, resulting in the release of cytochrome c and subsequent activation of intrinsic apoptosis. However, lysosome damage can trigger more than just apoptosis, and while this has not been established as a PDT-induced mechanism to yet, numerous characteristics of controlled necrosis have been related with LDCD. Indeed, the degradation of caspase-8 and recruitment of necroptosis machinery, as well as the alteration of iron homeostasis, resulting in an enhanced sensitivity to undergo ferroptosis, have been linked to lysosomal injury. Other porphyrins, including mTHPC and Hypericin, have been shown to target either the ER or both the ER and mitochondria. PDT can induce pro-death signalling via the unfolded protein response cascade when severe photodamage occurs in ER membranes. As a result of the ER stress, the pro-apoptotic transcription factor CHOP is activated, hence mediating mitochondrial death. Multiple cell death pathways activation is generally seen as a beneficial property of PDT, as it boosts photokilling in tumour cells resistant to a particular cell death route.

PDT and immune response as a strategy for metastasis control

The primary obstacle in the fight against cancer is the toxicity and drug resistance associated with insufficient tumour excision after surgery. Systemic chemotherapy has become an integral aspect of postoperative care in order to improve patient survival. However, medicines that are effective at both decreasing the disease's high mortality rate and enhancing patient quality of life remain undeveloped. Immunotherapy has been employed and developed as a strategy to manage cancer recurrence and metastases in an attempt to avoid the formation of a secondary disease. Due to the scarcity of effective treatments for metastases, interest in medicines that eradicate primary tumours and broadly trigger anticancer immune responses has surged. In this regard, PDT is emerging as a viable therapeutic to be employed alone or in combination with other approved or experimental techniques, as new data indicate that PDT can also induce systemic effects, including the reintroduction of immunosurveillance.

Immunotherapy may take the form of the use of monoclonal antibodies to inhibit cancer cells' immune checkpoint function, facilitating anti-cancer T cell responses, or the use of adoptive cellular therapy to prime the patient's own lymphocytes to attack cancer cells. Immunotherapy's objective is to elicit a robust immune response by boosting endogenous cytotoxic lymphocytes to kill tumour cells and thereby establishing long-lasting anticancer immunity. Thus, the ideal cancer treatment should combine direct cytotoxicity against tumour cells with the ability to boost the immune system via immunological detection of danger signals released by dying cells. In a typical immune response, dendritic cells (DCs) collect antigens and mature and transmit antigenic peptides to T cells in lymph nodes, resulting in effector T cells that travel to sites of infection, inflammation, or injury. IFN- and GM-CSF play critical roles in the development of DCs and activation of macrophages. DCs secrete cytokines such as IL-1β, IL-6, IL-12, and TNF, which influence the Natural Killer (NK) and T cell responses. T cells CD4+ and CD8+, as well as NK cells, can receive survival signals and stimulation from IL-2, resulting in the development of complete effector functions and the production of more IFN-. Normal immune regulation entails the use of cytokines such as IL-10 and TGF-β to suppress T cell and macrophage activity and decrease inflammation, thereby terminating immune responses and preserving the host from immunological-mediated damage. Certain tumours appear to have evaded identification by the immune system's numerous arms or have been able to limit the extent of immunological destruction, thereby evading elimination.

The most effective strategy to reestablish an immune response against tumours is to therapeutically trigger a cancer cell death pathway that is immunogenic and may be capable of inhibiting or reducing the influence of pro-tumorigenic cytokine signalling. Numerous research published in the last few years have indicated that a subset of selected anti-cancer therapy techniques is capable of inducing a promising type of cancer cell death called immunogenic cell death (ICD). The term "ICD" was used to refer to a mode of cell death that induces an immune response to antigens produced by dead cells. Following exposure to certain cytotoxic ICD-agents, alterations in the composition of the cell surface encourage the exposure or release of mediators, resulting in what are known as damage related molecular patterns (DAMPs). DCs then identify these signals and enhance the presentation of tumour antigens to T lymphocytes. It has been demonstrated that commencing a mode of tumour cell death in conjunction with the activation of signalling pathways that produce DAMPs significantly improves the immunogenicity of dying cancer cells. Until far, the primary DAMPs involved in ICD have been surface-exposed calreticulin (CRT), surface-exposed heat shock proteins (HSP) 70 and 90, secreted adenosine triphosphate, and passively released high-mobility group box 1 (HMG-1) (HMGB1). Numerous conventional anticancer medicines, including chemotherapies, radiotherapies, and targeted therapies, have been examined for their immunogenic potential, but only a few have been identified as ICD inducers. This exclusive inducer-induction link exists because ICD requires the induction of ER stress mediated by reactive oxygen species (ROS), which may or may not be predominantly ER-directed. PDT's potential for stimulating ICD appears to be fairly probable, and has been investigated, as a ROS-inducer treatment.

In general, mounting evidence indicates that the therapeutic efficacy of several anticancer agents, including PDT, is dependent on their ability to influence the tumor-host interaction, tipping the balance in favour of activation of an immune response specific for malignant cells, particularly metastasized cancer.

Instrumentation, disadvantages, and adverse effects

PDT has been demonstrated to be beneficial in treating several types of malignancies, particularly those with superficial localizations, because it significantly improves both the patient's quality of life and cost effectiveness when compared to palliative surgery or palliative chemotherapy. However, as is the case with other therapies, it has been observed that the predominant unfavourable anatomical and microenvironmental characteristics restrict its efficacy and contribute to the relatively sluggish transition of PDT for treating malignant malignancies from preclinical to clinical practice. Adjusting PDT parameters such as PS type and local concentration, light delivery and source, or dosimetry in a non-homogeneous environment is regarded as one of the major challenges of this therapeutic method.

The most frequently expressed worry regarding the therapeutic application of PDT is the low penetration of light. However, the conventional belief that PDT is a surface treatment is no longer accepted, as the use of external light can only treat superficial lesions. This issue is on the verge of being resolved due to the possibility of implanting fibres in specific spots within the tumour site. PDT can now be used in the clinic with interstitial, endoscopic, intraoperative, or laparoscopic light delivery devices, owing to advancements in fibre optics and microendoscopic technology. In this case, the laser light can be modified into thin optical fibres to transfer it to deeper and more difficult-to-reach therapy areas. Apart from delivering light, these fibres can also function as diagnostic sensors, monitoring essential PDT parameters that affect the treatment response, such as the fluence rate, PS concentration, PS photobleaching, and tissue oxygenation status. It is critical to keep in mind that the vascular collapse induced by PDT may result in decreased tumour oxygenation. Due to the fact that the treatment is successful because it utilizes preexisting ground state oxygen to generate singlet oxygen via a type II photochemical reaction [Figure 1], the oxygenation state of the tissue has a substantial effect on the efficiency of PDT. Additionally, during treatment, the production of ROS caused by high light fluence rates can rapidly deplete the oxygen levels in tumorigenic tissue, exacerbating tumour hypoxia and impairing treatment outcome. Thus, increasing the oxygen concentration is critical for PDT. Indeed, by changing the light and PS dosimetry, lowering the light fluence rate, or employing light fractionated techniques, oxygen depletion can be avoided and sufficient time for oxygen replenishment in the target tissue is allowed. However, it has been noted that different PS have varying effects on oxygen consumption rates, and so the outcome of PDT may vary. Taken together, these findings highlight the importance of additional research into how to maintain PDT performance. This issue was recently solved in an intriguing study that combined fractionated PDT with a PS capable of producing singlet oxygen during dark periods. Additionally, pre-existing hypoxia zones in tumours can be avoided using a variety of techniques, including increasing tissue oxygenation prior to PDT and creating radical species efficiently via type I photochemical processes.

In terms of light source technology, researchers have been working to develop light delivery systems that provide consistent illumination, which is critical for increasing light penetration and reproducibility. A good illustration of this is the use of bulb-shaped isotropic emitters in conjunction with light detectors in hollow organs. Additionally, light dosimetry can aid in optimizing the placement of light diffusers. Additionally, selectivity can be increased by adapting diffusers such as balloons and cylindrical applicators to the shape and dimensions of the target tissue.

Additionally, recent advancements in LED and diode laser technology have enabled the combination of their output potency, portability, and precision optical fibre coupling capabilities. These non-collimated, lower-cost light sources will undoubtedly facilitate the translation of PDT to clinical treatments. They are frequently used due to their robustness, narrow bandwidth, cheap maintenance requirements, and ability to be tuned to the PS's needed wavelength. In addition to Tungsten filament lamps, metal halide lamps, strong Xenon arc lamps, and pulsed lasers, the PDT field frequently employs other types of lights.

Apart from the light source itself, choosing the method for light application is critical, since different irradiation regimens employing the same source might provide very different results in PDT. Another issue to address in PDT prescriptions is light dose regimens, as they may interfere with the host's anti-tumor responses, and ideal solutions are likely case specific. As a result, a thorough grasp of light dosimetry is critical for PDT. The issue of light in PDT is being thoroughly investigated, and advancements and new technology in this field will undoubtedly result in overall PDT efficacy and protocols being adjusted. For instance, one technique for inducing phototoxicity in deep tissue is to execute recurrent PDT or metronomic PDT (slow infusion of PS and low dose light). Recent research indicates that fractionated PDT may generate a greater degree of necrosis than PDT alone. The possibility of continual accumulation of PSs at the treatment site contributed to a more favourable treatment response profile and boosted the feasibility of accessing deeper tissues using this method.

The most often reported adverse event linked with PDT is skin photosensitivity, particularly when PSs of the first generation are systemically delivered. In these instances, patients are need to abstain from sunshine and bright artificial light for several weeks. Another frequently reported adverse effect is discomfort. Although the primary cause of PDT-induced pain has not been identified, multiple studies have discovered that it is connected with the treated area's size, PS type, lesion type, gender, age, and light protocol. There is evidence that suggests that continuous activation of low PS levels utilizing lower irradiance and maybe shorter incubation durations results in decreased pain without compromising PDT efficacy. Additionally, inflammation, fever, and nausea are common but are frequently successfully controlled with medicine. Tumor recurrence is frequently observed in therapeutic trials, most likely as a result of insufficient tumour elimination. This may be due to poor light or PS penetration, but may also be due to the presence of PDT-resistant malignancies. Although the mechanisms for recurrence are frequently beyond the purview of clinical studies, there is an approach for overcoming insufficient tumour eradication with PDT that involves the combination of two or more PSs. The objective is to select PSs that target distinct cellular compartments within tumours, resulting in a more favourable overall therapy outcome. Another possibility is to combine PDT with already available chemotherapeutic agents. In a recent study, it was demonstrated that the combination of ferroptosis inducers and gemcitabine was capable of effectively overcoming the chemotherapeutic drug resistance that occurs commonly in pancreatic adenocarcinomas.

PDT in invasive cancer preclinical models: an updated report

Surgery is often necessary for getting rid of tumours in patients diagnosed with cancer, regardless of whether radiation, systemic therapy, or both are used. Tumor cells often make their way through the blood and lymphatic systems, moving from a primary tumour, and may be discovered in one or more sentinel lymph nodes before reaching another location. Identifying cancer cells in the lymph nodes is the most important prognostic indicator for evaluating whether a patient needs additional treatments like radiation or chemotherapy, and it is especially critical in patients with non-metastatic cancer. Once cancer has progressed to other parts of the body, the excision of tumours, while offering an increased chance of recovery, does not always mean an improved survival rate. Surgery may aid in the treatment of ulcerated tumours on the chest wall, and there are no particular treatments available at this time. For this reason, there is a demand for new and safe treatments that will address this stage of the disease.

Some studies have indicated a beneficial effect of combining PDT and ionizing radiation on cell death. Combining mild doses of radiotherapy (4 Gy) and indocyanine green (ICG) as well as light is surprisingly effective, yielding practically total survival reduction. A preclinical animal model found signs of enhanced trabecular structure in a PDT therapy procedure following radiation. In a comparison of radiotherapy alone to radiotherapy and photodynamic therapy (PDT), it was found that rats treated with PDT had increased osteoid formation and newly formed woven bone (versus the situation in rats who received radiotherapy alone). This was confirmed by a quantitative histological examination, which demonstrated a bone-to-marrow ratio increase due to the presence of newly formed woven bone. In follow-up experiments, PDT showed that it enhanced vertebral strength when used in combination with bisphosphonates or radiotherapy, which could mean that it can be useful for adjuvant treatment of spinal metastases. The studies found that using PS-mediated PDT combined with ionizing radiation treatment may be preferable to treatment with the two methods independently. To reduce radiation exposure and negative effects, PDT's systemic therapeutic impact can be strengthened with the combination of ionizing radiation.

Additional research and effort are required before PDT may be considered as a viable therapy option for breast cancer. While there is substantial evidence that PDT should be explored as an anticancer treatment, the true issue for PDT is translating improvements in understanding the effects shown in cell-line and animal model studies into clinical practice.

PDT applications in clinical practice; PDT in combination with other therapy; Ongoing trials

Despite the growing number of studies involving an increasing number of chemical compounds and their generally greater number of favourable characteristics when compared to more conventional treatments, only a few PS have been approved for clinical use and for the treatment of a limited number of diseases.

While the majority of PDT applications involve various types of cancer, ALA is already licensed for a variety of therapeutic indications, including mild to moderate actinic keratosis and non-hyperkeratotic actinic keratosis. Several of these medications are also used to treat Bowen's disease and basal cell carcinoma. Additionally, a clinically authorized PS called Verteporfin is currently being used to treat significant eye illnesses such as age-related macular degeneration and myopic choroidal neovascularization. Porfimer sodium (Photofrin) was the first PS licensed by the Canadian Health Agency for clinical use in the treatment of bladder cancer in 1993. Later, the Food and Drug Administration (FDA) and several other nations approved it for the treatment of several forms of cancer, including lung, esophageal, gastric, and cervical malignancies, as well as cervical dysplasia. This photosensitizer is still commonly used in photodynamic therapy (PDT) to treat a variety of illnesses. However, because porfimer sodium is a complex collection of molecules with low tissue selectivity and low light absorption, substantial doses are required, causing it to persist for up to two months after treatment, making people photosensitive. Following that, a second generation of PS was produced with increased purity, longer wavelength absorptions, and increased photosensitivity and tissue selectivity. Temoporfin was the second PS to get approval and is widely used to treat advanced squamous cell carcinomas of the head and neck. Temoporfin has also been tested in the treatment of breast, pancreatic, and prostate cancer, with inconsistent results. In all patients with breast cancer, there was a response with low invasiveness and minor adverse effects. Similarly, it proved to be a safe technique for prostate cancer, as the prostate specific antigen decreased by up to 67 percent after eight of ten PDT sessions, and biopsies of treated areas exhibited necrosis and fibrosis after 1-2 months. However, in patients with malignant biliary obstruction, endoscopically delivered Temoporfin-PDT was effective at necrosis and recanalization of blocked metal stents, but it was associated with a significant risk of complication, with one patient developing a fatal liver abscess and two developing haemobilia within four weeks of treatment, one of whom died of gall bladder empyema. Talaporfin, a mono-L-aspartyl chlorin, was licensed in Japan as a PDT for lung cancer but has also been used in patients with early head and neck cancer and is currently undergoing phase II testing for the treatment of colorectal neoplasms and liver metastases. Additionally, the FDA has approved additional medications as orphan pharmaceuticals for PDT therapy of Cutaneous T-cell lymphoma (SGX301) and biliary tract cancer (LUZ11).

Because PDT has the ability to have a local effect, it is free of the systemic side effects associated with other therapies. Additionally, due to how PDT works, it can be utilized in conjunction with other clinical procedures like as radiotherapy, chemotherapy, or surgery. At the moment, a variety of trials utilizing PDT with unique PS are being conducted for various forms of cancer. Approximately half of all ongoing clinical trials listed at clinicaltrials.gov (not yet ended) employ

PDT alone or in conjunction with other therapies for at least one ailment [Table 2]. PDT using a variety of different photosensitizers appears to be beneficial in reducing tumour size and enhancing patient survival in a number of treatments targeting a variety of different types of cancers [Table 3]. Interestingly, the vast majority of ongoing cancer trials employ photosensitizers that have previously been approved for clinical use, primarily Photofrin and ALA, but also Verteporfin and other yet-to-be-approved chemicals.

The majority of PDT regimens that have been approved are for the treatment of superficial skin and luminal organ lesions. However, as PS efficiency and light delivery have improved, interstitial and intra-operative techniques for the ablation of a wide variety of solid tumours have been examined. The initial therapeutic application of PDT in the treatment of breast cancer was to treat recurrence of skin metastases in the chest wall. Photofrin was used in the protocol studied, and it was found to be beneficial in 50% of patients. Subsequent studies using Photofrin, m-THPC, and Npe6 established PDT as an effective palliative treatment for breast cancer patients with chest wall recurrence. Additional applications of PDT as a treatment for breast cancer solid tumours and their sequelae are being investigated, most notably its role in combination with adjuvant radiation and chemotherapy. Regarding the metastatic problem in breast cancer, despite the fact that this systemic complication is the most difficult aspect of PDT treatment for this type of tumour, a study of fourteen patients with more than 500 truncal metastases revealed that all patients had tumour necrosis, and nine of them had complete responses. Finally, a clinical trial of late-stage breast cancer patients treated with a local intervention utilizing an 805 nm laser for non-invasive irradiation, indocyanine green, and an immunoadjuvant (glycated chitosan) for immunological stimulation demonstrated that the combined therapeutic approach was both safer and more effective than each individual strategy for treating metastatic breast cancer. This study indicated that adjuvant immunotherapy following PDT may enhance its effectiveness and may represent a feasible future therapeutic option for cancers in remote locations, as previously discussed, but requires additional clinical investigations.

The Bottom Line

Combating the disease presents difficulties due to intrinsic tumour resistant features, molecular heterogeneity, and metastasis. Considering all of the available facts, one may infer that one significant advantage of PDT over other cancer treatments is the possibility of causing less side effects in patients.

In summary, this study examined and summarized the current state of knowledge about the use of PDT as a therapeutic method in the treatment of primary cancer and metastases. We have discussed a variety of subjects, from the photochemical mechanisms involved to the many cell death pathways elicited by various photosensitizers to the more recent ongoing clinical trials. Additionally, we presented substantial evidence highlighting the importance of PDT as a novel treatment method capable of generating many mechanisms of cell death, some of them concurrently. This capability may be an intriguing way to circumvent the problem of death resistance displayed by many tumours, as one of the critical characteristics of an alternative therapy for cancer treatment is the ability to broaden the spectrum of cell death mechanisms gathered in order to circumvent the various resistance mechanisms displayed by malignant cells.

2.4 Copper-cysteamine nanoparticles as a novel photosensitizer for the treatment of hepatocellular carcinoma

Hepatocellular carcinoma (HCC) is one of the world's six most lethal cancers. According to the most recent global statistics report, 0.74 million cases of HCC occur each year, with 0.69 million deaths. Globally, China has the highest rate of HCC (54% of the worldwide total). Hepatocellular carcinoma is highly prevalent and has a dismal prognosis, with a 5-year survival rate of less than 5%. Among the most frequently used treatment modalities in HCC is drug therapy. 5-fluorouracil (5-FU) and doxorubicin are two commonly used chemotherapy agents. While drugs do have a curative effect in the treatment of HCC, some studies have revealed that these anticancer medications have adverse effects on the human body. As a result, new treatment methods and medications for liver cancer are critical.

Photodynamic therapy (PDT) is a novel and exciting technique that may one day replace conventional chemotherapy. When activated by light, photosensitizers used in PDT react with the oxygen molecules present in tissues, generating cytotoxic singlet oxygen. Several advantages of PDT over other techniques include the drug's selectivity for tumour tissue, the drug's lack of systemic toxicity, the ability to focus the light on the tumour region, the possibility of treating multiple lesions concurrently, and the ability to re-treat a tumour to improve the response. The outcome of the PDT is directly proportional to the efficiency of singlet oxygen generation, which is influenced by photosensitizer, light, and oxygen. To ensure that PDT works properly, the light must be delivered to the photosensitizer effectively. Lasers, light-emitting diodes, and in some cases halogen or arc lamps are used as light sources. However, light delivery is problematic for treating deep cancers due to light's inability to penetrate deeply into tissue. As a result, PDT is frequently utilized to treat superficial lesions (e.g., skin cancer). Apart from the light source, another factor affecting singlet oxygen efficiency is the photosensitizer itself. Traditionally used photosensitizers include hematoporphyrin derivatives, 5-aminolevulinic acid (5-ALA), and the organic dye phthalocyanine. These photosensitizers have some disadvantages in clinical applications due to their non-selectivity and biological toxicity. As a result, researchers are concentrating their efforts on developing new photosensitizers that have the potential to avoid or mitigate these adverse effects.

Nanomedicines have been extensively studied, as have nanoscale photosensitizers for cancer treatment. Chen et al. recently described a novel class of nanoparticle photosensitizers called copper-cysteamine (Cu-Cy). Two remarkable properties of this novel material are its strong red luminescence and its ability to generate singlet oxygen inducible by UV light, X-rays, ultrasound, and microwaves. As a result, Cu-Cy is a novel material that is being investigated for use in cancer treatment.

Cu-Cy's development as a new sensitizer for cancer treatment is still in its infancy, and numerous aspects of this novel material remain unknown. Cu-Cy NPs have not been tested for the treatment of liver cancer, and the efficacy of Cu-Cy NPs against liver cancer has not been determined. For the first time, we report the *in vivo* and *in vitro* PDT effects of Cu-Cy NPs on anti-HCC.

Outcomes

Characterization of Cu-Cy nanoparticles in their solid and soluble forms

Cu-Cy NPs have a high degree of crystallinity. Cu-Cy NPs include two distinct Cu atoms–Cu(1) and Cu(2) (both are Cu^+ ions), which attach to four and three additional atoms, respectively. Cu-Cy NPs exhibit strong photoluminescence (as seen in Figure 2-7(a)) as well as X-ray luminescence. Our earlier article detailed the crystal structure and optical characteristics of Cu-Cy NPs in detail. The samples employed in this investigation were coated with polyethylene glycol and have a diameter of approximately 100 nm, as determined by their TEM images, as shown in Figure 2-7(b). They exhibit an intense red luminescence, as illustrated in Figure 2-7 (c).

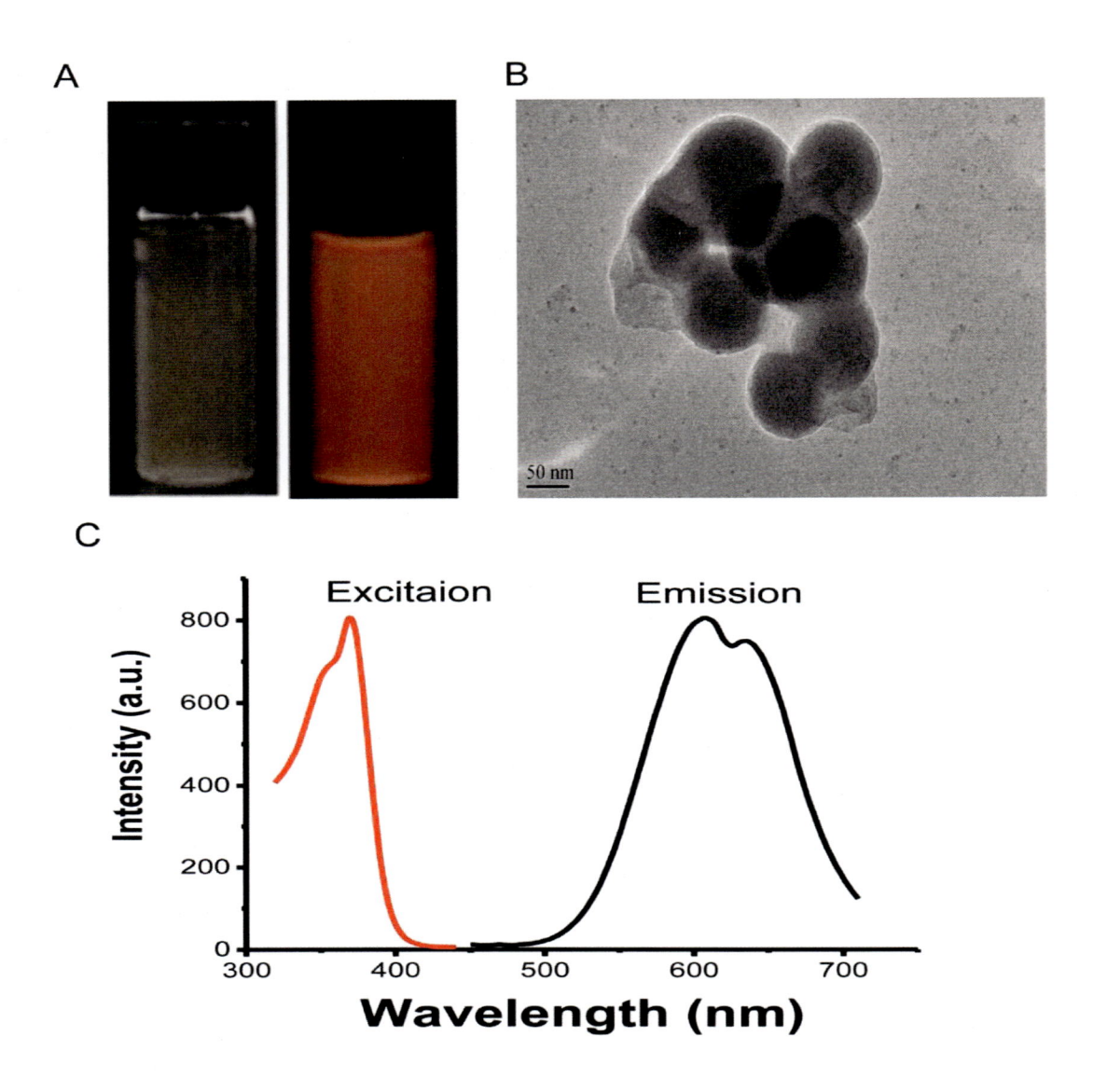

Figure 2-7. (A) Photo of the Cu-Cy NPs in aqueous solution (top left), (B) the TEM image, (C) and the excitation and emission spectra of Cu-Cy NPs; the excitation wavelength is 360 nm and the emission wavelength is 600 nm. Adopted from ref. 6 with permission

The generation of singlet oxygen in different time periods when exposed to UV light

We employed p-nitrosodimenthylaniline-imidazole to detect singlet oxygen after it was treated under UV light for various time durations. When ID is present, RNO is a water-soluble molecule that is irreversibly quenched by singlet oxygen. We noticed that the amount of singlet oxygen generated by Cu-Cy NPs was dependent on the irradiation duration time when comparing the quenching degree of RNO absorption with and without Cu-Cy NPs under UV irradiation. UV irradiation did not produce any singlet oxygen to quench the RNO absorption in the control group, RNO-ID alone. However, with UV irradiation with Cu-Cy NPs, the absorption of RNO was significantly reduced (0 min vs. 5 min: 0.749 ± 0.001 vs. 0.738 ± 0.006; P= 0.009). These findings revealed that Cu-Cy NPs were a novel class of photosensitizers capable of being activated by ultraviolet light to generate singlet oxygen for cancer treatment.

Viability of HepG2 cells after various UV irradiation times

Not only does ultraviolet radiation sterilize, but it also has an effect on cell proliferation. To determine the influence of UV light on cell activity, we employed 3-(4,5-dimethylthiazol-2-yl)-2,5-diphenyltetrazolium bromide (MTT) to determine the cellular survival of HepG2 cells after 24 hours of growth. The viability of cells was lowered following UV irradiation. It reduced significantly when the irradiation time was increased from 6 to 10 minutes. For less than 6 minutes, UV irradiation had no effect on cells. However, when the irradiation time was prolonged to 6 minutes (6 min vs. 0 min: 0.84 ± 0.03 vs. 1.00 ± 0.02; P = 0.001) or longer, cells were severely affected. As a result, we set a radiation time of 5 minutes (light dose = 6 J/cm^2) to avoid the side effect of UV irradiation.

Viability of HepG2 cells at various doses of Cu-Cy NPs

Toxicology is a critical element to consider when evaluating materials for biological applications. We used the MTT assay to determine the cytotoxicity of Cu-Cy NPs after 24 h of incubation against HepG2 cells. It was seen that increasing the concentration of Cu-Cy NPs decreased cellular activity. When the concentration of Cu-Cy NPs was increased from 0 to 200 µg/mL, the cellular viability steadily dropped from 100% to 85%. We observed an effect on cellular viability at a concentration of 50 µg/mL (0 µg/mL vs. 50 µg/mL: 1.00 ± 0.02 vs. 0.88 ± 0.01; P < 0.001). This finding revealed that Cu-Cy NPs were non-toxic at concentrations less than 50 µg/ml, and 25 µg/ml was employed in all subsequent studies in our investigation to prevent the nanoparticles' intrinsic cytotoxicity.

The binding of Cu-Cy NPs to HepG2 cells and their viability

Even when Cu-Cy NPs do not enter cells, they are effective at destroying cancer cells. We used the MTT assay and fluorescence staining to determine the killing effectiveness of Cu-Cy NPs on HepG2 cells over a three-day incubation period. The degree of Cu-Cy NPs (25 µg/mL) binding to cells was determined at three distinct phases. The proportion of Cu-Cy NPs binding to cells increased with increasing incubation time. When 5 minutes, 60 minutes, and 240 minutes were compared, the binding degree increased (60 minutes vs. 5 minutes: 0.36 ± 0.09 vs. 0.07 ± 0.02, $P = 0.006$; 240 minutes vs. 5 minutes: 0.91 ± 0.22 vs. 0.07 ± 0.02, $P < 0.001$; 240 minutes vs. 60 minutes: 0.91 ± 0.22 vs. 0.36 ± 0.09, $P < 0.001$). The cellular survival of these various cultivated stages was not significantly altered. These observations demonstrate that at a dosage of 25 µg/mL, there is no clear cytotoxic effect on cells.

However, we anticipate that if UV is used to irradiate the NPs, the cellular viability will be altered. The fluorescence images of HepG2 cells were acquired using an EVOS fluorescence microscope before and after UV irradiation. After 30 minutes of incubation, live cells were stained green and dead cells were stained red with calcein and ethidiumhomodimer-1 (EthD-1). As illustrated in Figure 2-8a, the numbers of cells dying at various degrees of Cu-Cy NPs binding to cells are nearly identical following 6 J/cm^2 UV irradiation. The statistical analysis revealed no statistically significant difference between the three stages of incubation. The control group's results demonstrated that UV irradiation alone was unable to destroy the cells (Figure 2-8b). MTT assay results further indicated that there was no difference in cellular viability between the three stages of Cu-Cy NPs incubation with cells following UV irradiation. This result established that the degree of binding of Cu-Cy NPs to cells was not a critical component in determining their killing power.

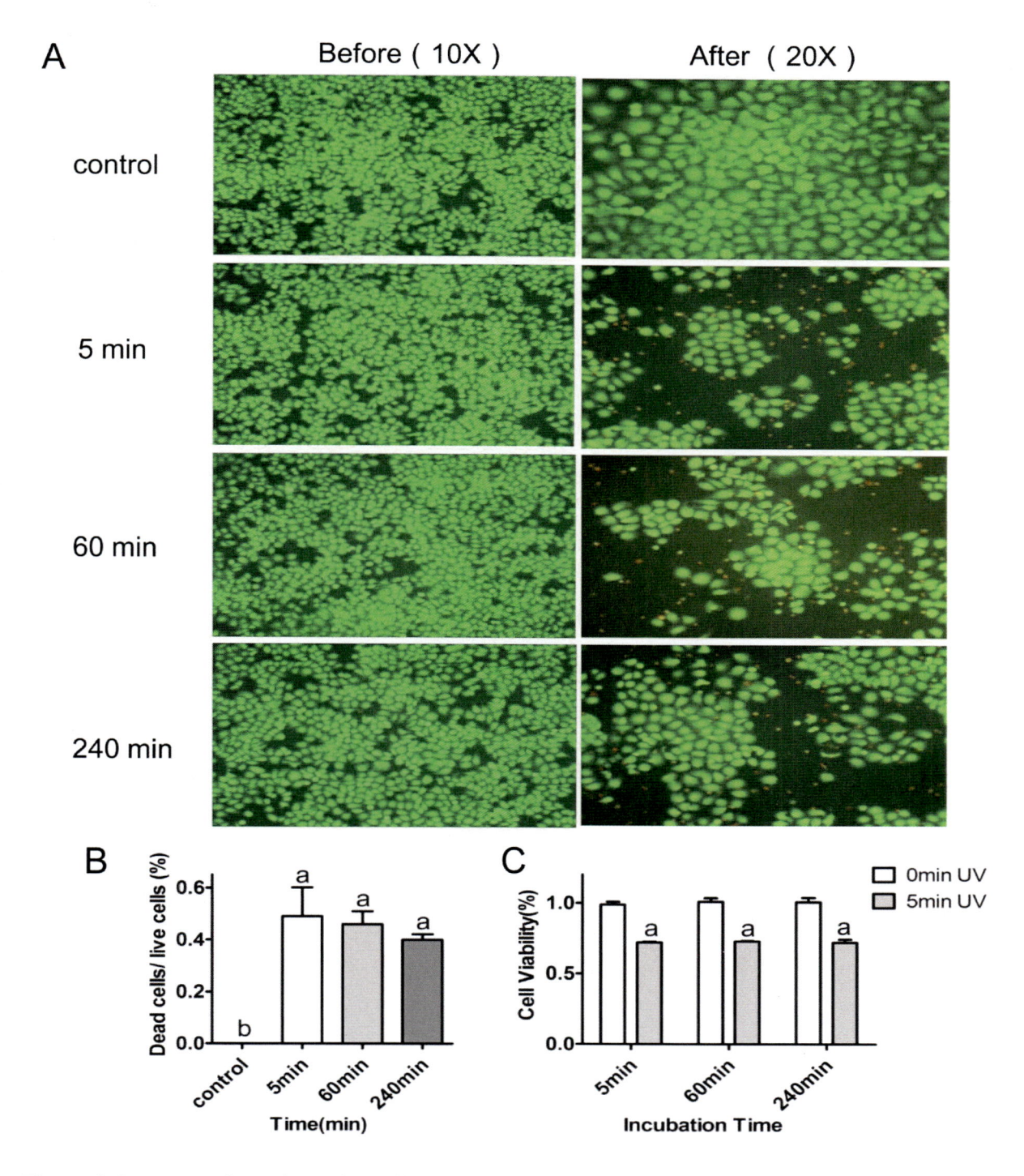

Figure 2-8. Destruction of HepG2 cells by Cu-Cy NPs (25 μg/ml) under different binding degree after UV irradiation. (A) Images of fluorescence staining show HepG2 live (green, calcein stain) and dead (red, EthD-1 stain) cells. Pictures (5 min), (60 min), and (240 min) show the damage of Cu-Cy NPs to cells in different binding degree (incubated with Cu-Cy NPs for 5, 60, and 240 min

respectively). (B) The proportion of dead and living cells in different incubation time after UV radiation. The data are expressed as the mean±SD of 3 random pictures. **a** $P < 0.05$ compared with control. (C) The viability of HepG2 cells at the same absorption/adhesion degree of Cu-Cy NPs with UV light in 24 h was determined using an MTT assay. **a** $P < 0.05$ compared with control. The data are expressed as the mean±SD of 3 independent experiments. Adopted from ref. 6 with permission

To assess the UV-induced PDT effects, we evaluated cellular viability before and after exposure to Cu-Cy NPs with the same binding degree. The results suggest that UV irradiation considerably decreased cellular viability when compared to a control (Figure 2-8c), indicating that Cu-Cy NPs had a considerable inhibitory effect on cellular viability following UV exposure. Regardless of whether Cu-Cy NPs are absorbed by cells or not, once they are bound to them, a severe killing effect on cancer cells would manifest following 6 J/cm^2 UV activation.

Cu-Cy NPs caused apoptosis in HepG2 cells

We compared the apoptosis caused by Cu-Cy NPs to that induced by 5-FU, a commonly used chemotherapeutic agent for HCC. The data in Figure 2-9(a) and (bi) demonstrated that, in comparison to the other three groups, Cu-Cy NPs + UV elicited apparent apoptosis at a concentration of 25 μg/mL (Cu-Cy NPs + UV vs. control: 12.32 ± 0.53 vs. 3.35 ± 1.51, P< 0.001; Cu-Cy NPs + UV vs. 5-FU: 12.32 ± 0.53 vs. 4.86 ± 1.60, Cu-Cy NPs and Cu-Cy NPs + UV significantly improved the rate of cellular death at a high dose (50 μg/mL) (Cu-Cy NPs vs. control: 9.10 ± 0.69 vs. 1.09 ± 1.51, P< 0.001, Cu-Cy NPs vs. 5-FU: 9.10 ± 0.69 vs. 0.50 ± 0.51, P 0.001, Cu-Cy NPs + UV vs. control Cu-Cy NPs + UV vs. 5-FU: 6.09 5.80 vs. 0.50 0.51, P = 0.002) (Figure 2-9(a) and (bii)). These findings suggest that both 5-FU and Cu-Cy NPs + UV can induce apoptosis in HepG2 cells. In comparison to 5-FU, UV-irradiated Cu-Cy NP had a greater effect on HepG2 cell death.

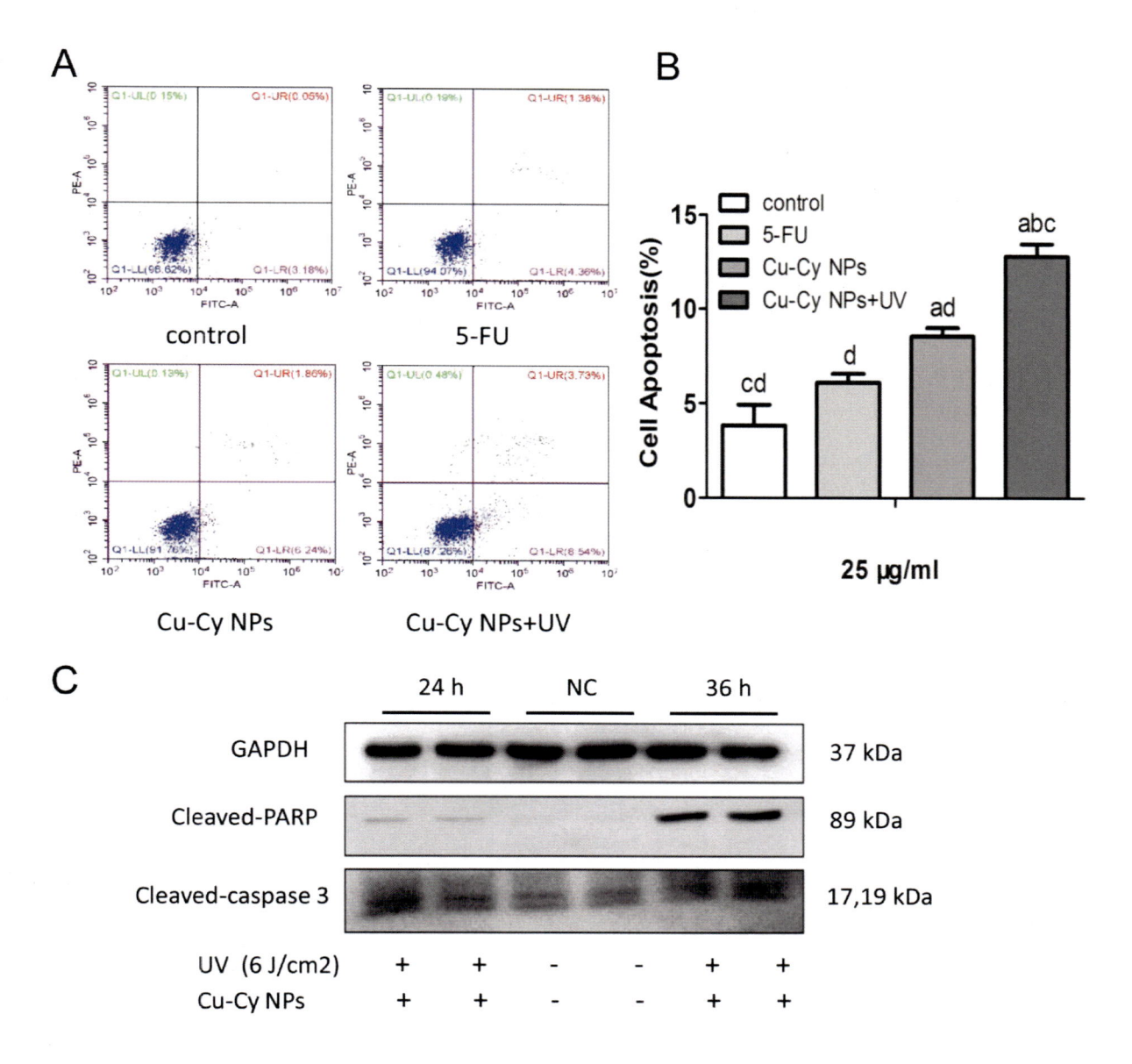

Figure 2-9. Comparison of Cu-Cy NPs and 5-FU induced HepG2 cells apoptosis. (A) Cell apoptosis profiles were measured by flow cytometry following treatment of different groups with the concentration of 25 μg/ml for 24 h. (B) Cellular consequence was quantified by apoptosis. The data are expressed as the mean±SD of 3 independent experiments. **a** $P < 0.05$ compared with control, **b** $P < 0.05$ compared with 5-FU group, **c** $P < 0.05$ compared with Cu-Cy NPs group, and **d** $P < 0.05$ compared with Cu-Cy NPs+UV group. (C) The expression levels of the proteins including cleaved- caspase 3 and cleaved-PARP in HepG2 cells.

Additional data was gathered to establish that Cu-Cy NPs trigger apoptosis. Western blotting was used to determine the expression of the apoptotic protein (cleaved-PARP) in HepG2 cells treated with Cu-Cy NPs + UV (6 J/cm^2) for 24 and 36 hours. Consistent with the previous results, UV dosage had no effect on the expression of cleaved-PARP when compared to control; however, elevated expression levels of cleaved-PARP were seen in the group treated with Cu-Cy NPs. Additionally, when stimulated with UV (6 J/cm^2), Cu-Cy NPs increased the expression of cleaved-PARP. Additionally, 36 h after the addition of Cu-Cy NPs and 6 J/cm^2 UV irradiation, the expression of apoptosis-related protein increased much more than 24 h after the addition of Cu-Cy NPs (Figure 2-10). This study suggested that the rate of cell apoptosis increases gradually when the action time is increased.

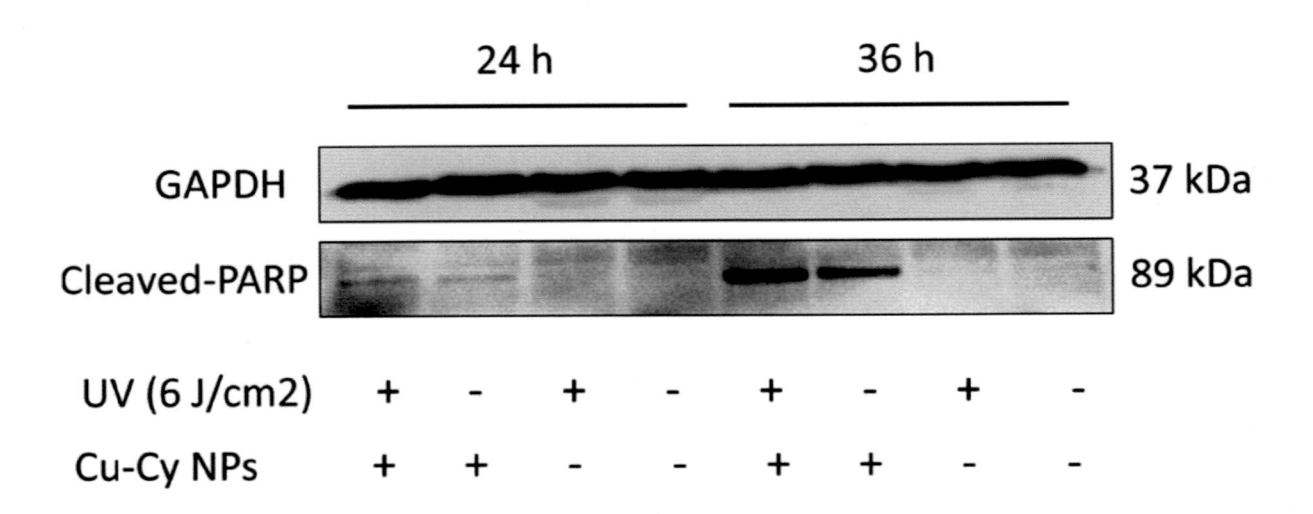

Figure 2-10. Protein expression levels in HepG2 cells, including cleaved-PARP

Anti-HepG2 tumour activity of Cu-Cy NPs in vivo

To further assess the therapeutic potential of Cu-Cy NPs, UV-irradiated Cu-Cy NPs were examined in an in vivo subcutaneous tumour model. Subcutaneous injection of a suspension of 1 × 10^6 HepG2 cells into the flank and shoulder of mice was used to assess tumour growth daily. Two weeks after injection, mice were randomly assigned to one of five groups: control (saline), 5-FU, UV, Cu-Cy NPs, or Cu-Cy NPs + UV (Figure 2-11a). The Cu-Cy NPs+UV group received daily UV irradiation at a dose of 6 J/cm^2, and all trials were studied for one month. As illustrated in Figure 2-11b, the tumour grew successfully in each group of naked mice. H&E staining was used to confirm the formation of tumours as seen in Figure 2-11c for the characteristic morphological characteristics of tumour cells: the volume and nucleus of tumour cells were larger than normal cells, the cellular shape and arrangement were irregular, the nuclei of cells were deeply stained and varied in shape, and a large number of multinucleated cells were visible. These variables indicated that the tumour model in naked mice had been generated successfully.

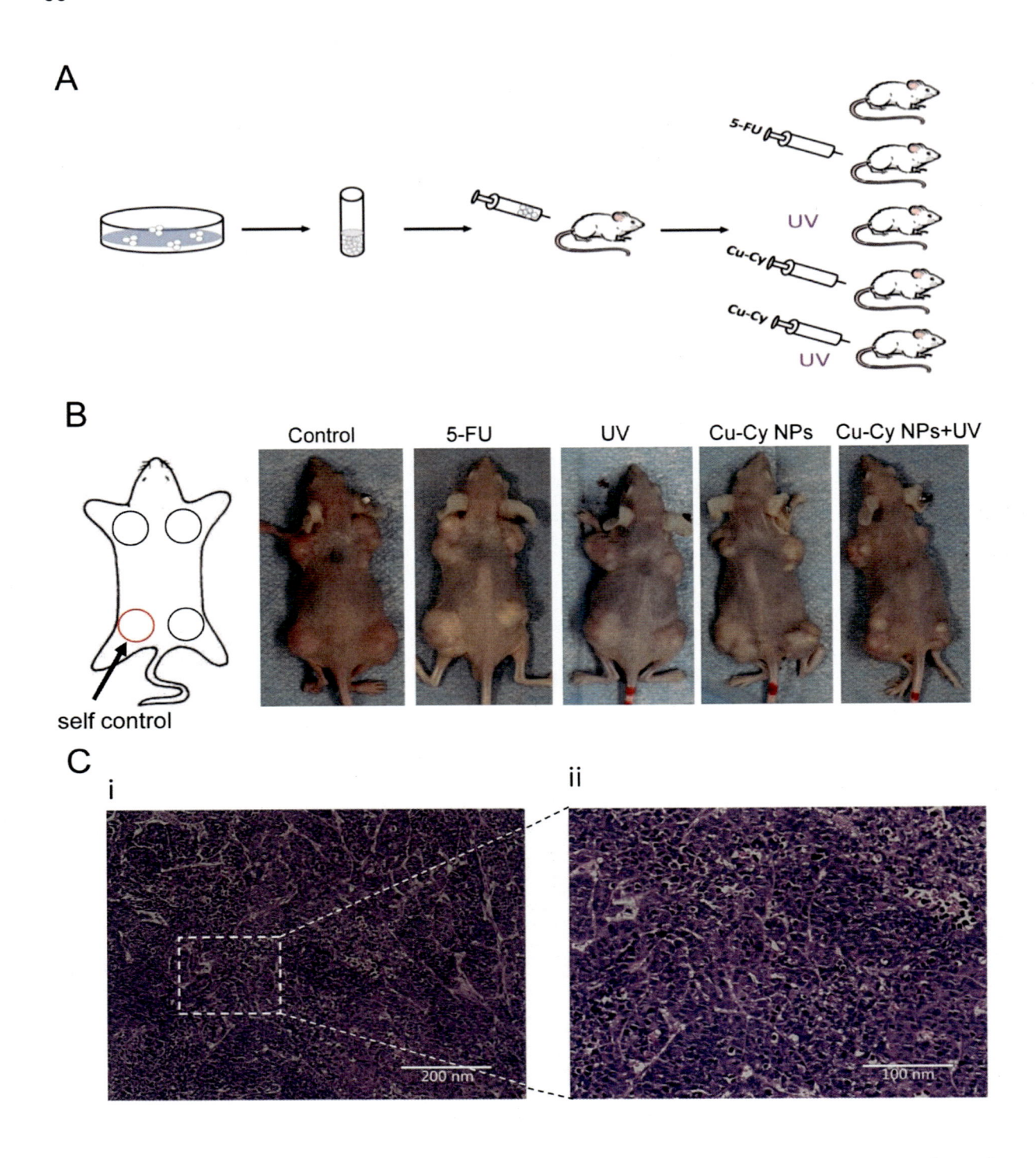

Figure 2-11. Establishment of tumor model. (A) The process and grouping of experiment in nude mice. (B) Images of nude mice with different sized HepG2 tumors after different treatment. The left leg of each mouse is the control. (C) HE staining of HepG2 tumor in mice.

As illustrated in Figure 2-12a, the UV group had no influence on tumour growth, the Cu-Cy NPs alone marginally suppressed tumour growth, and the 5-FU and Cu-Cy NPs + UV groups grew tumours at significantly slower rates than the control. These findings suggested that UV-irradiated Cu-Cy NPs had the same tumour growth inhibitory impact as 5-FU.

The tumours were surgically dissected after a month of treatment. The tumour volumes were substantially less in 5-FU than in control (control vs. 5-FU: 793.16 ± 425.33 vs. 518.40 ± 327.11, P = 0.026). Cu-Cy NPs + UV volumes were also smaller than control volumes (793.16 ± 425.33 vs. 515.99 ± 323.98, P = 0.004). However, there was no difference in volume between the 5-FU and Cu-Cy NPs + UV groups. Additionally, no differences were seen between the control, UV alone, or Cu-Cy NPs alone (Figure 2-12b and c). These findings revealed that UV-irradiated Cu-Cy NPs had the same tumour growth inhibitory effect as 5-FU.

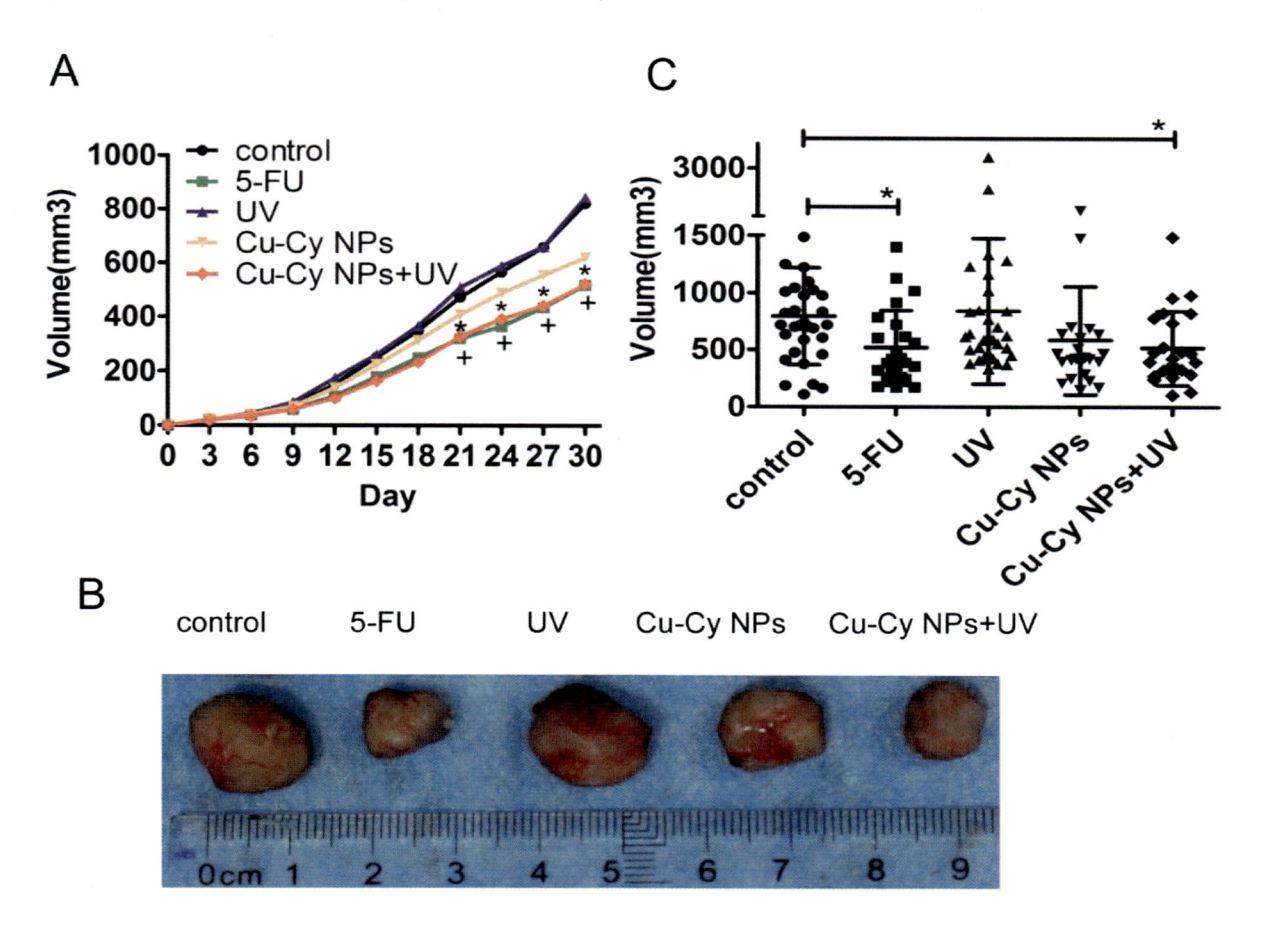

Figure 2-12. Images of tumors sized after treatment. (A) Image of growth curve of tumor in different groups of mice. The results are presented as the mean of 8 mice per group from the

experiment. * $P < 0.05$ Cu-Cy NPs+UV compared with the control, $^+P < 0.05$ 5-FU compared with the control. (B) Images of tumor size in different group after different treatment. (C) Scatter plots of tumor volume after treatment with different groups of mice. The results are presented as the mean±SD of 8 mice per group from the experiment. *$P < 0.05$ compared with the control. Adopted from ref. 6 with permission

Analysis

PDT has gained considerable attention in recent years as a novel cancer treatment method. It works by activating a photosensitizer that reacts with oxygen molecules found in tissues when exposed to light. This reaction produces cytotoxic singlet oxygen and results in oxidative damage. The photosensitizer, one of the three components of PDT (photosensitizer, light source, and tissue oxygen), is critical in this process because it contributes to the production of singlet oxygen. When activated with UV light, Cu-Cy NPs produced significant amounts of singlet oxygen. At greater UV exposures, more singlet oxygen was produced. Singlet oxygen's cell-killing impact was required to rule out the influence of UV and Cu-Cy NPs. UV can be used to sterilize, and other studies have demonstrated that NPs are very non-toxic to cells at low concentrations. Our MTT assay revealed that UV irradiation for 5 minutes (6 J/cm^2) had no significant effect on cellular viability, as did incubation with 25 µg/mL Cu-Cy NPs, and that the combination of UV irradiation and Cu-Cy NPs had a strong killing effect on the cell.

At the time of writing, there were three possible explanations for PDT's anti-tumor mechanism: (i) ROS directly killing tumour cells via apoptosis or necrosis; (ii) destruction of blood vessels in the tumour stroma, resulting in tumour ischemic necrosis; or (iii) inflammatory cells releasing immune mediators to enhance a specific immune function necessary for promoting the anti-tumor effect. The majority of researchers believe that ROS directly kill tumour cells by triggering apoptosis and that singlet oxygen is the primary cytotoxic agent. Emens discovered that the photosensitizer accumulates in subcellular organelles including the lysosome, mitochondria, and other membrane organelles. Singlet oxygen enhances the lysosome's permeability and releases a variety of enzymes that cause cell damage. Additionally, it disrupts mitochondria and induces the release of apoptotic agents such as caspase-3. We discovered that both Cu-Cy NPs and 5-FU were capable of inducing cellular death in our investigation using flow cytometry. 5-FU is a traditional Chinese medication used to treat liver cancer. It is used alone or in combination with other medications to treat liver cancer in clinical trials. Additionally, we noticed an increase in the expression of apoptosis-related proteins as the duration of action of Cu-Cy NPs (after UV irradiation) increased. Fortunately, *in vitro* experiments revealed that at the optimal concentration of Cu-Cy NPs (25 μg/mL), which was significantly less than the IC-50 value of 5-FU (226.84 μg/mL for HepG2), Cu-Cy NPs could initiate significantly more cellular apoptosis than 5-FU, indicating that the mechanism of action of Cu-Cy NPs in tumour treatment was induction of cellular apoptosis. We discovered that the anti-cancer activity of Cu-Cy NPs + UV was as effective as 5-FU *in vivo*, demonstrating that Cu-Cy NPs possessed anti-cancer potential. Nevertheless, there was no difference between the Cu-Cy NPs and the Cu-Cy NPs + UV groups *in vivo*. The explanation for this was that Cu-Cy NPs have a unique capacity to kill cancer cells. Due to the limitations of this experiment, we used UV rather than X-ray as the light source, as UV had a limited effect on penetrating the skin. As a result, the Cu-Cy NPs + UV reaction was altered. According to a previous study by Lun Ma, the optimal light source for irradiating Cu-Cy NPs was X-ray. If we employed X-rays instead of UV, the *in vivo* investigation would yield a more favourable result.

Two challenges must be resolved before this novel form of photosensitizer may be used in practical applications. The first is that the photosensitizer must reach the target tissue, and the second is that it must avoid being cleared by the reticuloendothelial system. Exosomes are a natural vehicle for the delivery of cancer drugs. They act as a buffer between the tissue and the medication. This protective layer not only assists in avoiding the reticuloendothelial system but also reduces tissue damage caused by the singlet oxygen produced by Cu-Cy NPs. We hypothesized that the soluble Cu-Cy NPs may enter the exosomes released by HepG2 cells based on the findings of the singlet oxygen detection. This discovery suggested a possible solution to the two concerns stated previously.

PDT is a highly successful treatment option that can be used in conjunction with surgery or radiation therapy to treat some types of cancer and precancerous lesions. Unlike other forms of conventional therapy (radiation, hormone therapy, or chemotherapy), PDT seldom causes DNA damage and is helpful in treating cancers that have established tolerance to other cytotoxic agents. PDT, on the other hand, continues to have some limits in clinical application. One of the drawbacks is the requirement for direct light supply to activate the photosensitizer. Thus, for some tumours that are anatomically distant, the supply of light is what makes PDT difficult to use for deep cancer treatment. The other constraint is the photosensitizer's biotoxicity. Numerous conventional photosensitizers, such as 5-aminlevulinic acid (5-ALA), have been shown to induce adverse effects in the human body during treatment. Cu-Cy NPs, as proposed in this research, may give a novel approach to overcoming these two restrictions. Cu-Cy NPs are a novel Cu-Cy complex that differs from conventional Cu-Cy complexes. They are being used as model compounds to advance our fundamental understanding of copper-containing enzymes. These Cu-Cy NPs exhibit several distinctive properties: (i) minimal cytotoxicity; (ii) can be activated immediately by UV radiation, X-rays, microwaves, and ultrasound; and (iii) soluble Cu-Cy NPs were able to penetrate exosomes, establishing a new route for nanoparticle targeting. Additionally, Cu-Cy NPs are inexpensive to produce.

The Bottom Line

In summary, we describe the anti-HCC activity of Cu-Cy NPs in this study. Cu-Cy NPs drastically reduced the activity of HepG2 cells at a very low dose following a brief exposure to ultraviolet radiation, and Cu-Cy NPs triggered cell death, which is associated with cellular apoptosis. Additionally, we discovered that Cu-Cy NPs suppressed tumour growth *in vivo*. Cu-Cy NPs can be incorporated into tumour cells' exosomes, and exosomes could be exploited to deliver Cu-Cy NPs to tumour cells. All of these findings show that Cu-Cy NPs as a novel class of medications have a bright future in cancer treatment.

2.5 Copper-Cysteamine Nanoparticles as a Novel Class of Antimicrobial Photodynamic Inactivation Agents

Antimicrobial photodynamic inactivation (aPDI) has gained popularity as a non-antibiotic alternative method for destroying pathogenic germs of all types, including Gram-positive and Gram-negative bacteria, fungal cells, viruses, and parasites. Its efficiency is not dependent on the bacteria' antibiotic resistance status, and despite repeated attempts, it has not been demonstrated to generate resistance. Because the germ-killing effect is active only in the presence of light, aPDI is safer than disinfectants and can also be used *in vivo* to treat localized illnesses. aPDI is a process that generates reactive oxygen species (ROS) when molecular oxygen reacts with the photosensitizer's excited state (PS). The majority of PS are dyes with an extensively conjugated system of unsaturated double bonds, which results in a strong absorption peak in the visible range and a high quantum yield of the excited singlet state. Intersystem crossing to a long-lived excited triplet state enables interaction with oxygen, either via energy transfer (Type II PDT) to generate

$^1O_2$ or via electron transfer (Type I PDT) to produce $O_2^{\cdot -}$, H_2O_2, and •OH. Both singlet oxygen and •OH are extremely reactive and have the potential to cause damage to lipids, proteins, and nucleic acids, ultimately resulting in cell death.

Gram-positive bacteria were discovered to be extremely susceptible to aPDI mediated by a wide variety of PS in 1990, whereas Gram-negative bacteria were only sensitive to PS with a strong cationic charge. Gram-negative bacteria's double cell wall acts as a barrier against the passage of anionic and neutral charged PS, as well as extracellularly produced $^1O_2$. Along with classic PS (phenothiazinium dyes, porphyrins, and phthalocyanines), there is another light-activated mechanism known as photocatalysis that can kill microbial cells. Photocatalysis utilizes NPs as large band-gap semiconductors that are stimulated by short wavelength light (mostly UVA and blue light) to generate ROS (hydroxyl radicals, hydrogen peroxide, and singlet oxygen) that are used to destroy bacteria. The best-studied example is titanium dioxide (TiO_2) nanoparticles with a diameter of 25 nm, such as the P25. TiO_2 nanoparticles have been proven to destroy a range of pathogenic bacteria by photocatalysis.

A novel kind of sensitizer was invented in our group in 2014, called copper-cysteamine (Cu-Cy). Cu-Cy is different from the other photosensitizers, and its various features make it a promising candidate for use in real-world scenarios. First, Cu-Cy, a novel sensitizer, generates $^1O_2$ in three ways: UV light, X-rays, and other methods such as microwaves and ultrasound and because of this, Cu-Cy NPs could be employed for both treating skin diseases and combating tumours. The second positive feature of Cu-Cy NPs is that they produce a strong luminescence, useful for both diagnostics and treatment. Cu-Cy has, however, never been proven to kill microorganisms. The first study we have reported on this shows whether light-activated sensitizers (killing bacteria) may be in the Cu-Cy NPs. To test for it, we experimented on two Gram-positive and two Gram-negative bacterial species, both of which are linked to multi-drug resistance.

Procedures

A 365-nm UVA light-emitting diode (LED) light source was used in this study (Larson Electronics LLC, Kemp, TX). A spectroradiometer (SPR-01; Luzchem Research, Inc., Ottawa, Ontario, Canada) was used to determine the emission spectra, which revealed a peak at 365 ± 5 nm. For all trials, the irradiance was set at 16 mW/cm^2 (1 J/cm^2 given in 1 minute), as determined by an International Light, Inc. model IL-1700 research radiometer-photometer (Newburyport, MA).

Gram-positive bacteria included Staphylococcus aureus (MRSA) US300 and Enterococcus faecalis ATCC 29212; Gram-negative bacteria included Escherichia coli (E. coli) K-12 (ATCC 33780) and Acinetobacter baumannii ATCC BAA 747 (ATCC, Manassas, VA). A colony of bacteria was suspended in 10 mL of BHI and cultivated overnight at 37°C and 120 rpm in an aerobic shaker incubator (New Brunswick Scientific, Edison, NJ, USA). A 1 mL aliquot from an overnight suspension was refreshed for 2 hours at 37°C in fresh BHI to mid-log phase. The optical density (OD) at 600 nm was used to calculate the cell concentration (OD of 0.8 = 10^8 CFU cells/mL).

Suspensions of bacteria (10^8 cells/mL) were incubated in the dark at room temperature for 30 minutes with various doses of Cu-Cy (1 µM, 10 µM, 50 µM, 100 µM). A 100 µL aliquot was obtained as the dark control from each sample; another 200 µL aliquot was transferred to a 96-well plate and lit from the top of the plates with 10 J/cm^2 of UVA light at 365 nm at room temperature. After illumination (or dark incubation), aliquots (100 µL) of each well were obtained to determine the colony-forming unit (CFU). Prior to sampling, care was taken to thoroughly mix the contents of the wells, as germs can settle to the bottom. The aliquots were serially diluted tenfold in pH 7.4 phosphate-buffered saline (PBS) to obtain dilutions of 10^{-1}–10^{-5} times the original concentration, and 10 µL aliquots of each dilution were streaked horizontally on square BHI agar plates. Plates were incubated at 37°C in the dark for 12–18 hours to allow colony development. Each experiment was repeated a minimum of three times. A control group of cells exposed to light alone (without the addition of Cu-Cy) exhibited the same number of CFU as the control (data not shown). Survival fractions were frequently represented as ratios of the number of CFU of microbial cells treated with light and Cu-Cy (or Cu-Cy alone) to the number of CFU of microorganisms treated with neither.

The generation of H_2O_2 from Cu-Cy mediated PDT was detected using an Amplex Red hydrogen peroxide/peroxidase assay. In the presence of peroxidase, the coloured probe Amplex Red (10-acetyl-3,7-dihydroxy phenoxazine) interacts with H_2O_2 to create resorufin (7-hydroxy3H-phenoxazin-3-one). The detection procedure was carried out according to the manufacturer's instructions following Cu-Cy-mediated PDT. The reaction systems containing 10 µM Cu-Cy were illuminated with increasing fluences of UVA (365 nm) light, and aliquots were taken and added to 50 µM Amplex Red reagent and 0.1 U/mL horseradish peroxidase (HRP) in Krebs-Ringer, phosphate (contains 145 mM NaCl, 5.7 mM Na$_3$PO$_4$, 4.86 mM KCl, 0.54 CaCl$_2$, 1.22 mM MgSO$_4$,

5.5 mM glucose, pH 7.35). After 30 minutes of incubation, an incremental fluorescence of 365 nm light was given using a fluorescence microplate reader (excitation 530 nm; emission 590 nm). There were two groups: (1) Cu-Cy + light; and (2) Amplex Red reagent alone. Each experiment was repeated a minimum of three times.

Outcomes

Cu-Cy NPs include two distinct Cu atoms—Cu(1) and Cu(2) (both are Cu^+ ions), which attach to four and three additional atoms, respectively. Cu-Cy NPs exhibit strong photoluminescence and X-ray luminescence. Our earlier article detailed the crystal structure and optical characteristics of Cu-Cy NPs in detail. The samples employed in this investigation were coated with polyethylene glycol and have a diameter of approximately 70–110 nm, as determined by their TEM images displayed in Figure 2-13a. The image shows a lattice spacing of 0.227 nm (Figure 2-13b). As illustrated in Figure 2-13c-e, the particles exhibit a strong red luminescence. As illustrated in Figure 2-13e, the emission spectrum has doublet peaks at 607 and 633 nm (bottom). Two emission peaks correspond to two distinct types of copper ions, namely Cu(1) and Cu(2), which differ in their degree of coordination. The longer wavelength (633 nm) emission is attributed to Cu(1) since it has shorter distances to surrounding copper ions (2.81 Å and 2.89 Å) than Cu(2) does (3.31 Å and 3.74 Å); so, the 607 nm emission is attributed to Cu(2) ions.

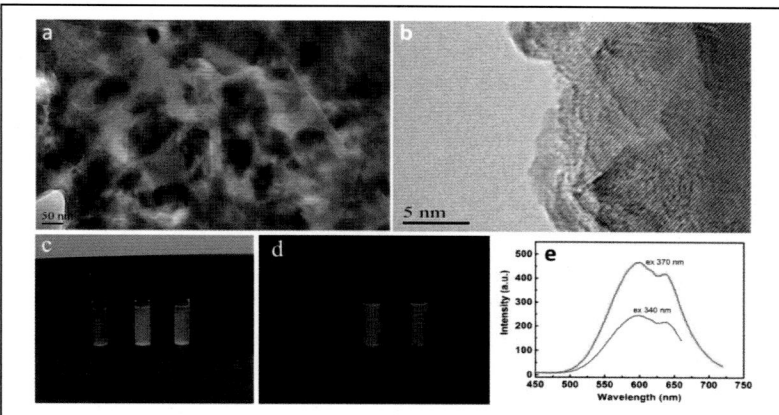

Fig. 2-13 The TEM images (a,b), the picture of the samples at room light (c) and under a UV light (d) as well as the emission spectra of Cu-Cy nanoparticles. The particle size is about 100 nm. Adopted from ref. 7 with permission

It is critical to establish in vitro ROS generation during *in vitro* aPDI investigations. There are several different ROS assays that can be employed, each with a distinct range of ROS species that can be detected and a varied level of specificity. We were able to quantify the dose-dependent generation of H_2O_2 in the present investigation by irradiating 10 μM with 360 nm UVA radiation and utilizing the Amplex Red assay, as shown in Figure 2-14. Additionally, sodium azide at a concentration of 50 mM was added to the mixture in order to better understand the photochemical reaction process. Azide suppressed H$_2$O$_2$ generation by more than 80% at higher light exposures. The fact that the rate of H$_2$O$_2$ production remains linear even at relatively high light doses (up to 80 J/cm^2) indicates that Cu-Cy NPs are relatively resistant to photobleaching. Azide is used to physically quench ^{1}O$_2$. The discovery that azide greatly inhibited H$_2$O$_2$ generation shows that H$_2$O$_2$ is formed when ^{1}O$_2$ undergoes a two-electron oxidation in the following manner:

$$^1O_2 + 2H^+ + 2e^- \rightarrow H_2O_2 \quad (1)$$

Cu-Cy NPs activated by UV radiation, X-rays, microwaves, or ultrasound produced ROS that were identified as ^{1}O$_2$ using the p-nitrosodimethylaniline (RNO)-imidazole (ID) technique and fluorescence activation of DCFH-DA. All of these findings suggest that Cu-Cy NPs are potentially useful and effective photodynamic activators.

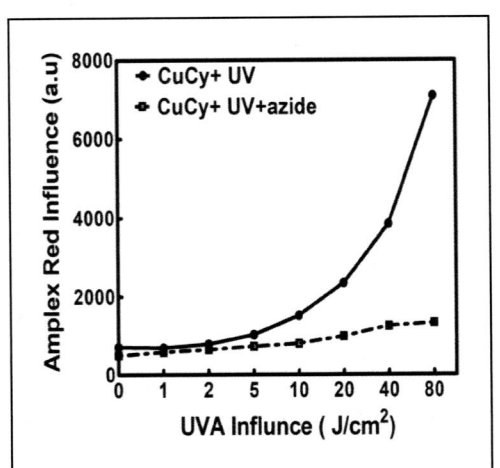

Figure 2-14. Production of H$_2$O$_2$ from UVA (360 nm) illuminated Cu-Cy NPs and inhibition by azide. Cu-Cy was used at 10 μM and azide at 50 mM. After each incremental dose of light an aliquot of the reaction mixture was removed and added to the Amplex red reagent. Adopted from ref. 7 with permission

The death curves for four distinct bacteria are shown in Figures 2-15. They were incubated with increasing concentrations of Cu-Cy NPs and illuminated with 10 J/cm^2 of 360 nm light. Gram-positive MRSA is depicted in Figure 2-15(A), and nearly two logs of killing were observed with 50 μM Cu-Cy, with total eradication (>6 logs of killing) accomplished with 100 μM Cu-Cy. The other Gram-positive species, E faecalis (Fig. 2-15(B)), was slightly more sensitive to death, with 10 μM Cu-Cy killing 1 log, 50 μM killing 3 logs, and 100 μM killing completely. In comparison, Gram-negative E. coli was hardly killed at all (Fig. 2-15(c)), with less than a log of death detected at 100 μM. Similarly, even at 100 μM, Gram-negative A. baumannii (Fig. 2-15(d)) was only minimally destroyed.

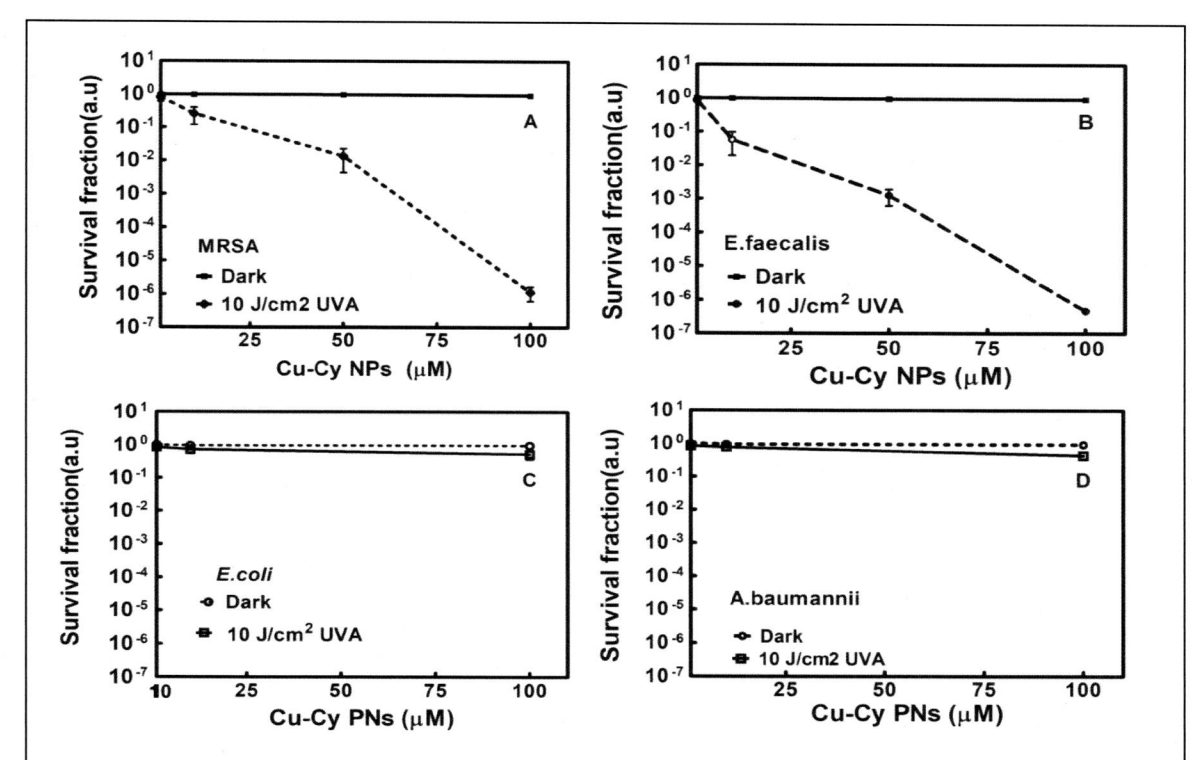

Figure 2-15. aPDI killing curves of bacteria incubated with increasing concentrations of Cu-Cy NPs and irradiated or not with 10 J/cm² of UVA light. (A) Gram-positive MRSA; (B) Gram-positive *E. faecalis;* (C) Gram-negative *E. coli;* (D) Gram-negative *A. baumannii.* Adopted from ref. 7 with permission

Analysis

The findings indicate that Cu-Cy NPs are highly effective at inactivating gram-positive bacteria but are ineffective against gram-negative bacteria. This is consistent with the majority of photosensitizers reported on bacteria inactivation thus far. Gram-negative bacteria are more resistant to antibiotics than Gram-positive bacteria, which should come as no surprise to those working in the aPDI sector. This observation has been reported numerous times over a broad spectrum of various PS. The difference in how gram-positive and gram-negative bacteria are killed is due to their structural differences.

The distinctions between Gram-positive and Gram-negative bacteria are mostly based on the structure of their cell walls. Gram-positive bacteria have cell walls composed primarily of a material called peptidoglycan that is peculiar to bacteria. Gram-negative bacteria have cell walls composed entirely of peptidoglycan and an outer membrane composed entirely of lipopolysaccharides, which are absent from Gram-positive bacteria. Gram-negative bacteria are composed of three distinct layers: an outer membrane (OM), a peptidoglycan cell wall, and an inner membrane (IM). They account for the majority of drug-resistant infections and have a complex envelope consisting of an outer (OM) and inner (IM) membrane delimiting a periplasmic gap. This cellular structure leads to the presence of many protein channels that regulate the transport, absorption, and efflux of a wide variety of substances, nutrients, and harmful molecules (sugars, medicines, short peptides, and chemicals). Gram-negative bacteria's outer membrane serves as their first line of defense against harmful chemicals. This barrier is completely impenetrable to big, negatively charged molecules. Porins, which are water-filled open channels that cross the outer membrane and allow passive penetration of hydrophilic molecules, are mostly responsible for flow control. Bacterial pathogenicity is mostly determined by the surface features of the bacteria. Outer membrane proteins (OMPs), such as the porins, are critical components of the bacterial outer membrane and represent promising targets for therapeutic development. Porins are crucial in the exchange of nutrients across the Gram-negative bacteria's outer membrane, but they are also implicated in pathogenesis. The OM is a distinctive feature of Gram-negative bacteria; in fact, Gram-positive bacteria lack this structure, which helps differentiate the two bacteria's behaviours.

Bacterial cells have a negative charge on their walls. The explanation for the negative charge in Gram positive bacteria is the presence of teichoic acids that connect the peptidoglycan to the underlying plasma membrane. Due to the inclusion of phosphate in their structure, these teichoic acids are negatively charged. Gram negative bacteria are covered in phospholipids and lipopolysaccharides on the outside. Lipopolysaccharides negatively charge the surface of Gram-negative bacteria. As a result, cationic NPs are superior at killing Gram-negative cells, whereas cationic PS are frequently far more effective at killing Gram-positive bacteria. It has been proposed that cationic PS enter the outer membrane of Gram-negative bacteria via a "self-promoted uptake pathway" in which the divalent metal cations Ca^{2+} and Mg^{2+} are gradually displaced by the PS and the lipopolysaccharide in the outer membrane permeability barrier is destabilized. Cu-Cy NPs are negatively charged due to their coating with poly(ethylene glycol) methyl ether thiol, making them difficult to adhere to bacterial membranes or cell walls. This is one of the reasons why gram-negative bacteria are resistant to antibiotics. Second, due to their huge size, the Cu-Cy NPs were unable to permeate the cell walls. General bacterial porins are a family of proteins found in Gram-negative bacteria's outer membranes. Porins function as a molecular filter for hydrophilic molecules. They are responsible for the outer membrane's 'molecular sieve' characteristics. Porins are broad, water-filled channels that allow hydrophilic molecules to diffuse into the periplasmic region. The inner membrane is the primary permeability barrier in gram-negative bacteria. Due to the presence of porins, the outer membrane is more permeable to hydrophilic molecules. Porins have transportable molecule thresholds that vary according to the kind of bacteria and porin. Generally, only compounds with a diameter of less than 600 Daltons, or approximately 2 nm, can diffuse through. The Cu-Cy particles used in this study are 70–110 nm in size, which is significantly larger than the channels of porins and so cannot pass through them. Thus, the bulk of killing may be due to the ROS created by Cu-Cy NPs during light activation.

Our results established that when UV light at 360 nm was used to activate Cu-Cy NPs, the combined treatment produced $^1O_2$ and H_2O_2. The damage caused by $^1O_2$ and/or H_2O_2 could be a significant factor in the bacteria's death, as $^1O_2$ or H_2O_2 has been shown to directly kill both gram-positive and gram-negative bacteria. The lipopolysaccharide coat (LPS) on the gram-negative bacterial cell wall provides some protection against the harmful effects of external substances. The majority of gram-positive bacteria lack a protective structure comparable to the gram-negative LPS and the outer membrane to which it is attached. Additionally, to acting as a structural barrier to penetration, this outer membrane may operate as a chemical trap for $^1O_2$; it is made of unsaturated fatty acids and proteins, both of which react chemically with $^1O_2$. However, the outer membrane and LPS of gram-negative bacteria are not critical targets for singlet oxygen's fatal action, as they can be removed without killing the cells (spheroplast formation). Because the cell wall structure of gram-positive and gram-negative bacteria is fundamentally different, once the barrier is passed by $^1O_2$, the targets and processes for cell killing would be comparable or identical for both gram-positive and gram-negative bacteria. As mentioned in Reference 10, $^1O_2$ hitting the outer membrane-LPS section of the gram-negative bacteria's cell wall may collide without causing any response or penetration, react with the outer membrane's components, or penetrate through the various layers to the essential target. Reactions with the outer membrane components may result in the formation of reactive secondary products such as peroxy radicals, which may cause deadly damage to the essential target. The total toxicity would then be the sum of the $^1O_2$ that enters the inner membrane and the deadly effects of secondary reaction products that exit the outer membrane. $^1O_2$ may easily diffuse through the comparatively open structure of the peptidoglycan layer of the gram-positive bacteria's cell wall to react with the critical target. The pace of killing should then be entirely determined by direct singlet oxygen-vital target interactions, with no need for additional reaction mechanisms such as those found in the gram-negative outer membrane. This explains pretty well why Cu-Cy NPs are far more effective in killing gram-positive bacteria than gram-negative bacteria, as $^1O_2$ is the major ROS product produced by Cu-Cy NPs during the energy transfer process during UV excitation. While H_2O_2 was discovered using the Amplex Red test, it is not the predominant result because it is a byproduct of $^1O_2$. As demonstrated in Eq. (1), the process described only possible in acidic circumstances, such as those seen in tumours. Additionally, it was observed that, similar to other ROS, H_2O_2 has a restricted ability to diffuse through membranes. As depicted in Figure 2-16, the observations demonstrate that Cu-Cy nanoparticles are extremely effective as a novel class of therapeutics for photodynamic inactivation of bacteria and related infectious illnesses.

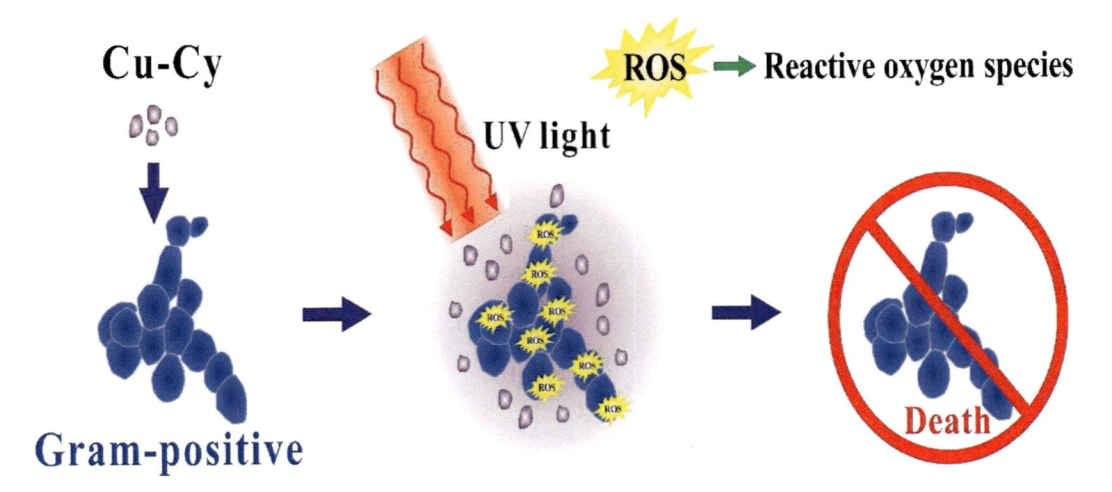

Figure 2-16 Copper Cysteamine nanoparticles as a new type of agents for photodynamic inactivation of bacteria and infectious diseases by producing reactive oxygen species for bacterial destruction Adopted from ref. 7 with permission

The Bottom Line

In summary, we demonstrated that copper-cysteamine NPs, a novel class of sensitizers, are quite effective against gram-positive bacteria but are quite ineffective against gram-negative bacteria at the moment. The primary mechanism of action is the interaction of $^1O_2$ and H_2O_2. Gram-positive bacteria are more susceptible to ROS assault from Cu-Cy NPs due to the comparatively open structure of their peptidoglycan layer. Cu-Cy NPs are promising anti-bacterial and associated disease agents due to their effective generation of various ROS such as $^1O_2$ and H_2O_2. Cu-Cy NPs exhibit properties extremely similar to TiO_2 NPs, which have been extensively researched for their ability to inactivate microorganisms. Both TiO_2 and Cu-Cy NPs can be activated using X-rays or microwaves to generate ROS. PS that can be activated by X-rays or microwaves is pretty unique. Cu-Cy NPs appear to have a high potential for bacteria inactivation, which warrants further investigation.

2.6 Highly Effective Combination of Copper-Cysteamine Nanoparticles and Potassium Iodide for the Killing of Bacteria

Preface

Bacterial and viral diseases have always posed a significant hazard to human beings. Excessive consumption and reliance on antibiotics increase the likelihood of antibiotic resistance developing in many bacterial species, prompting numerous academics to discuss the 'end of the antibiotic epidemic.' Antibiotic resistance is a public health issue. Finding more effective antibiotic medicines to tackle resistant strains is a pressing issue that could help avert an outbreak. For instance, a pathogenic Gram-negative bacterial species such as E. coli, which possesses an unmatched ability to survive on surfaces for extended periods of time, poses a risk to patients. As a result, researchers are concentrating their efforts on developing novel remedies that are effective against multidrug-resistant bacteria that cause fatal illnesses.

Photodynamic treatment utilizes photosensitizers (PS) that, when activated by a proper light source, generate reactive oxidative species (ROS) that can destroy bacteria and viruses. These ROS are capable of neutralizing a wide variety of biomolecules found in microbes independent of their structure or resistance. The photodynamic efficiency of a PS is dependent on a number of elements, including the PS concentration, the oxygen level, the wavelength of the light, and the intensity of the light. It is well established that a PS may be highly selective for bacteria through careful chemical design, ensuring that molecules stick to bacteria rather than normal human cells during brief incubation durations. We recently invented copper-cysteamine (Cu-Cy), Cu$_3$Cl(SR)$_2$ (R = CH$_2$CH$_2$NH$_2$), as a novel form of sensitizer with high luminescence and the ability to generate ROS when exposed to UV light, X-rays, microwaves, and ultrasound. All of these findings suggest that Cu-Cy is a new sensitizer with anti-infection and anti-tumor potential. Our earlier study demonstrated that while Cu-Cy NPs can successfully kill gram-positive bacteria such as MRSA, they are ineffective against gram-negative bacteria such as E. coli when exposed to UV radiation. The present work demonstrates that when KI is added to Cu-Cy NPs, both Gram-positive MRSA and Gram-negative E. coli are considerably inactivated. Additionally, to demonstrate the phenomenon, the interaction of KI with Cu-Cy NPs and the killing mechanisms were explored in detail. The mechanistic studies demonstrated that when Cu-Cy NPs + KI are exposed to UV radiation, they create singlet oxygen, hydrogen peroxide, and triiodide ions, which kill both gram-positive and gram-negative bacteria.

G2. Components and Procedures

Strains and cultures of bacteria

As microbiological strains, Gram-positive (methicillin-resistant Staphylococcus aureus (MRSA) US300) and Gram-negative (E. coli K-12 (ATCC 33780)) bacteria were used. Bacteria were colonized by suspending in 25 mL of BHI broth and incubating overnight at 37 °C and 120 rpm in a shaker incubator. 1 mL of this suspension was added to freshly prepared BHI and incubated at 37 °C for 2 hours to reach the mid-log growth phase. To determine the cell concentration, the suspension's optical density (OD) at 600 nm was determined (OD of 0.8 = 10^8 colony-forming unit (CFU) cells/mL). The suspension was then centrifuged, washed, and resuspended in PBS to inhibit microbial growth before being employed (10^8 CFU).

Studies on photodynamic treatment (PDT)

We performed PDT experiments on MRSA and E. coli cells (10^8 CFU; 500 L) that were cultured for 30 minutes with or without UV radiation with various concentrations of Cu-Cy NPs (1, 10, 50, and 100 μM). Afterwards, 10 μL of the suspension from each sample was used as a control, while 200 μL of the suspension was placed to a 96 well plate and irradiated with UV radiation (365 nm, 10 J/cm^2). To determine the survival fraction, cell samples were serially diluted in PBS up to 10^{-5}

times their initial concentration, and 10 µL of each dilution streaked horizontally on square BHI agar plates for bacteria. Plates were then streaked in triplicate and incubated at 37 °C in the dark for 12–18 hours. The survival fractions were calculated as the ratio of CFU of experimental and control microbial cells. To examine the influence of KI on bacterial inactivation, we repeated the experiment with a mixture of Cu-Cy NPs (10 and 50 µM) and KI (0, 50, and 100 mM). Finally, we examined the bactericidal activity of Cu-Cy NPs on MRSA and E. coli in the presence or absence of KI-mediated PDT therapy under UV light.

Cu^{2+} detection

Cu^{2+} was determined using electron spin resonance (ESR) at the X band on a Bruker ER-200DSRC Analytic ESR spectrometer at room temperature in order to better understand the likely mechanism of bacteria-killing. The experiment was conducted at a frequency of 9.64 GHz with a microwave power of 63 µW. 1 mL Cu-Cy (1 mg/mL), and 1 mL Cu-Cy (1 mg/mL) + KI (600 mg/mL) solutions were prepared and stored overnight in liquid nitrogen.

Detection of singlet oxygen ($^1O_2$)

We measured $^1O_2$ using the RNO-ID technique. Specifically, 0.225 mg of RNO and 16.34 mg of ID were added in DI water (30 mL). The solution was then oxygenated by air bubbling for approximately 20 minutes. The sample was prepared by diluting 2 mL of the aforesaid RNO-ID solution with 0.5 mL of Cu-Cy (200 µM) and 0.5 mL of KI (50 mM). The control experiment was conducted by substituting 0.5 mL DI water for 0.5 mL KI while maintaining all other experimental conditions. Meanwhile, the two groups were exposed to UV radiation (10 J/cm^2) at intervals ranging from 0–8 minutes. A Shimadzu UV-2450 spectrophotometer was used to determine the RNO absorbance at 440 nm.

Determination of hydrogen peroxide using the Amplex red assay

The formation of H_2O_2 from Cu-Cy NPs plus KI-mediated PDT was determined using the Amplex Red hydrogen peroxide test. Amplex Red, which is not fluorescent, can react with H_2O_2 to form fluorescent resorufin in the presence of peroxidase. UV light was used to illuminate reaction systems containing Cu-Cy NPs with or without KI (365 nm). The illuminated samples were then transferred to Krebs–Ringer phosphate and incubated with Amplex Red reagent (50 µM) and horseradish peroxidase (0.1 U/mL). After a half-hour incubation period, a fluorescence microplate reader (Exi/Emi at 530 nm/590 nm) was used to quantify the fluorescence intensity changes on Cu-Cy NPs and Cu-Cy NPs + KI upon UV stimulation (365 nm). To establish whether H_2O_2 was involved in the generation of singlet oxygen in the mixture, sodium azide (NaN_3), a physical scavenger of singlet oxygen, was utilized.

Test for Iodine starch

Cu-Cy NPs (100 µM) and Cu-Cy NPs (100 µM) + KI (100 mM) were irradiated with UV light at various intensities for 5 minutes, and aliquots (50 µL) were taken following each illumination to determine iodine concentration by adding 50 µL of the starch indicator. Following that, absorbance at 610 nm was determined using a microplate reader.

Detection of superoxide radicals using the nitroblue tetrazolium (NBT) assay

The superoxide assay NBT (20 mM), Cu-Cy NPs (10 µM), and KI (50 mM) were combined in PBS immediately prior to the experiment. After UV illumination of Cu-Cy and Cu-Cy + KI, the absorbance of the resultant blue product was measured at 560 nm using an optical microplate reader.

Analysis of Statistics

To determine statistical significance, a one-way analysis of variance (ANOVA) was utilized. P less than 0.05 was considered significant statistically. At least three independent analyses of the data indicated by the mean and standard deviation were done.

G3. Outcomes

Cu-Cy Characterizations

Cu-Cy NPs dispersed in DI water are shown in Fig. 2-26a under ambient light (left) and UV irradiation (right). As illustrated in Fig. 1a and b, the Cu-Cy NPs exhibit a bright red glow. As illustrated in Fig. 2-26b, the emission spectrum contains doublet peaks at 607 and 633 nm. Two emission peaks correspond to two distinct copper ions—Cu(1) and Cu(2) that differ in their coordination. The emission peak at 633 nm relates to Cu(1) because it has shorter distances to nearby copper ions (2.81 Å and 2.89 Å) than Cu(2) does (3.31 Å and 3.74 Å); hence, the emission at 607 nm corresponds to Cu(2) ions. TEM images of the Cu-Cy NPs employed in this work are shown in Fig. 2-26c and d. The size distribution of Cu-Cy NPs with an average diameter of 93 ±

41 nm is shown in Fig. 2-26e. The electron diffraction pattern (Fig. 2-26f) demonstrates the Cu-Cy NPs are single crystals.

Measurement of Reactive oxygen species (ROS)

The absorption spectrum of Cu-Cy NPs in DI water is shown in Fig. 2-17a. Cu-Cy absorbs strongly in the ultraviolet region (peak at 365 nm), but relatively little in the visible range. This property distinguishes Cu-Cy NPs from typical photosensitizers, which exhibit significant absorption in both the UV and visible ranges. Due to its high absorption in the UV region, Cu-Cy can be utilized to cure bacterial infections when exposed to UV radiation. Meanwhile, there was no drop in RNO absorbance in the control group (DI water) (Fig. 2-17b), demonstrating that UV radiation alone is incapable of generating singlet oxygen.

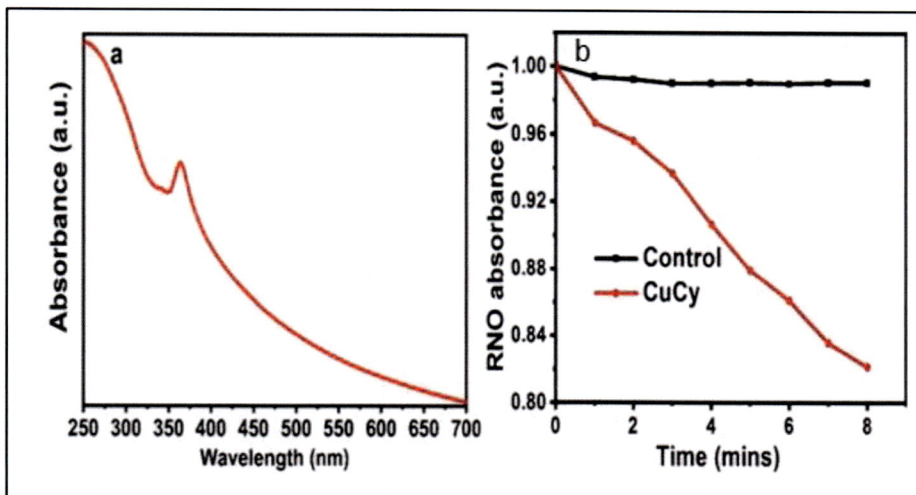

Figure 2-17. (a) Optical absorption spectrum of Cu-Cy NPs in aqueous solution. **(b)** RNO absorption curves of DI water (control) and Cu-Cy NPs upon UV light irradiation. Adopted from ref. 8 with permission

Cu-Cy NPs had a PDT effect on MRSA and E.coli when exposed to UV radiation

We tested the PDT effect of Cu-Cy in the presence of UV radiation, and the results are shown in Fig. 2-18. The results indicated that in the absence of light, Cu-Cy NPs posed no discernible toxicity to any type of bacterium. However, when exposed to UV light, the Cu-Cy NPs demonstrated clear antibacterial activity against MRSA in a dose-dependent manner (Fig. 2-18a). As seen in Fig. 2-18a, even at 50 μM Cu-Cy, the cytotoxic effect increased dramatically. When 100 μM Cu-Cy was applied, the cytotoxicity against MRSA increased by more than five logs. Cu-Cy NPs, on the other hand, were unable to significantly kill E.coli; even at a concentration of 100 μM Cu-Cy, the survival fraction decreased by less than 1 log (Fig. 2-18b). So, we may conclude that Cu-Cy exposed to UV radiation has a considerable effect on MRSA but essentially little effect on E. coli, as previously reported.

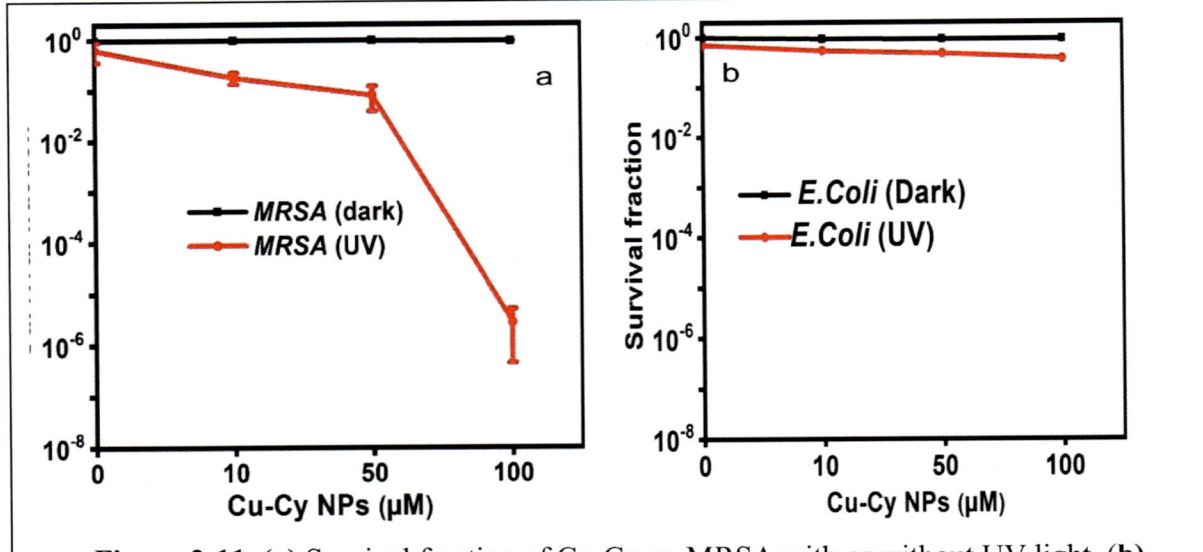

Figure 2-11. (a) Survival fraction of Cu-Cy on MRSA with or without UV light. (b) Survival fraction of Cu-Cy on *E. coli* with or without UV light. Adopted from ref. 8 with permission

Cu-Cy NPs plus KI have a PDT effect against MRSA

To assess the PDT effect of Cu-Cy with KI, MRSA was inoculated with 10 µM of Cu-Cy NPs containing varying doses of KI (Fig. 2-19a). The results indicated that as the concentration of KI is increased, the bactericidal action becomes increasingly significant. Additionally, when 50 µM Cu-Cy NPs were used, the bactericidal ability enhanced considerably when 50 mM KI was added ($P < 0.01$). The results indicate that KI can improve the lethal impact of Cu-Cy NPs mediated by PDT. Notably, no significant variation in the survival fraction of bacteria was reported when 100 mM KI was utilized instead of 50 mM, demonstrating that KI is non-toxic. These findings prompted us to investigate the PDT effect of Cu-Cy + KI on gram-negative bacteria such as E. Coli.

Cu-Cy NPs plus KI have a PDT effect on MRSA and E.coli

MRSA and E. coli bacteria were treated with UV, Cu-Cy + UV, and Cu-Cy + UV + KI. As illustrated in Fig. 2-19b, UV light (10 J/cm^2) alone had no effect on the survival proportion of bacteria. UV irradiation, on the other hand, had a considerable killing effect on MRSA bacteria in the presence of Cu-Cy NPs (50 μM) (MRSA vs. E.coli: 0.08 0.025 vs. 0.52 0.127; P 0.005). Additionally, Cu-Cy NPs + UV killed significantly more MRSA than UV alone, but not E. coli, which is consistent with our prior result. Most intriguingly, when KI (50 mM) was added to Cu-Cy NPs, the killing impact on MRSA and E.coli was dramatically increased, with the latter being more pronounced (>6 log). MRSA (Cu-Cy alone vs. Cu-Cy + KI: 0.143 ± 0.065 vs. $e^{-9} \pm e^{-10}$; P= $0.014 < 0.05$); E.coli (Cu-Cy alone vs. Cu-Cy + KI: 0.523 ± 0.127 vs. 0.029 ± 0.016; P < 0.001). Additionally, the Cu-Cy + KI group had a statistically equivalent killing effect on gram-negative and gram-positive bacteria (P > 0.05) (MRSA vs. E.coli: $e^{-9} \pm e^{-10}$ vs. 0.029 ± 0.016; P= $0.575 > 0.005$), implying that Cu-Cy NPs + KI was effective against both types of bacteria. This finding

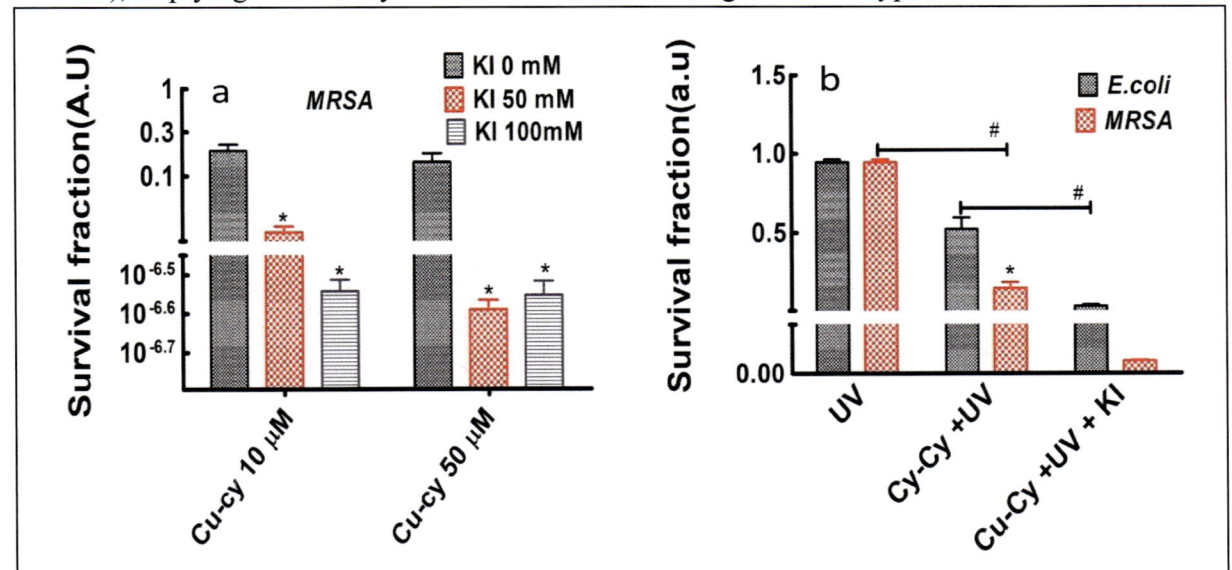

Figure 2-19. PDT effect study of Cu-Cy + KI. **(a)** Killing effect of Cu-Cy NPs (10 μM) and (50 μM) with or without KI on PDT against MRSA. *versus control, P < 0.01, #versus in group, P < 0.05. **(b)** Killing effect of Cu-Cy NPs (50 μM) with or without KI (50 mM) against MRSA and *E. coli*. *versus MRSA and *E. coli* in group, P < 0.01, #versus in different group, P < 0.01. Adopted from ref. 8 with permission

demonstrates that the bactericidal activity of Cu-Cy NPs was significantly enhanced by the addition of KI, particularly against E.coli.

Analysis

We conducted a number of experiments to elucidate the mechanisms underlying the powerful combination of Cu-Cy NPs and KI. Due to the presence of phospholipids and lipopolysaccharides, Gram-negative bacteria have a significant negative charge on their outer membrane. Thus, cationic NPs are superior at killing Gram-negative organisms, whereas cationic PS are frequently superior at killing Gram-positive bacteria. It has been claimed that the cationic PS enter the outer membrane of Gram-negative bacteria via a "self-promoted uptake pathway" in which the divalent metal cations Ca^{2+} and Mg^{2+} are gradually displaced by the PS and the lipopolysaccharide in the outer membrane permeability barrier is destabilized. Cu-Cy NPs were coated with a negatively charged poly (ethylene glycol) methyl ether thiol, which makes them insoluble in bacterial membranes or cell walls. This is one of the reasons why gram-negative bacteria are resistant to antibiotics. Second, because of the huge size of the Cu-Cy NPs, they were unable to enter the cell walls. Gram-negative bacteria contain an outer membrane protein family called porins. Porins act as molecular filters for water-soluble compounds. At the outer membrane, they act as molecular sieves. Porins can typically disperse particles up to 600 Da or around 2 nm in size. Cu-Cy NPs in this study are 93 ± 41 nm in size, which is significantly larger than the channels of porins, and so cannot pass through them. As a result, the bulk of killing may be due to the ROS and other toxins created when Cu-Cy NPs interact with KI in response to light activation.

ESR detection of Cu^{2+}

One theory is that when Cu-Cy NPs interact with KI, copper ions are liberated from Cu-Cy NPs, resulting in a Fenton reaction that generates ROS capable of killing bacteria. Copper is a redox-active transition metal that can promote the generation of ROS. Cu^{2+} can be reduced to the strong and reactive Cu^+ ion under reducing circumstances, which can produce ROS such as hydroxyl radicals (•OH), which can cause tissue damage. Copper ions produced from Cu-Cy NPs have been demonstrated to promote ROS production via the Fenton and Haber-Weiss reactions:

$Cu^+ + H_2O \rightarrow Cu^{2+} + •OH + {}^-OH$ (Fenton Reaction) - (1)

$O_2^- + H_2O_2 \rightarrow O_2 + •OH + {}^-OH$ (Haber–Weiss Reaction) - (2)

If the aforementioned Fenton reactions occurred, Cu^{2+} ions would be identified through ESR, as previously described. As illustrated in Fig. 2-20a, the ESR spectra for Cu-Cy and Cu-Cy + KI both exhibit a very faint Cu^{2+} signal near g = 2.06. In comparison to the signal strength of a 1 mM Cu^{2+} standard, this signal would account for 8 μM and 2 μM total Cu^{2+} concentrations, respectively, in Cu-Cy and Cu-Cy + KI samples. The result implies that KI does not induce copper release from Cu-Cy NPs in aqueous solution, and hence that copper release and thus Fenton reaction is not one of the mechanisms by which Cu-Cy NPs + KI generate cytotoxicity for bacterial inactivation. As stated below, there must be some other toxic species formed during the interaction of Cu-Cy NPs with KI that are fatal to bacteria.

The effect of KI on the formation of singlet oxygen from Cu-Cy NPs

As mentioned in our earlier work, the RNO-ID approach was employed to determine singlet oxygen ($^1O_2$). To ascertain if $^1O_2$ plays a significant role in the potentiated microbial death, we examined the generation of $^1O_2$ from Cu-Cy NPs with and without KI. As illustrated in Fig. 2-20b, KI effectively quenched the $^1O_2$ produced by Cu-Cy NPs. As a result, it is reasonable to conclude that $^1O_2$ does not play a significant role in PDT-mediated apoptosis.

Other probable results of the interaction between Cu-Cy NPs and KI

The generation of H_2O_2 was further examined using the Amplex red assay. As shown in Fig. 2-30c, the fluorescence intensity of the Amplex red increased linearly with increasing UV light fluence to a solution of Cu-Cy NPs (50 μM) and KI (400 mM), whereas without KI, the fluorescence intensity increased only slightly. As a result, we determined that a large amount of H_2O_2 was generated when KI was added to Cu-Cy NPs. Interestingly, when $^1O_2$ was quenched with NaN_3, nearly little H_2O_2 was created, demonstrating that $^1O_2$ plays a critical role in H_2O_2 generation.

ROS formed during the photodynamic reaction have the potential to oxidize the iodide anion to molecular iodine. Additionally, we performed a starch iodine assay to determine whether molecular iodine was produced when Cu-Cy NPs and KI were mixed (Fig. 2-20d). However, the experiment identified no molecular iodine at various light intensities (0–32 J/cm^2).

Oxidation of iodine and production of H_2O_2

In Eqs. (3)–(5), one proposed method of H_2O_2 generation is provided. $^1O_2$ can oxidize the iodide ion through this manner, generating iodide radical and superoxide radical ($O_2^{\cdot-}$) (Eq. (3)). The iodide radical dimerizes to form diiodine (Eq. (4)), whereas the $O_2^{\cdot-}$ dismutates to form H_2O_2 (Eq (5)).

$$^1O_2 + I^- \rightarrow O_2^{\cdot-} + I^\cdot \qquad - (3)$$

$$2I^\cdot \rightarrow I_2 \qquad - (4)$$

$$2O_2^{\cdot-} + 2H^+ \rightarrow O_2 + H_2O_2 \qquad - (5)$$

To ascertain that the procedure was followed, we performed the nitro blue tetrazolium (NBT) assay to assess whether $O_2^{\cdot-}$ was created in the Cu-Cy + KI. However, no $O_2^{\cdot-}$ was identified using the NBT assay, showing that the postulated process for H_2O_2 production did not occur. (Equations (3)–(5))

The interaction of $^1O_2$ and iodide is a second proposed process for H_2O_2 generation.

$$^1O_2 + I^- + H_2O \rightarrow IOOH + HO^- \qquad - (6)$$

$$IOOH + I^- \rightarrow HOOI_2^- \qquad - (7)$$

$$HOOI_2^- \rightarrow I_2 + HO_2^- \qquad - (8)$$

$$I_2 + I^- \rightarrow I_3^- \qquad - (9)$$

$$HO_2^- + H_2O \rightarrow H_2O_2 + HO^- \qquad - (10)$$

The reaction schemes (Eqs. (6)– (10)) outline the stages involved in the generation of H_2O_2 in the Cu-Cy + KI mixture. These reactions can be merged into a single equation (Eq. 11). The interaction of $^1O_2$ and iodide is a second proposed process for H_2O_2 generation.

$$^1O_2 + 3I^- + 2H_2O \rightarrow I_3^- + 2H_2O_2 \qquad - (11)$$

It has been stated that absorptions at 288 and 352 nm are due to a portion of the I_3^- anion in solution and that all molecular iodine has been transformed to I_3^-. As a result, we analyzed the absorbance of the Cu-Cy NPs + KI mixture in the UV wavelength area to confirm the presence of triiodide species. As expected, introducing KI to Cu-Cy NPs resulted in the appearance of a new absorption peak at 280–290 nm, which became increasingly prominent over time (Fig. 2-20e). In the presence of $^1O_2$, the iodine molecule exists only in a transitory state and promptly changes to the triiodide species. As a result, the iodine molecule was not detectable using a starch assay. As a result, $^1O_2$, biocidal triiodide (I_3^-), and H_2O_2 may be the results of Cu-Cy NPs + KI solution that contribute to the improved antimicrobial activity. Our findings corroborate a prior observation that triiodide can enhance microbial death when combined with H_2O_2.

Influence of KI on the luminescence of Cu-Cy NPs

To investigate the influence of KI on the luminescence of Cu-Cy NPs, different concentrations of KI were added with the same amount of Cu-Cy NPs. After two hours of incubation, the emission spectra were measured using a spectrofluorophotometer. We discovered that as the amount of KI increased, the luminescence intensity decreased (Fig. 2-20f). This may be due to the interaction of iodide ions with Cu-Cy NPs, as iodide ions have the potential to decrease the fluorescence of several luminous dyes.

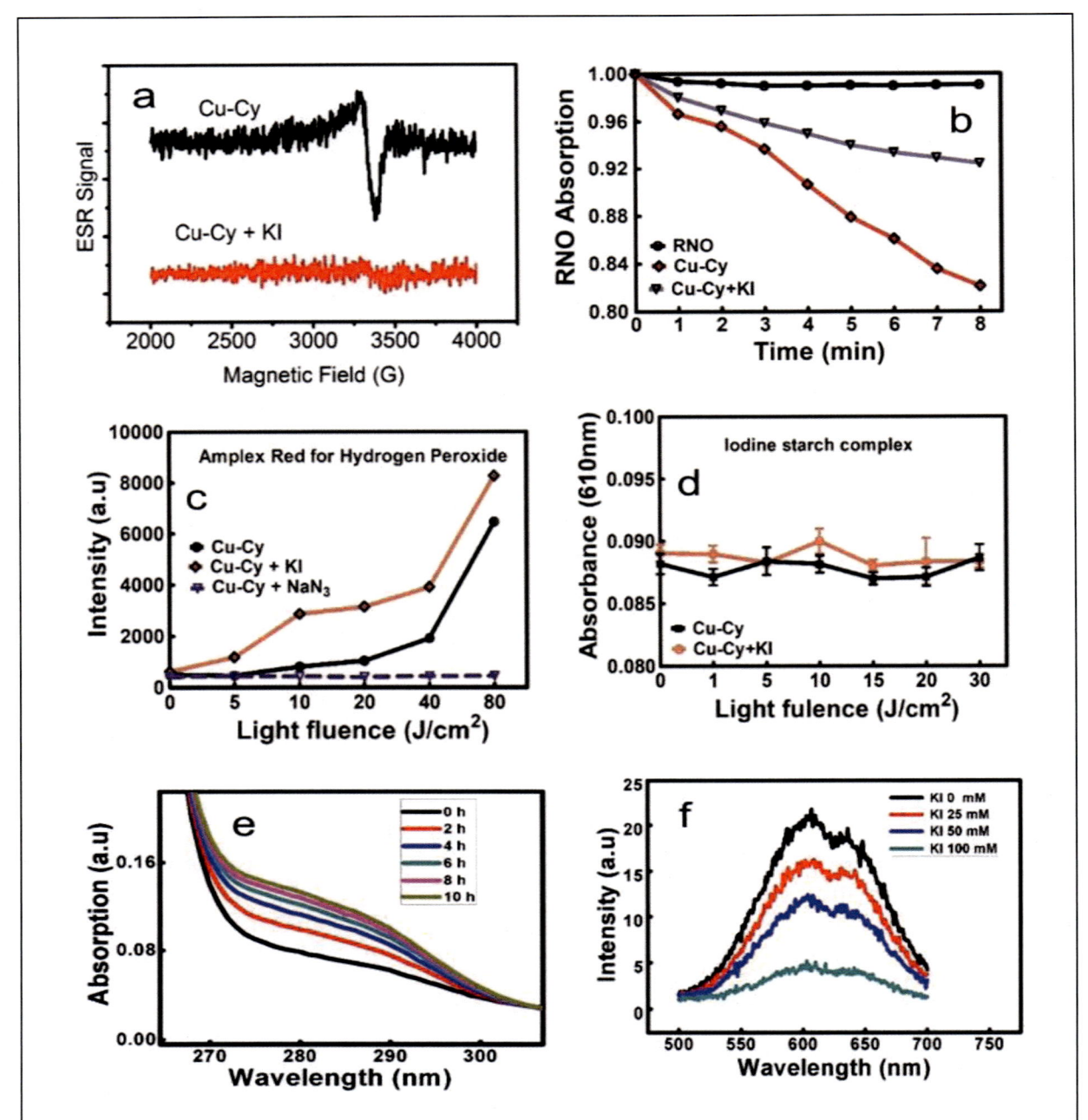

Figure 2-20. (a) ESR spectra of Cu-Cy NPs (black) and Cu-Cy NPs + KI (red). (b) RNO absorption curves of DI water (control), Cu-Cy NPs (100 μM) + KI (100 mM), and Cu-Cy NPs (100 μM) under UV irradiation. (c) Cu-Cy NPs, Cu-Cy NPs + KI, and Cu-Cy + NaN$_3$ irradiated with UV light and aliquots were withdrawn and added to Amplex Red reagent. (d) Cu-Cy NPs (100 μM) and Cu-Cy NPs (100 μM) + KI (100 mM) were illuminated with increasing fluence of UV light and aliquots were withdrawn and added to starch solution. (e) Absorption spectra of Cu-Cy NPs + KI after different incubation time. (f) The photoluminecence spectra of Cu-Cy NPs after adding different concentration of KI to Cu-Cy NPs after 2 h. Adopted from ref. 8 with permission

KI's interaction with Gram-positive and Gram-negative bacteria

KI is a safe and nontoxic health food supplement that has been shown to be effective in the treatment of bacterial infections. We observed that the inclusion of KI significantly enhances the antibacterial activity of Cu-Cy NPs when exposed to UV light, but Cu-Cy NPs alone have no effect on negative bacteria. The mechanism through which KI increases potentiation is intriguing but not totally understood yet. Numerous possibilities exist. First, iodide anions may oxidize photoexcited Cu-Cy NPs via electron transfer, forming iodide radicals and other bactericidal reactive radical species. Iodide anions could be employed as an electron source to enhance the type-1 electron-transfer photochemical pathway, resulting in increased ROS production. Additionally, both types-1 and type-2 are capable of rapidly oxidizing iodide anion to molecular iodine I_2 or I_3^-, which are poisonous to bacteria and are capable of successfully killing them, as illustrated in Fig. 2-21.

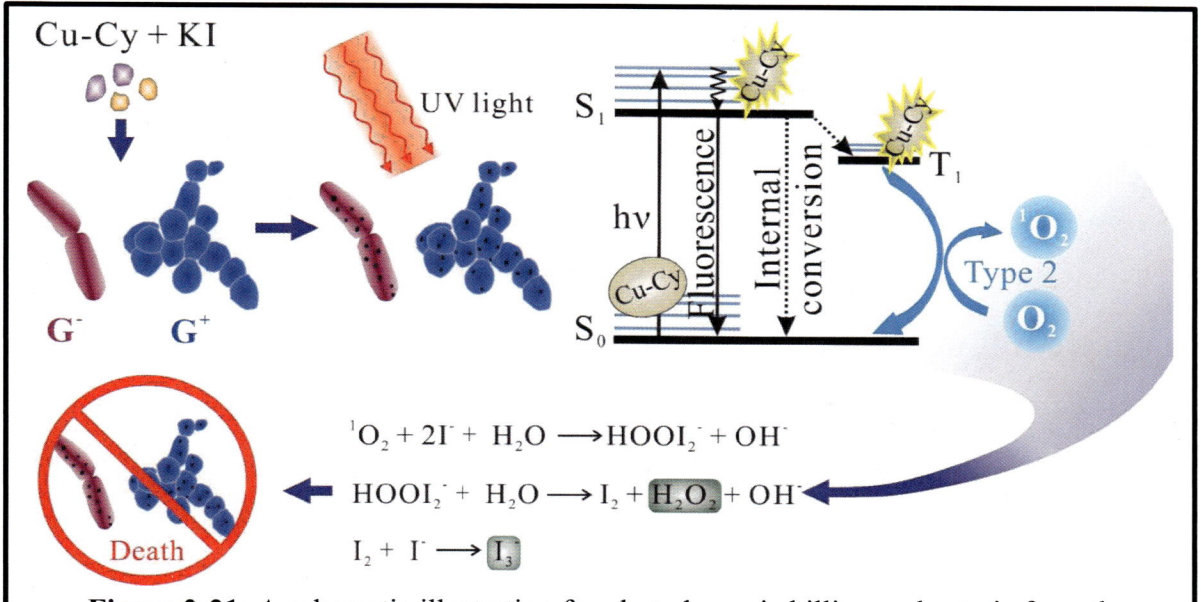

Figure 2-21: A schematic illustration for photodynamic killing on bacteria from the combination of Cu-Cy NPs with KI under UV light activation. Adopted from ref. 8 with permission

As previously reported, Photofrin (PF) is inefficient at killing Gram-negative bacteria by PDT and PF is not taken up by E.coli. The ineffectiveness of PF against Gram-negative bacteria is due to its neutral or slightly anionic composition, which prevents it from attaching to the Gram-negative bacteria's outer membrane. Gram-negative bacteria, particularly in solution, are shielded from extracellularly generated $^1O_2$. This is also supported by our findings: Cu-Cy NPs (50 μM) and UV radiation (10 J/cm^2) had no effect on Gram-negative E.coli species. However, when KI was added to Cu-Cy NPs and exposed to UV light, over >6 log of cells was killed. Cu-Cy NPs are inert against Gram-negative bacteria because they are neutral or negatively charged, which prevents them from attaching to the Gram-negative bacterium's outer membrane.

For Gram-positive bacteria, the situation is different: intrinsic cytotoxicity was present with or without KI in Cu-Cy-mediated photodynamic anti Gram-positive MRSA treatment. Cu-Cy NPs and $^1O_2$ are both neutrally charged molecules that are highly permeable to Gram-positive bacteria. Additionally, the porous structure of the Gram-positive cell wall allows for the penetration of different particles or radicals. Gram-positive bacteria, without a doubt, are more susceptible to extracellularly generated $^1O_2$. The permeability of microorganisms to iodide anions has received little attention. We assume in this study that Cu-Cy NPs generate $^1O_2$ via PDT, and that $^1O_2$ or another ROS reacts with iodide to form triiodide ions, which enhances the bactericidal activity. These findings suggest that the combination of Cu-Cy NPs and KI exposed to UV light could be used to develop a new antibiotic drug for the prevention and treatment of a variety of infectious diseases caused by bacteria and/or viruses, including wound healing, skin diseases such as lupus and vitiligo, wastewater treatment, and blood or medicine sterilization.

The Bottom Line

In summary, we discovered for the first time that the combination of Cu-Cy NPs and KI is extremely effective at killing Gram-positive MRSA and Gram-negative E.coli bacteria. Due to the fact that the NPs are substantially larger than the channels found on the exterior members of bacteria, Cu-Cy NPs are unable to enter the cell walls and reach the inner cytosols to kill them. After adding KI to Cu-Cy in DI water, no copper ions were produced, indicating that the Fenton reaction induced by copper ions may not be responsible for bacterial death. To elucidate the likely mechanism, we studied the interaction of KI with Cu-Cy NPs in detail and discovered the results of their interaction. We conclude from our findings that the primary mechanism of death is the formation of toxic species such as H_2O_2, triiodide ions, and $^1O_2$. The combination of Cu-Cy and KI has the potential to act as a stand-alone treatment or as an additional method in the treatment of infectious illnesses.

References for this chapter

1. **Michael R Hamblin, Antimicrobial photodynamic inactivation: a bright new technique to kill resistant microbes, Curr Opin Microbiol. 2016, 33: 67–73**

2. Baskaran, R., Lee, J. & Yang, SG. Clinical development of photodynamic agents and therapeutic applications. *Biomater Res* **22**, 25 (2018). https://doi.org/10.1186/s40824-018-0140-z

3. **Mallidi, S., Anbil, S., Bulin, A.L., Obaid, G., Ichikawa, M., Hasan, T,. Beyond the Barriers of Light Penetration: Strategies, Perspectives and Possibilities for Photodynamic Therapy. Theranostics, 2016, 6(13), 2458-2487. https://doi.org/10.7150/thno.16183.**

4. Niculescu, A.-G.; Grumezescu, A.M. Photodynamic Therapy—An Up-to-Date Review. Appl. Sci. **2021**, 11, 3626. https://doi.org/10.3390/app11083626

5. dos Santos AF, de Almeida DRQ, Terra LF, Baptista MS, Labriola L. Photodynamic therapy in cancer treatment - an update review. J Cancer Metastasis Treat 2019;5:25. http://dx.doi.org/10.20517/2394-4722.2018.83

6. Xuejing Huang, Fengjie Wan, Lun Ma, Jonathan B. Phan, Rebecca Xueyi Lim, Cuiping Li, Jiagui Chen, Jinghuan Deng, Yasi Li, **Wei Chen**, Min He Investigation of Copper-cysteamine Nanoparticles as A New Photosensitizer for Anti-hepatocellular Carcinoma, *Cancer Biol. Ther.* 2019, 20 (6): 812–825

7. Liyi Huang, Lun Ma, Weijun Xuan, Xiumei Zhen, Han Zheng, Wei Chen, and Michael R. Hamblin, Exploration of Copper-Cysteamine Nanoparticles as a New Type of Agents for Antimicrobial Photodynamic Inactivation, *J. Biomed. Nanotechnol.* 2019, 15: 2142–2148

8. Xiumei Zhen, Lalit Chudal, Nil Kanatha Pandey, Jonathan Phan, Xin Ran, Eric Amador, Xuejing Huang, Omar Johnson, Yuping Ran, **Wei Chen**, Michael R Hamblin and Liyi Huang, A Powerful Combination of Copper-Cysteamine Nanoparticles with Potassium Iodide for Bacterial Destruction, *Mater. Sci. Eng. C.* 2020, 110:110659 1-8

Chapter 3

X-ray induced photodynamic therapy

3.1 The Concept of X-PDT

Photodynamic therapy (PDT) involves the use of light and a photosensitizer that induces the production of reactive oxygen species at the tumor site after the absorption of light energy to kill nearby tumor cells. Singlet oxygen has a short lifetime in biological systems, less than 0.04 µs, and therefore has a short radius of action of less than 0.02 µm. Thus, PDT is minimally invasive, and when used with light and a photosensitizer to selectively target cancerous cells, can minimize side effects to surrounding healthy tissues. PDT is also unlikely to cause genotoxicity, rarely leads to DNA damage, and is effective at treating tumors that have already developed resistance to other cytotoxic treatments such as radiotherapy, hormone therapy, or chemotherapy.

Despite these advantages, one major drawback of PDT is the limited penetration depth of light. PDT agents generate reactive oxygen species after the interaction with light, and the wavelengths of light for most of the clinically approved photosensitizers are in the UV/visible range. This limits the use of conventional PDT methods to skin (surface) tumors only, and it is not effective for deep tumors. Recently, possible solutions to treat deep tumors with PDT have been proposed, for example: 1) the use of agents activatable by near-infrared (NIR) light with relative longer wavelengths, 2) the use of upconversion nanoparticles that absorb NIR light and emit visible light to activate conventional photosensitizers, 3) the use of fiber optics that transmit light deep into tissue and 4) the use of ionizing X-rays for photosensitizer activation. However, NIR light with enough energy to activate photosensitizers can penetrate only 5 mm into tissue. Similarly, upconversion nanoparticles are also limited by the penetration depth of NIR. The use of fiber optics is invasive, inconvenient and cannot effectively and homogenously activate the photosensitizers. Furthermore, the treatment of metastatic sites or lymph nodes is difficult as these sites are located in regions where light delivery is challenging. In contrast, the use of X-rays to activate photosensitizers may overcome the challenges of light penetration as X-rays, already used in medical imaging and therapy, can easily penetrate as deeply as necessary into patients. X-ray induced PDT (X-PDT) was proposed in 2006 by Wei Chen, which has become a hot and popular area on cancer treatment as illustrated in Figure 3-1. X-PDT is not only a good solution for PDT penetration but also a good strategy to reduce X-ray dose and side-effects for X-ray radiology.

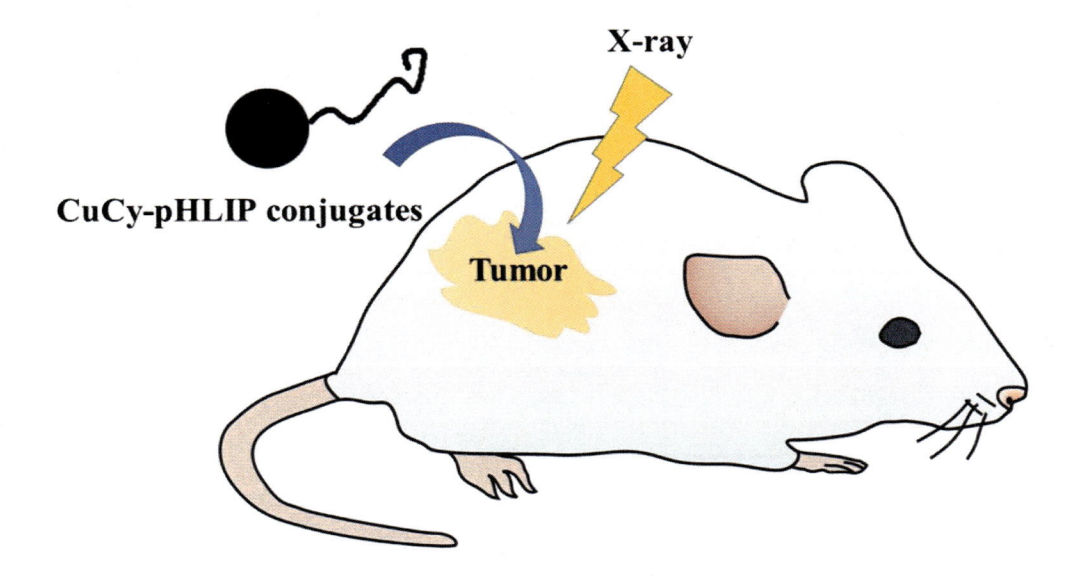

Figure 3-1 A schematic illustration of X-ray induced PDT with pHLIP-conjugated Cu-Cy nanoparticles in mice. Adopted from ref. 9 with permission

As an ionizing radiation with photon energies ranging from kiloelectronvolts (keV) to megaelectronvolts (MeV) and an excellent tissue penetration depth, RT is the most widely used method of cancer treatment, meeting the demands of more than 70% of cancer patients. Ionizing radiation can cause DNA damage in cancer cells, resulting in a very efficient method of destroying cancer cells. However, in order to effectively destroy cancer cells and slow tumour growth, a large dose of X-rays (50-80 Gy) is often required, particularly for deep-seated tumours, increasing the radiation's toxicity to healthy tissue adjacent to the target tissue.

Thus, researchers believed that by combining PDT with X-rays rather than laser light and haematoporphyrin derivatives (HPD), the potential of PDT may be expanded. Due to X-rays' high tissue penetration, researchers proposed X-ray induced photodynamic therapy (X-PDT) to improve therapeutic outcomes and minimize radiation damage to normal tissue while treating deep-seated cancer. X-PDT works on the premise of converting X-rays to optical luminescence and initiating the RT and PDT processes via an energy transducer. Since the notion of nanoparticle-mediated X-PDT was presented in 2006 by Wei Chen, X-PDT has been developed in vitro and in vivo for more than a decade, with multiple reviews concentrating on the creation of nanosensitizers and references mentioned therein. Here we introduce the basic principle of X-PDT and its potential applications on cancer treatment.

The X-PDT principle

X-PDT technique

X-rays utilized in clinical RT have energies ranging from hundreds of keV to MeV. As a result, the majority of conventional photosensitizers used in cancer PDT cannot be activated successfully with X-rays. A physical transducer is required in this case to absorb the X-ray energy and pass it to photosensitizers, which generate the deadly singlet oxygen ($^1O_2$) required for tumour elimination. This energy transfer occurs in the classical X-PDT model by transforming the absorbed x-ray energy to optical photons of the proper wavelength that can be successfully absorbed by photosensitizers. These transducers are referred to as scintillators and exhibit optical luminescence when activated by X-rays (XEOL). Additionally, there are additional energy transfer pathways between X-ray absorbers and photosensitizers. For example, acridine orange is a potent photosensitizer that has been demonstrated to be successful in cancer models and sarcoma patients when exposed to low-dose X-rays without the use of a specialized scintillator transducer.

As indicated in Figure 3-2, the conventional X-PDT method consists of three distinct stages: (1) X-rays are used to irradiate the nanoscintillators, generating XEOL. (2) The resulting XEOL is absorbed by nearby, well-matched photosensitizers to form $^1O_2$, which can directly damage tumour cell membrane phospholipids while also generating radical species and breaking DNA double strands. (3) To accomplish effective cancer treatment, the produced ROS trigger cancer cell death by a combination of PDT and RT processes. Thus, X-rays can be used as the excitation light source to activate PDT for the treatment of deep-seated cancers, owing to the efficient energy transfer in the photosensitizer-loaded nanoscintillators (dubbed nanosensitizers).

Due to the unique mechanisms of cell death, each component of X-PDT inhibits the cell repair mechanism of the other, resulting in improved treatment outcomes. As illustrated in Figure 3, X-PDT generated considerable cell death and decreased clonogenicity at all doses as compared to RT (0-5 Gy). At 24 hours, an apoptotic/necrotic assay (Figure 3A) revealed that cells treated with RT had a low degree of apoptosis and no apparent necrosis, but cells treated with X-PDT exhibited significant necrosis. These findings demonstrated that a membrane-targeted PDT mechanism is capable of degrading unsaturated lipids and surface proteins via oxidative degradation. A lipid peroxidation analysis demonstrated that both X-PDT and RT exhibited considerable lipid peroxidation, with X-PDT exhibiting 1.5-fold greater lipid peroxidation than RT alone (Figure 3B). Additionally, the obvious, comet-like appearance of the cells and loosening of the nucleus revealed that both X-PDT and RT generated significant DNA damage (Figure 3C). A western blot experiment validated the effects further. As illustrated in Figure 3D, both COX-2 (cyclooxygenase-2) and -H2AX (phosphorylated histone H2AX) levels increased following X-PDT therapy, owing to membrane oxidation and DNA double-strand breaks, respectively. These data imply that X-PDT integrates the RT and PDT processes. Recent research has verified this mode of action for X-PDT.

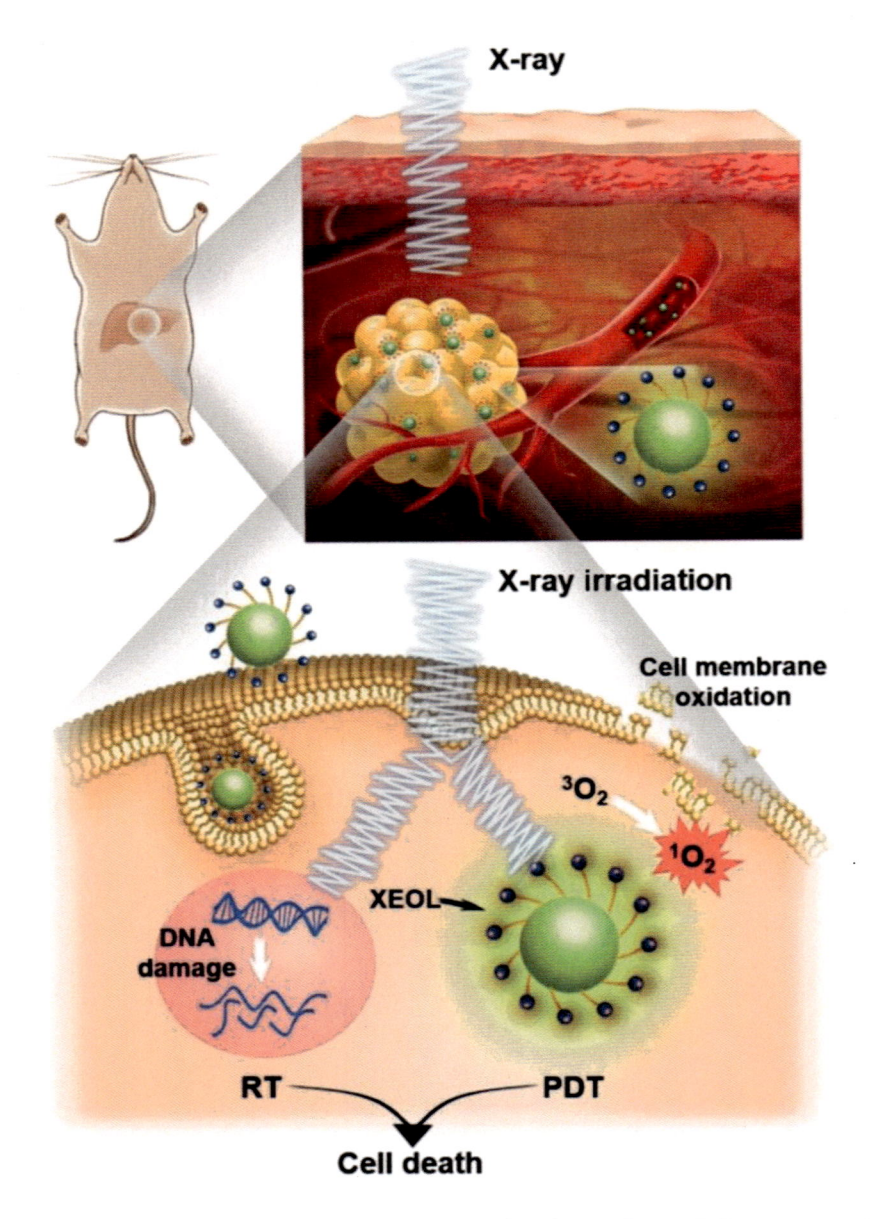

Figure 3-2. Schematic illustration showing the mechanism of X-PDT Adopted from ref. 3 with permission

Cellular experiments established that X-PDT is not only a PDT derivative but also a sort of RT derivative. PDT has the ability to stimulate photosensitizers, thereby producing $^1O_2$. Rapid radiolysis of water can result in the production of hydroxyl radicals (•OH). The combination of RT and PDT, dubbed X-PDT, can generate a substantial amount of ROS, which is critical for inducing damage to the cell membrane and DNA. The X-PDT approach has a number of advantages over traditional RT. To begin, X-PDT is capable of killing cells that are resistant to RT alone (e.g., glioblastoma cells, prostate cancer cells, and colorectal cancer cells). Together, the PDT-induced cell membrane damage and the radiation-induced DNA damage promote tumour cell death and necrosis simultaneously. Second, the low dose of irradiation (typical total dose: 5 Gy) used in X-PDT is significantly less than that used in conventional clinical RT (typical total dosage: 60-80 Gy). As a result, X-PDT would have fewer adverse effects on healthy tissue. Third, compared to conventional RT, the X-PDT process can be triggered with a single dosage and at a lower dose rate. It is well established that the toxicity caused by irradiation is positively associated with the dosage rate. A common amount of irradiation required for treatment in X-PDT is in the range of 2-5 Gy, which is frequently comparable to a fraction of the total dose utilized in conventional RT (e.g., 50-80 Gy in 2-Gy quantities).

Current advancements in the development of the traditional X-PDT

As mentioned above, the notion of X-PDT mediated by nanoparticles was first presented in 2006. There have been numerous attempts since then to progress the development of X-PDT. Initially, studies established that X-PDT may create $^1O_2$ in solution utilizing fluorides and oxides as transducers at the same doses as RT (i.e., 6-8 Gy). Then, the studies concentrated on *in vitro* demonstrations using a specific dose of RT. Until 2015, there had been no demonstration of this technology *in vivo* utilizing a low-dose of X-rays. The advancement of nanosensitizer design and modification has resulted in more comprehensive investigations.

Initial studies on X-PDT in solution

During the early stages, the majority of experiments established the possibility of $^1O_2$ generation using scintillator fluorides and oxides as transducers. As one of the most extensively researched scintillators, rare-earth-element doped nanomaterials may absorb and transport high-energy radiations to luminescent centres, resulting in efficient visible light luminescence. Porphyrin is a photosensitizer that is frequently used in clinical PDT, and Tb^{3+} has an effective green luminescence that is well matched to porphyrin's absorption band. Chen's group generated meso-tetra(4-carboxyphenyl) porphine (MTCP) coupled LaF_3:Tb nanoparticles (LaF_3:Tb-MTCP) in 2008 to explore the formation of $^1O_2$ following the X-PDT process. The nanoparticles were around 10-15 nm in size and emitted green XEOL with a central wavelength of 540 nm. The luminescence of 9,10-anthracenedipropionic acid (ADPA) was suppressed by both MTCP and LaF_3:Tb-MTCP under X-ray irradiation (0.44 Gymin^{-1}, 13.2 Gy), with the latter quenching more than doubling the luminosity (Figure 3-3A). Another study demonstrated X-PDT effects utilizing mesoporous LaF$_3$:Tb nanoparticles. The green XEOL of LaF$_3$:Tb might be absorbed by an adsorbed rose Bengal (RB) under X-ray irradiation (Figure 3-3B). Under X-ray irradiation, RB alone was capable of suppressing approximately 40% of the fluorescence of 1,3-Diphenylisobenzofuran (DPBF), but quenching caused by RB-adsorbed LaF$_3$:Tb was approximately two-fold that of RB alone (Figure 3-3C). The same group then covered the mesoporous LaF$_3$:Tb scintillators with a layer of silica. After incorporation with RB, the nanosensitizers demonstrated an efficient production of $^1O_2$ in the presence of X-rays. Apart from fluorides, oxides were also used to assess the efficiency of X-PDT. The Dujardin group coupled porphyrin with silica-coated Tb$_2$O$_3$ (Tb$_2$O$_3$@SiO$_2$) core-shell nanoparticles (Figure 3-3D). The absorption of porphyrin was effectively matched by the XEOL (Figure 3-3E), and $^1O_2$ was created in the presence of X-rays (5.4 mGys-1), as evidenced by a rise in the emission of 3-p-(amino phenyl) fluorescein (APF) (Figure 3-3F). Following the concept of nanoparticle-mediated X-PDT proposed by Chen in 2006, these early initiatives accelerated the development of feasible methods for designing nano sensitizers and their application in cancer management.

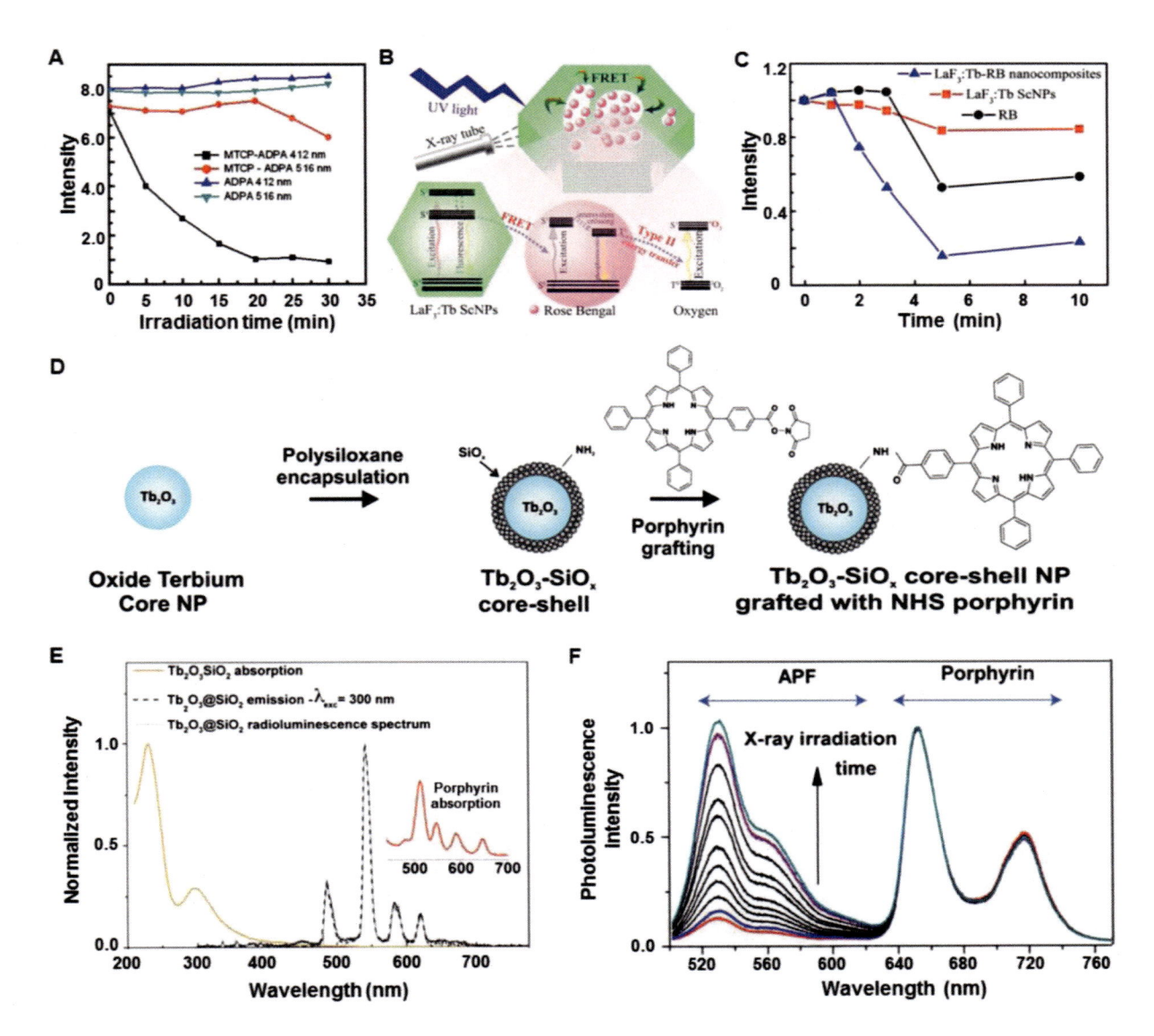

Figure 3-3. Fluorides and oxides for use with of X-PDT. (A) Quenching of ADPA with X-ray irradiation. Adapted with permission from Ref [33]. Copyright 2008 American Institute of Physics. (B) Scheme of LaF3:Tb-RB-mediated X-PDT. (C) Decrease in the emission of DPBF treated with LaF3:Tb-RB and X-rays. Adapted with permission from Ref [34]. Copyright 2015 American Chemical Society. (D) Synthesis of porphyrin-Tb2O3@SiO2. (E) XEOL of Tb2O3@SiO2. (F) 1O2 generation of porphyrin-grafted Tb2O3@SiO2 under X-ray irradiation. Adapted with permission from Ref [3].

X-PDT for the eradication of malignant cells

The preceding investigations established the X-PDT strategy's ability to generate ROS in solution. This method was subsequently extended to the death of cancer cells, where it is necessary to consider effective cellular absorption in order to generate lethal ROS intracellularly.

The radiosensitizers, which included TiO_2, ZnS:Ag, CeF_3, and quantum dots (CdTe and CdSe), were designed to create ROS either inside or outside HeLa cells in particulate form. With increasing concentrations of TiO_2, ZnS:Ag, CeF3, and CdSe quantum dots, a corresponding rise in ROS generation was seen under high-dose X-ray irradiation. Additionally, the survival fraction of HeLa cells, as determined by a cell proliferation kit, demonstrated that the sensitizing materials had a negligible effect as compared to the control group (i.e., cells irradiated directly by X-ray). To increase the sensitization effect, the radiosensitizers' surfaces were modified to aid in their internalization into HeLa cells and decrease cell survival. However, the method by which these radiosensitizers induced cell damage was distinct from that of conventional RT, which is characterized by double-strand breaks in DNA. Further investigation is required on the mechanism by which these radiosensitizers cause cell damage when exposed to X-rays.

Persistent luminescence (also known as afterglow) phosphors can produce light for an extended period after illumination and have been utilized as nanoprobes in small animal optical imaging to eliminate background autofluorescence interference. Persistent luminescence enables the host to retain excitation energy and then gradually release it via trapped charge carriers to produce a long-lasting phosphorescence. This one-of-a-kind characteristic has the potential to be employed as an energy mediator in PDT treatment.[ ] The Chen group initially investigated the efficiency of X-PDT in vitro using ZnS:Cu,Co afterglow nanoparticles. ZnS:Cu generates green light as a first generation persistent luminescence material, which coincides well with the absorption of tetrabromorhodamine-123 (TBrRh123) and PPIX (Figure 3-4). Additionally, the XEOL afterglow of ZnS:Cu,Co can persist for more than 10 minutes following the cessation of X-ray irradiation. The nanosensitizers were readily absorbed by cancer cells, resulting in a significant decrease in cell survival following X-ray irradiation (2 Gy). However, X-ray irradiation alone showed a modest effect on cancer cell death. Afterglow nanoparticles were identified as a possible light source for triggering PDT for deep-seated cancers in this investigation.

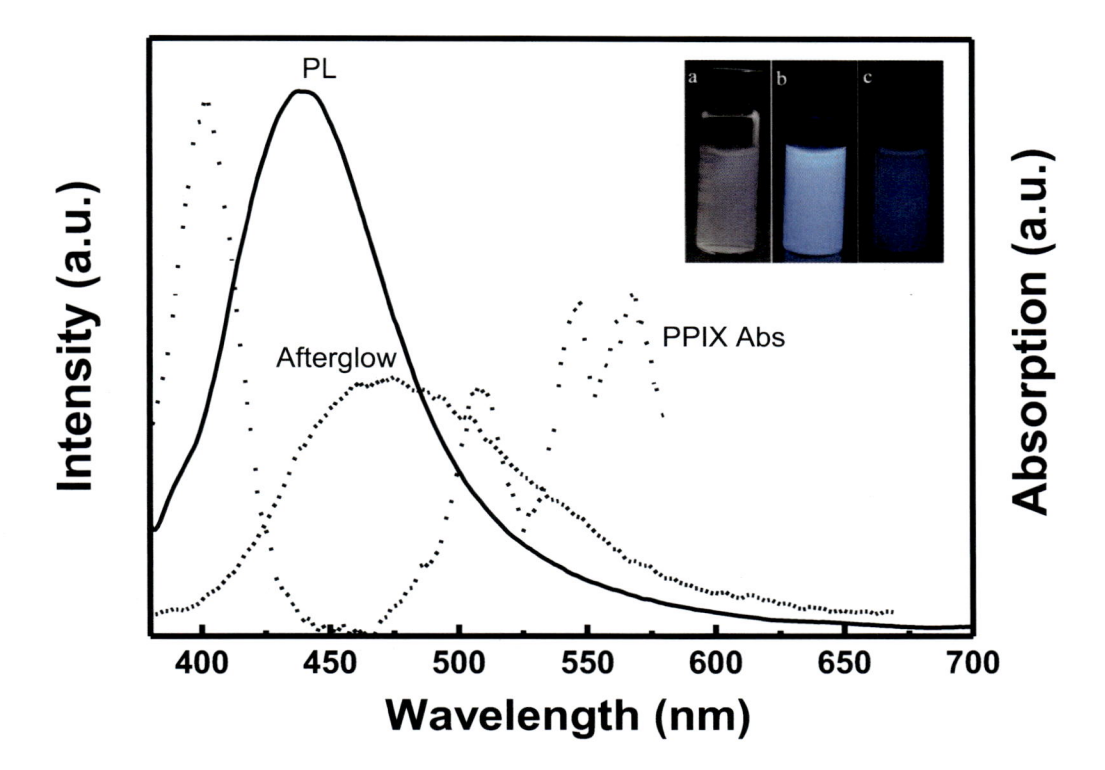

Figure 3-4. The photoluminescence (solid curve) and afterglow (dash curve) spectra of ZnS:Ag,Co nanoparticles in water (λ_{exc} = 360 nm). The afterglow spectra were recorded after 2 min exposure by the UV lamp (360 nm). The inset images are photo pictures of ZnS:Ag,Co nanoparticles redispersed in water under room light (a), UV lamp (b), and afterglow (c). The afterglow image was taken after the UV lamp was off for 2 seconds. The dot curve displays the absorption spectrum of a photosensitizer PPIX in water. Adopted from ref. 4 with permission

As seen above in solution and at the cellular level, these results demonstrate that when exposed to X-rays, transducers can transfer irradiated energy to bound photosensitizers, generating ROS and inducing cell death. While not all examples closely reflect the mechanistic cell death caused by X-PDT, we can still learn from these findings and develop some tactics for *in vivo* applications.

X-PDT *in vivo* for cancer treatment

During the first decade of development, essentially no in vivo X-PDT research were conducted. The inventor of X-PDT stated in 2014 that "prior attempts to activate photosensitizers with X-rays were not very effective, as traditional PDT photosensitizers could not be activated properly by X-rays." It is vital to demonstrate that nanosensitizers can be activated by external X-ray irradiation to generate XEOL and activate X-PDT in vivo in order to advance X-PDT technology. This section will highlight the progress toward developing more realistic in vivo applications for the X-PDT idea.

Apart from commenting on past research, the Chen group examined the X-PDT performance of copper-cysteamine complex (Cu-Cy) microparticles (3-10 μm) for in vivo cancer treatment. In vitro studies utilizing Cu-Cy particles activated by X-rays demonstrated considerable cell death, while in vivo treatment using a subcutaneous tumour model suppressed tumour development following intertumoral injection of Cu-Cy particles and X-ray irradiation (5 Gy). These findings indicated that Cu-Cy particles can be effectively activated by X-rays to ROS for cancer treatment. Although the results were favourable, the precise mechanism of ROS formation remained unknown due to the absence of a photosensitizer in the Cu-Cy structure. Cu-Cy nanoparticles were shown to be capable of regulating the tumour microenvironment during in situ glutathione (GSH)-activated and H_2O_2-reinforced chemodynamic treatment for drug-resistant breast cancer in a recent study. By reacting with local GSH and H_2O_2, the Cu-Cy nanoparticles could create poisonous •OH via a Fenton-like reaction.

Others and we have demonstrated the efficacy of X-PDT in vivo. The Shi and Bu groups coated a semiconductor layer of ZnO onto Ce-doped LiYF$_4$ nanoparticles (LiYF4@ZnO) and then examined the in vivo efficacy of X-PDT with low oxygen dependence (Figure 3-5A). Ce-doped LiYF$_4$ displayed significant UV emission bands (305 and 325 nm) that matched the bandgap of the surface-bound ZnO layer. The subsequent formation of excitons (the electron-hole (e^--h^+) pairs) resulted in the formation of free radicals when they interacted with water and oxygen molecules (Figure 3-5B). These ROS were mostly generated via an oxygen-independent PDT (type I reaction) mechanism and were capable of causing permanent oxidative damage to DNA, lipids, and proteins, even in low oxygen environments. Under X-ray irradiation (3 Gy), considerable ROS generation was seen regardless of the oxygen tension, supporting the X-excellent PDT's efficiency in normoxic (21% O_2) and hypoxic (2% O_2) cells (Figure 3-5C). Additionally, the in vivo investigation demonstrated that intertumoral injection of LiYF4@ZnO into subcutaneous tumours and irradiation with X-rays (8 Gy) significantly suppressed tumour growth (Figure 3-5D). The Bu group expanded on this method by including scintillators and heavy metals to absorb X-rays and pass the energy to photosensitizers. LiLuF$_4$:Ce created X-ray excited UV luminescence in this design, which was absorbed by the photosensitizers (Ag$_3$PO$_4$) to form •OH. To maximize the production of •OH by segregating the electrons and holes in Ag$_3$PO$_4$, a cisplatin prodrug Pt(IV) was used as a sacrificial electron acceptor. Additionally, cisplatin was formed during the reduction of Pt(IV), enhancing the toxicity of •OH. LiLuF$_4$:Ce@Ag$_3$PO$_4$@Pt(IV) nanoparticles (LAPNP) increased the therapeutic benefits of X-PDT via a two-step amplification technique.

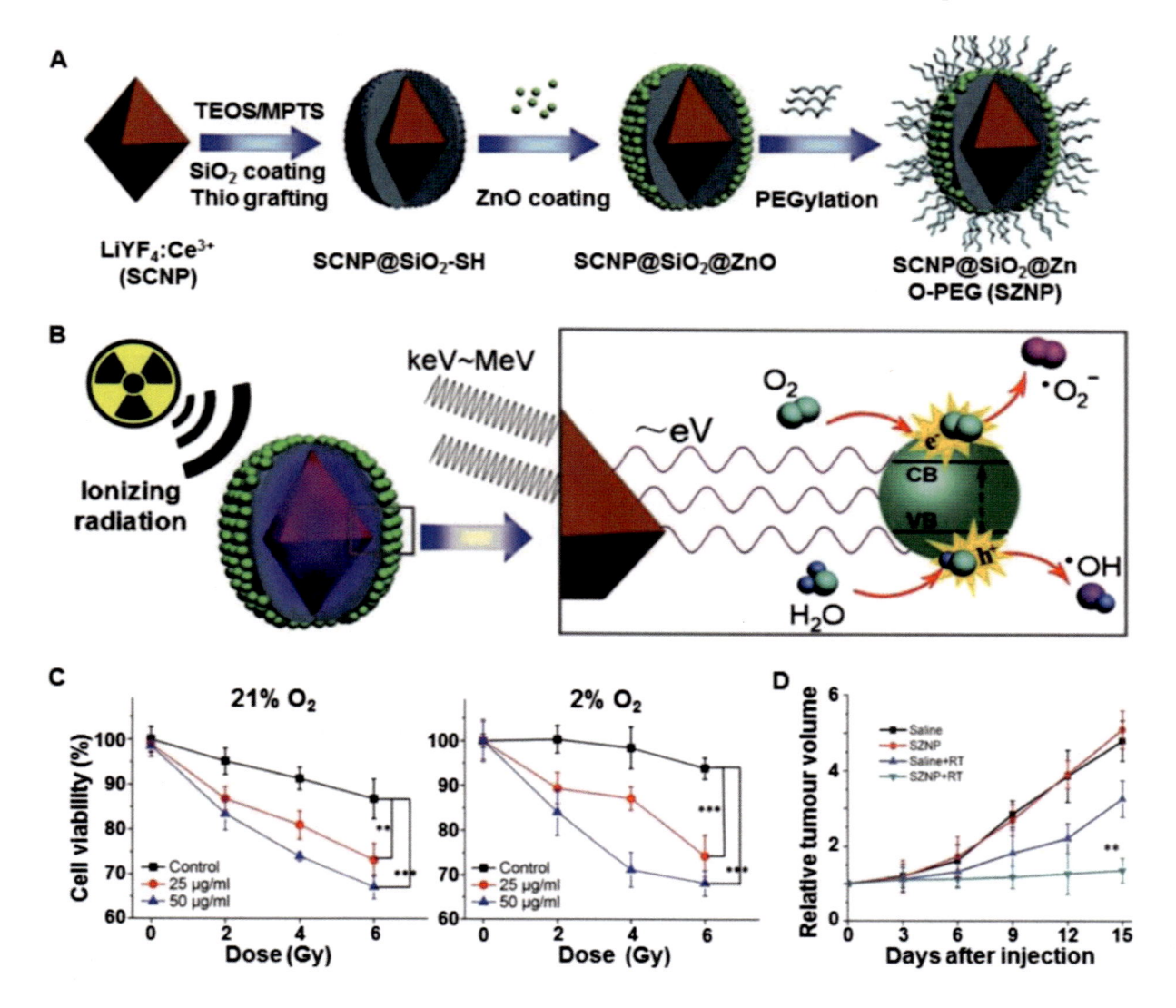

Figure 3-5. (A) Schematic illustration of the synthetic route to ZnO coated LiYF4:Ce (SZNP). (B) The mechanism of SZNP-mediated X-PDT. (C) Viabilities of normoxic and hypoxic HeLa cells treated with SZNPs for 24 h under X-ray radiation (0, 2, 4, 6 Gy). (D) *In vivo* evaluation of SZNPs-mediated synchronous RT and PDT. Adapted with permission from Ref [3].

Furthermore, Dou et al. synthesized a radiation-responsive scintillating nanotheranostic system (NSC@mSiO$_2$-SNO/ICG) by covalently attaching S-nitrosothiol groups (SNO, a NO donor) and indocyanine green (ICG, a photosensitizer) to mesoporous silica-coated Eu^{3+}-doped NaGdF$_4$ scint (Figure 3-6A). The energy transferred from NSC to ICG triggered the X-PDT process, which generated a considerable amount of ROS. Meanwhile, the S-N bond in SNO was activated to generate a high NO concentration in tumours when irradiated with X-rays, which reduces tumour hypoxia due to increased vasodilation (Figure 3-6B).

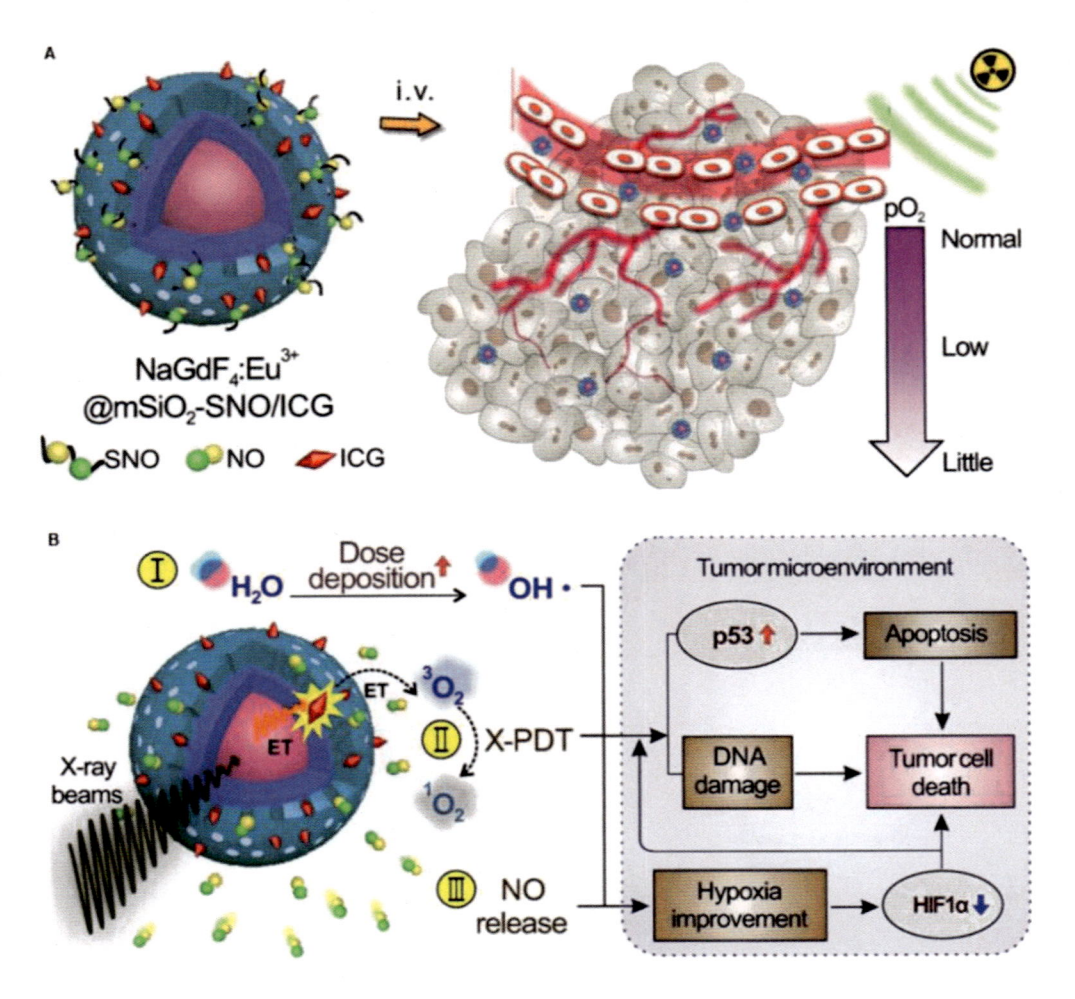

Figure 3-6. (A) Schematic of the structure of NSC@mSiO2-SNO/ICG NPs and their passive accumulation in tumors via the EPR effect. (B) X-ray radiation on this system would trigger multiple tumoricidal responses by: (I) increasing dose deposition to accelerate radiolysis, (II) producing cytotoxic ROS by activating ICG based on the scintillation effect of NSC, and (III)

releasing high levels of NO due to radiation fracture of S-N bonds. Adapted with permission from Ref [3].

As a method of traditional clinical therapy, RT has developed into a critical strategy for cancer management. Immunotherapy has piqued the interest of researchers, doctors, and pharmaceutical businesses in recent years. Parallel to this, new ways for combining classic radiotherapy and developing immunotherapy for cancer treatment have been investigated. Recently, the Lin group confirmed a synergistic impact when nano-MOFs were used with cancer immunotherapy. The Lin group bridged the gap between Hf/Zr-MOF-enabled X-PDT and checkpoint blockade immunotherapy in that study to produce radio enhancers for X-ray irradiation for both local and systemic tumour elimination (Figure 3-7A). Intratumorally delivery of 5,15-di(p-benzoato)porphyrin (DBP)-Hf and 5,10,15,20-tetra(p-benzoato)porphyrin (TBP)-Hf nano-MOFs resulted in efficient tumour suppression in all radioresistant head and neck squamous cell carcinoma (SQ20B), glioblastoma (U87MG), prostate cancer (PC-3), and Consistent abscopal responses were reported in all CT26 and TUBO tumour models treated with low-dose X-rays when loaded with an inhibitor of the immunological checkpoint molecule indoleamine 2,3-dioxygenase (IDOi) (Figure 3-7B). Not only did the treatment mitigate the adverse effects of local RT, but it also stimulated systemic immunity to effectively suppress tumour growth. By combining the benefits of local radiation therapy and systemic tumour rejection via synergistic X-ray-induced in situ vaccination and indoleamine 2,3-dioxygenase inhibition, MOF-based nanoplatforms may overcome some of the limitations of radiation therapy and checkpoint blockade therapy in cancer treatment. A Phase 1 research of RiMO-301 in patients with advanced cancers has been commenced using this radio-immuno metal-organic (RiMO) technology.

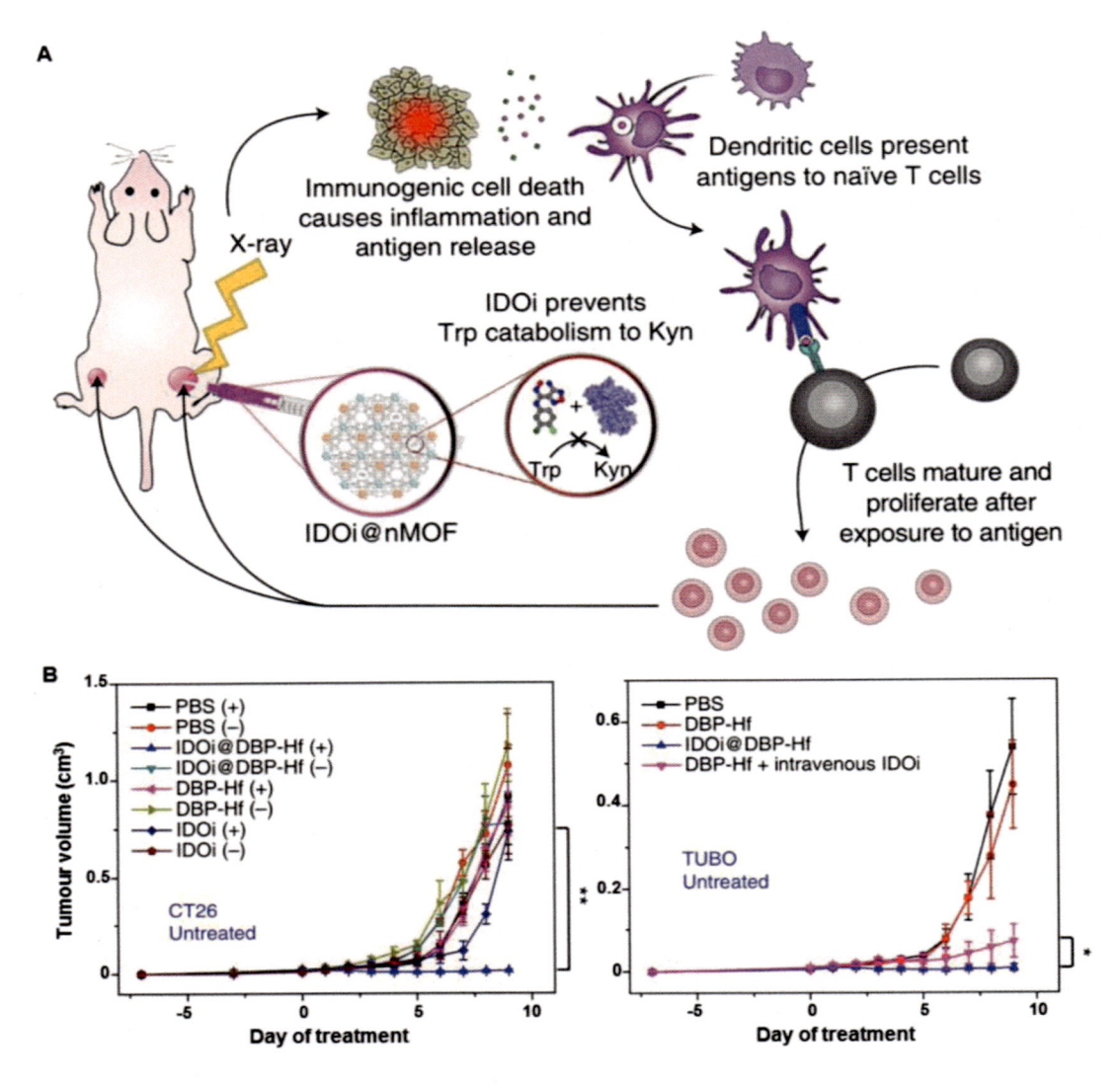

Figure 3-7. (A) Scheme of nano-MOF enabled synergistic X–RDT and immunotherapy using extremely low doses

of X-rays. (B) Growth curves of CT26 and TUBO tumor-bearing mice intravenously administered with PBS, DBP-Hf, IDOi@DBP-Hf, or DBP-Hf + IDOi, with or without X-ray irradiation. Adapted with permission from Ref [3].

Perspectives for the future

While X-PDT has showed efficacy and advantages, its development is still in its infancy. As mentioned previously, X-PDT is effectively a combination of PDT and ionizing irradiation. However, resolving the interplay between the two approaches and enhancing this synergy further by tweaking irradiation settings and/or altering the targeting capabilities of a transducer remain significant challenges.

Only two simulations have been proposed thus far. These simulations used the photon and electron cross-section models. Both simulations employed fluorides as a model and determined that irradiation levels greater than 60 Gy were required to create a sufficient amount of $^1O_2$ per cell to provide a lethal dosage. In vivo studies using xenograft tumour models (subcutaneous and orthotopic tumors) indicated that low-dose X-rays (5 Gy) were adequate to slow or eradicate tumour growth when administered intratumorally or systemically. These in vivo experimental data contradicted the simulations' conclusions. Thus, there may be more mechanisms at action in addition to the PDT and RT processes. Additional research into the role of X-ray luminescence and fluorescence in cell lethality should be conducted. During the scintillation process, ultraviolet and other types of ionizing radiation were created. Deep-UV light alone can be used to cause cell death and malignant tissue destruction. To summarize, it is reasonable to acknowledge that X-PDT is an organically intricate process and that cell death is the outcome of a variety of causes. These unexplored variables may contribute to the disparity between theoretical models and experimental findings. Thus, based on the experimental data, the mechanism by which X-PDT triggers cell death should be thoroughly studied.

It is critical to note that optimizing the energy conversion and safety profiles of scintillators is critical for X-PDT. When engineering scintillators, several factors must be considered, including the following: (1) constructing scintillators with a large X-ray absorption cross-section, a high conversion efficiency of X-rays to visible photons, and optimized spatial positioning of the molecular entities involved; (2) reducing the overall size of the transducers, which must be balanced against the loss of energy conversion efficiency; and (3) It is worth noting that many of the reported X-PDT transducers are relatively big, which is inefficient for tumour targeting; and (3) achieving a balance between short-term stability and rapid biodegradation of scintillators. Initially, the high XEOL efficiency of transducers exposed to low-dose X-rays should be evaluated. Additionally, transducers with a regulated size distribution in the range of 50-200 nm should demonstrate prolonged blood circulation, a low rate of absorption by reticuloendothelial or mononuclear phagocyte systems, and an elevated rate of tumour uptake due to improved permeability and retention effects. Additionally, coating stealth components (e.g., polyethylene glycol, zwitterionic compounds) on the surface of nanoparticles can help prevent the creation of nonspecific protein coronas in vivo. Most significantly, the nanosensitizers should be non-toxic, quickly digested, and have a low potential for long-term toxicity. When exposed to water, the majority of excellent scintillator candidates, such as aluminate and all-inorganic perovskites, are hydrolytic in nature and rapidly disintegrate into their constituent ions. One solution to this challenge is to coat hydrolytic scintillator cores with coating polymers to increase their physiological stability in media. Materials/coating methods should be used to control scintillator stability and degradation in vivo. Additionally, the amount of photosensitizers put in scintillators and their spacing impact the efficiency of energy transmission from scintillators to photosensitizers. As a result, a covalent conjugation strategy for combining photosensitizers and scintillators that allows for control of the intra-component distance may be more appropriate than a physical loading method. There have been few studies that have examined them on a systematic basis in terms of X-PDT efficacy.

X-PDT has been demonstrated primarily in vitro or in vivo using subcutaneous tumour models. This technique is likely to cure a large number of therapeutically relevant tumour models, particularly those with deep-seated malignancies. Additionally, the majority of in vivo investigations use intertumoral injections of nanosensitizers, which precludes non-invasive therapeutic therapy of deep orthotopic cancer. This would necessitate a high degree of selectivity in the X-PDT nanoplatforms' absorption by these cancer cells. It could be completed by conjugating it with various cancer targeting agents such as folic acid, RGD (for integrin $a_v\beta_3$), cetuximab and panitumumab (for epidermal growth factor receptor), herceptin (for human epidermal growth factor receptor 2), and bevacizumab (for vascular endothelial growth factor), among others. For instance, mitochondria-targeting drugs accumulated highly in mitochondria, and X-ray irradiation generated ROS that dramatically increased mitochondrial collapse and cellular death compared to X-ray alone. Thus, modifying the energy deposition profile in cells may contribute to X-cell-killing PDT's process.

Low-dose irradiation activated X-PDT has the potential for clinical translation as a non-ionizing irradiation therapy alternative. It is critical to evaluate the two approaches in a clinical setting in order to determine the advantages and disadvantages of X-PDT in terms of therapeutic efficacy and side effects. It is necessary to assess X-ability PDT to treat radiation-refractory malignancies. Pre-treatment functional imaging (e.g., positron emission tomography) is frequently used in RT to help stage tumours and plan irradiation. Functional imaging, on the other hand, is not permitted in an irradiation room, and a change in the patient's state from pre-scans may occur, resulting in setup problems. Numerous scintillators contain elements with a high-Z value, which makes them visible under on-board CT. Thus, these scintillators can be used to not only regulate PDT, but also to guide irradiation in order to avoid harm to normal tissue. These avenues should also be explored in order to expedite the clinical translation of X-PDT.

The Bottom Line

Over the last decades, there has been a dramatic increase in the viability of X-PDT as a revolutionary cancer treatment technology. By combining PDT and RT techniques, X-PDT has demonstrated promising therapeutic results in the treatment of deep-seated cancers. We have attempted to present an overview of the research developments in the X-PDT strategy in this study, including the concept, associated design parameters, the combination therapeutic mechanism, biomedical applications, and concluding prospects. As a combined PDT and RT technique, X-ray-activated PDT overcomes the depth constraint of classic light-activated PDT, and requires less irradiation for tumour ablation than traditional RT. However, X-true PDT's biomedical uses are still in their infancy. We believe that this assessment will provide an up-to-date snapshot of the current state of the field and show the way forward in the fight against cancer.

3.2 New Development in X-PDT

A. X-ray Induced Nanoparticles Based Photodynamic Therapy of Cancer

In this study LaF$_3$:Ce nanoparticles were synthesized by a wet-chemistry method in dimethyl sulfoxide (DMSO) and their application as an intracellular light source for photodynamic activation was demonstrated. The LaF$_3$:Ce^{3+}/DMSO nanoparticles have a strong green emission with a peak at around 520 nm which is effectively overlapped with the absorption of protoporphyrin IX (PPIX). The nanoparticles were encapsulated into poly (D,L-lactide-co-glycolide) (PLGA) microspheres along with PPIX. Upon irradiation with X-rays (90 kV), energy transfer from the LaF$_3$:Ce/DMSO nanoparticles to PPIX occurs and singlet oxygen is generated for cancer cell damage. The LaF$_3$:Ce/DMSO/PLGA or LaF$_3$:Ce/DMSO/PPIX/PLGA microspheres alone caused only sublethal cytotoxicity to the cancer cells. Upon X-ray irradiation, the LaF$_3$:Ce/DMSO/PPIX/PLGA microspheres induced oxidative stress, mitochondrial damage and DNA fragmentation on prostate cancer cells (PC3). The results indicate that X-rays can activate LaF$_3$:Ce^{3+} and PPIX nanocomposites, which can be a novel method for cancer destruction.

These nanoparticles made in DMSO have intense green emission at around 520 nm (Fig. 3-8). The green emission is not from the d – f transition of Ce^{3+} but from the metal-to-ligand charge transfer states. The PLGA microspheres synthesized in this work are spherical in shape with their average diameter about 2 μm (Fig. 3-9, A). The shape and size of the PLGA microspheres loaded with the LaF$_3$:Ce^{3+}/DMSO nanoparticles are almost the same as that of the blank PLGA microspheres (Fig. 3-9, B). Fluorescence imaging shows that the nanoparticles colocalize with the microspheres (Fig. 3-9, B3). The emission and excitation spectra of the LaF$_3$:Ce^{3+}/DMSO nanoparticles and LaF$_3$:Ce^{3+}/DMSO/PPIX/PLGA microspheres are almost identical with the excitation and emission peaks at 468 nm and 528 nm, respectively. The imaging and spectroscopic data show that the LaF$_3$:Ce^{3+}/DMSO nanoparticles were successfully encapsulated into the PLGA microspheres.

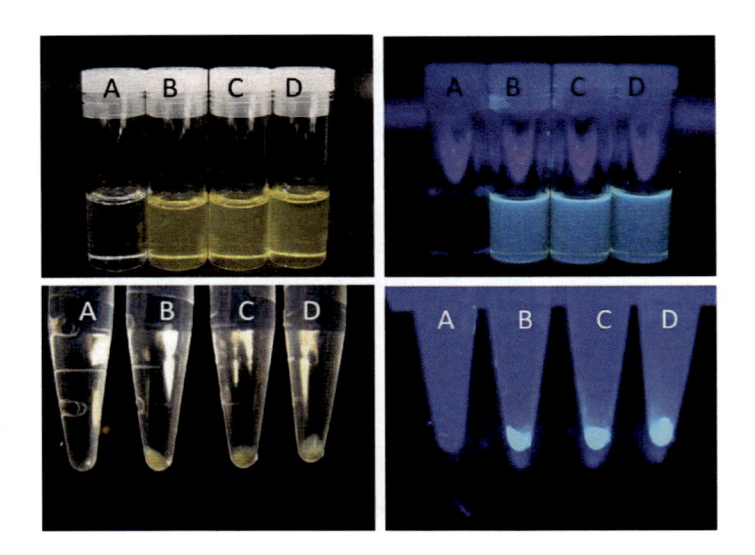

Figure 3-8. Optical (left panel) and fluorescence (right panel) photographs of the LaF$_3$:Ce^{3+}/DMSO nanoparticles. A: PLGA (10 μg/ml) microspheres without the LaF$_3$:Ce^{3+}/DMSO nanoparticles. B: LaF$_3$:Ce^{3+}/DMSO nanoparticles (1 μg/ml). C: LaF$_3$:Ce^{3+}/DMSO/PLGA (10 μg/ml) microspheres. D: LaF$_3$:Ce^{3+}/DMSO/PPIX/PLGA microspheres. Adopted from ref. 5 with permission

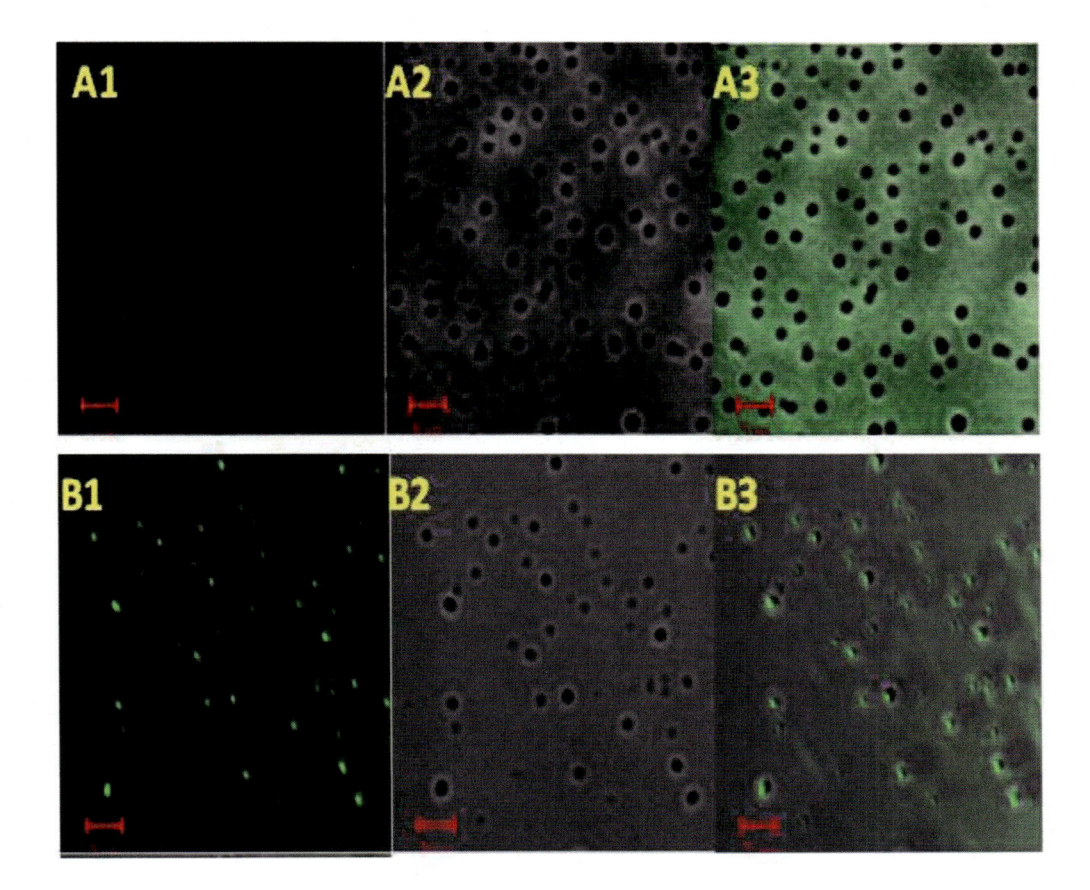

Figure 3-9. Fluorescence microscopy images of the LaF$_3$:Ce^{3+}/DMSO//PLGA microspheres. 1: Fluorescence detected through the 505-550 nm filter. 2: Photograph of the microspheres in the same field using bright-field mode. 3: Overlay of the bright-field and fluorescence images. A: PLGA (10 µg/ml) microspheres without the LaF3:Ce3+ /DMSO nanoparticles. B: LaF$_3$:Ce^{3+}/DMSO/PLGA microspheres. The LaF$_3$:Ce^{3+}/DMSO nanoparticles were excited with the argon–krypton laser (λ_{ex} = 488 nm). Scale bar is 5 µm. Adopted from ref. 5 with permission

Further, the PLGA microspheres were loaded with the LaF$_3$:Ce^{3+}/DMSO/PPIX nanoparticles. Fluorescence imaging shows that the LaF$_3$:Ce^{3+}/DMSO/PPIX nanoparticles were successfully encapsulated into the PLGA microspheres (Fig. 3-10). This is particularly clear from the enlarged images (Fig. 3-10, D). In the PLGA microspheres loaded with the LaF$_3$:Ce^{3+}/DMSO/PPIX conjugates, both the green fluorescence from the LaF$_3$:Ce^{3+} nanoparticles and red fluorescence from PPIX are observed. In the LaF$_3$:Ce^{3+}/DMSO/PPIX conjugates, the fluorescence of the LaF$_3$:Ce^{3+}/DMSO nanoparticles decreases in intensity and that of PPIX increases as the concentration of PPIX is increasing (Fig. 3-11). The fluorescence intensity from the LaF$_3$:Ce^{3+} nanoparticles is decreased in the LaF$_3$:Ce^{3+}/DMSO/PPIX conjugates comparing to that in the LaF$_3$:Ce^{3+}/DMSO nanoparticles. This is an evidence for the energy transfer from the LaF$_3$:Ce^{3+} compound to PPIX molecules. Furthermore, the fluorescence spectrum from the LaF$_3$:Ce^{3+}/DMSO nanoparticles is different from that in the microspheres containing PPIX. The LaF$_3$:Ce^{3+}/DMSO nanoparticles show one broad emission band from about 450 to 600 nm while in the LaF$_3$:Ce^{3+}/DMSO/PPIX/PLGA microspheres it possesses four bands with the peaks at 480, 525, 560 and 590 nm. This is caused by the optical absorption of PPIX; the positions of the spectral dips of the microspheres at 505, 540, 575 and 615 nm (Fig. 3-11) match the peaks of the Q-bands of PPIX in water.

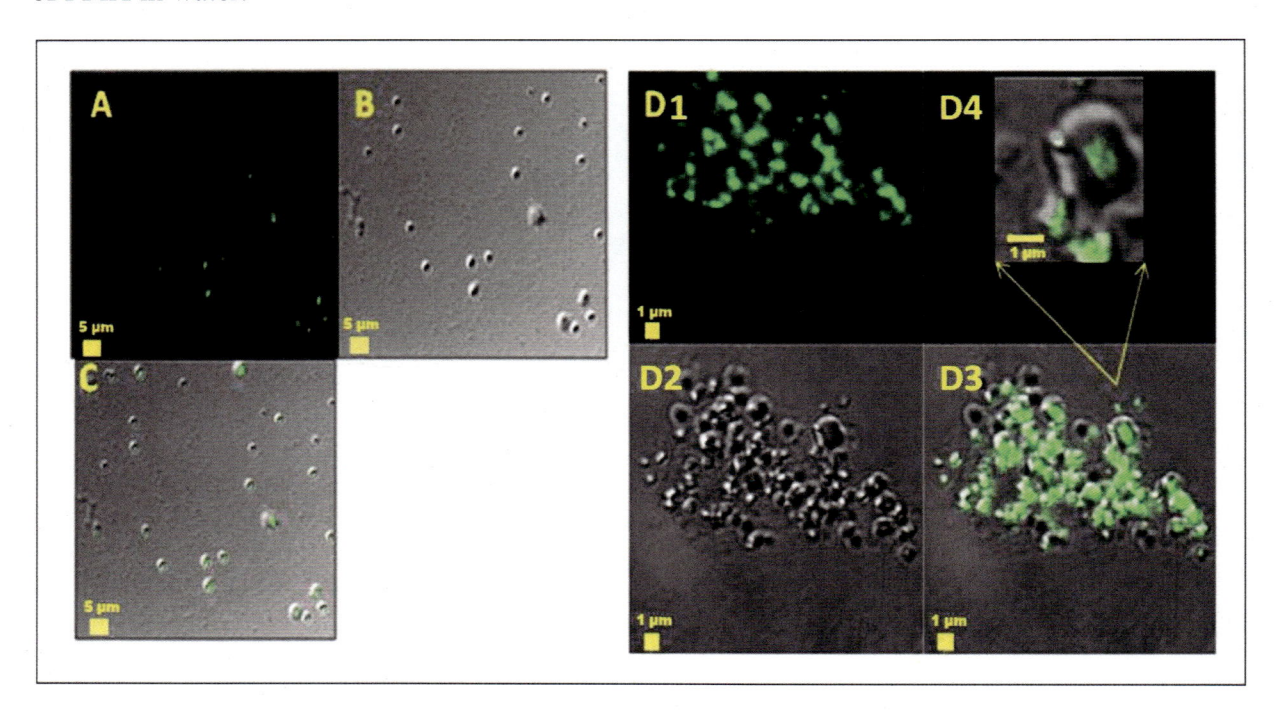

Figure 3-10. Fluorescence microscopy images of the LaF$_3$:Ce^{3+}/DMSO/PPIX/PLGA microspheres. A: Fluorescence detected through the 505-550 nm filter. B: Photograph of the microspheres in the same field using a bright-field mode. C: Overlay of the bright-field and fluorescence images. The LaF$_3$:Ce^{3+}/DMSO nanoparticles with the argon–krypton laser (λ_{ex} = 488 nm). Scale bar is 5 μm. D: High resolution fluorescence images of the LaF$_3$:Ce^{3+}/DMSO/PPIX/PLGA microspheres.(D1: fluorescence. D2: bright-field. D3: Overlay of the bright-field and fluorescence. Arrow in D3 is pointing at single particles in D4. Scale bar is 1 μm. Adopted from ref. 5 with permission

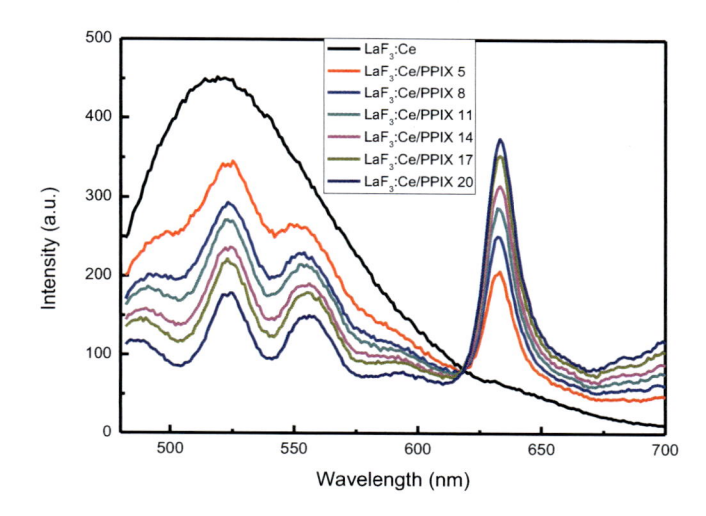

Figure 3-11. Fluorescence spectra of the LaF$_3$:Ce^{3+}/DMSO nanoparticles and LaF$_3$:Ce^{3+}/DMSO/PPIX/PLGA microspheres with different concentrations of PPIX. The nanoparticles were excited at 468 nm. Adopted from ref. 5 with permission

The fluorescence microscopy shows the uptake of the LaF$_3$:Ce^{3+}/PPIX-loaded PLGA microspheres into the cytoplasm of the cancer cells at 1, 4 and 24 hours (Fig.3-12) as well as 48 hours (Fig. 3-13) after incubation. As seen from the images, the loaded microspheres reach the cytoplasm but they did not get into the cell nucleus even at 48 hours. Further, we have conducted experiments with fluorescent dye combinations to see if oxidative injury can be observed in the cells. Healthy cells (negative control) showed blue nuclei and red cytoplasm staining indicating healthy mitochondria (Fig. 3-14). At the same dose of X-ray treatment (2 Gy), the percentage of the cells with mitochondrial perturbation was the highest in the cells treated with the LaF$_3$:Ce^{3+}/DMSO/PPIX/PLGA microspheres. Treatment with the LaF$_3$:Ce^{3+}/DMSO/PLGA microspheres also resulted in a small population of the cells with unhealthy mitochondria, while the negative control (treatment with PBS only) showed no sign of mitochondrial toxicity (Fig. 3-14). All these indicate that X-rays can activate the LaF$_3$:Ce/DMSO/PPIX/PLGA microspheres for cancer treatment.

We found that X-ray treatment with the LaF$_3$:Ce^{3+}/PLGA microspheres resulted in a small population of cells with damaged mitochondria. This could be possible that under X-ray irradiation, the nanoparticles produce a small amount of singlet oxygen because when

particles are smaller, their surface areas increase and the chance for them to generate singlet oxygen or other oxygen free radicals is increased.

The concept for enabling PDT for deep cancer treatment via nanoparticles and the combination of PDT with radiation treatment was proposed by Chen in 2006.[34] Comparing with the previous results, these nanocompounds reported here are more effective and the dose for the treatment is much lower. In addition, the encapsulation of the nanoparticles and PPIX into PLGA is easier than nanoparticle-PPIX conjugation. The only downside is that the PLGA microspheres are large and cell uptake is lower than small size nanoconjugates. Therefore, reducing PLGA microsphere size and functioning with cancer targeting ligands may enhance their targeting and the treatment efficacy.

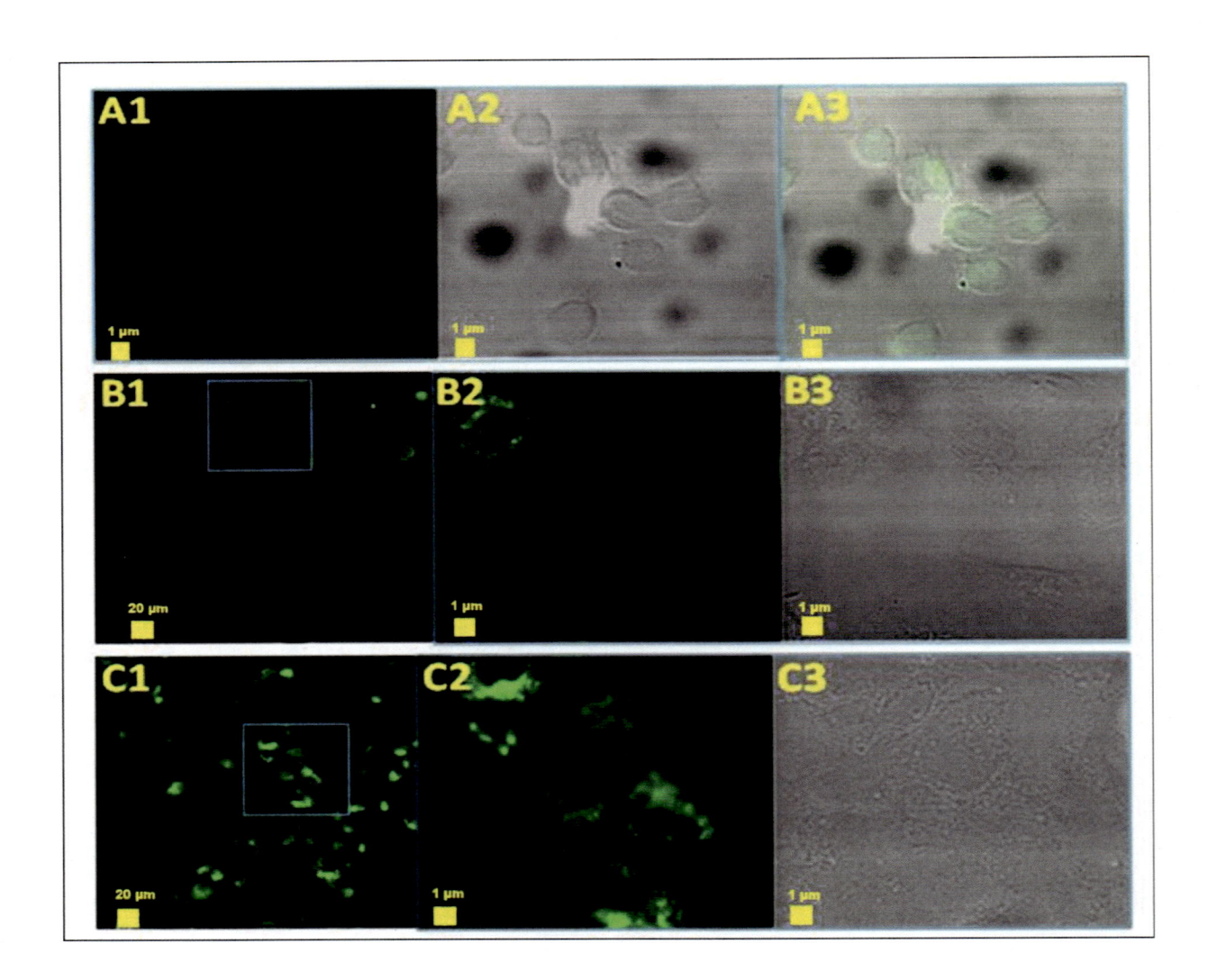

Figure 3-12. Uptake of the LaF$_3$:Ce^{3+}/DMSO/PPIX/PLGA microspheres (1µg/ml) into the cytoplasm of the PC3 cells during different incubation times: 1 h (first row), 4 h (second row) and 24 h (third row). Green color represents the LaF$_3$:Ce^{3+}/DMSO/PPIX/PLGA microspheres (excited with the argon–krypton laser, λ_{ex} = 488 nm). The cell nuclei remain dark since the PLGA microspheres did not penetrate into the nuclei. The cytoplasm shows intense fluorescence after 24 h. B2 and C2: images in high magnification. A3: merge images of A1 and A2(with translation channel). B3 and C3 show bright field images. Adopted from ref. 5 with permission

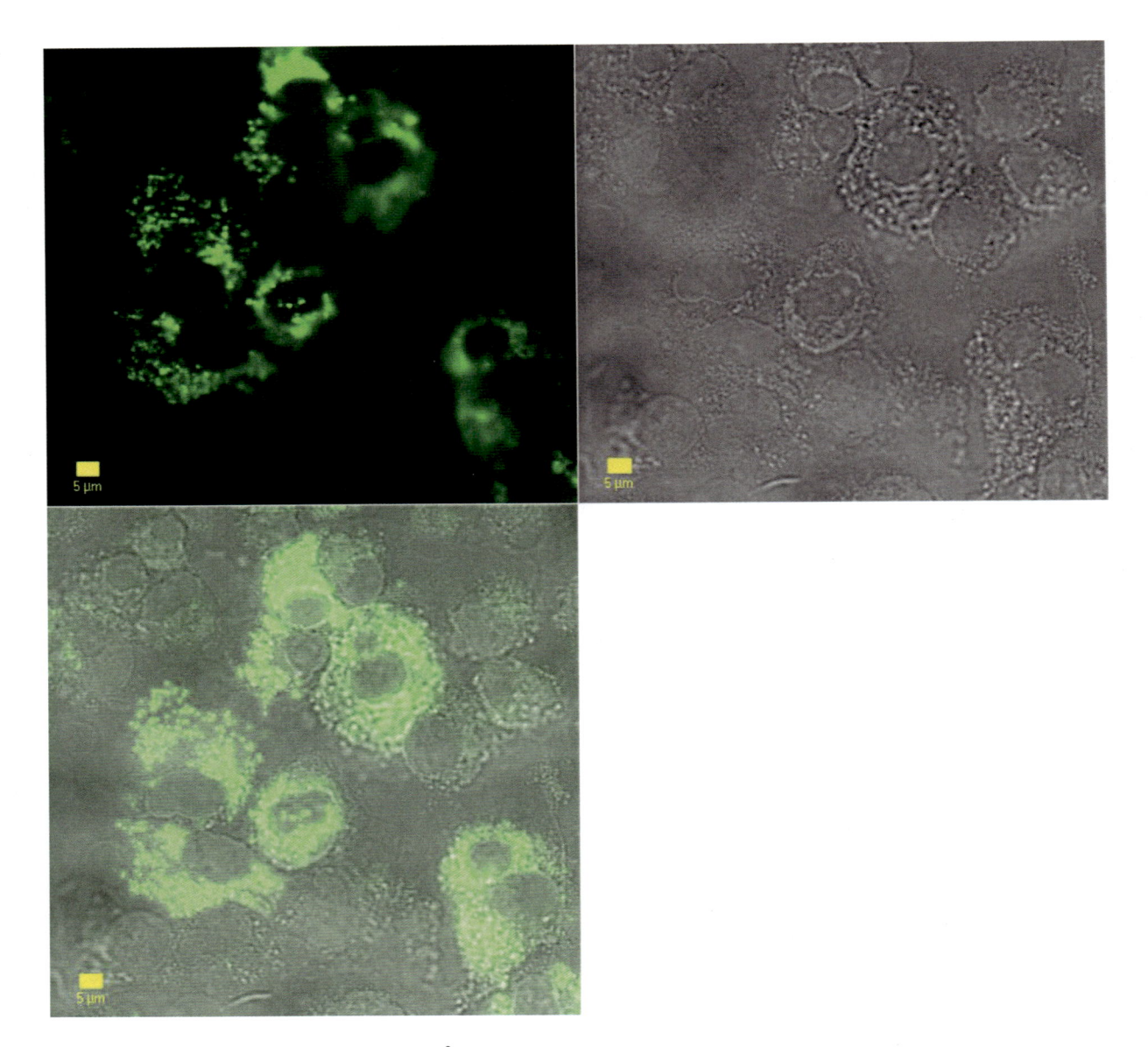

Figure 3-13. Uptake of the LaF$_3$:Ce^{3+}/DMSO/PPIX/PLGA microspheres (1µg/ml) into the cytoplasm of the PC3 cells during incubation time of 48 hours. Green color represents the LaF$_3$:Ce^{3+}/DMSO/PPIX/PLGA microspheres (excited with the argon–krypton laser, λ_{ex} = 488 nm). The cell nuclei remain dark since the PLGA microspheres did not penetrate into the nuclei. Adopted from ref. 5 with permission

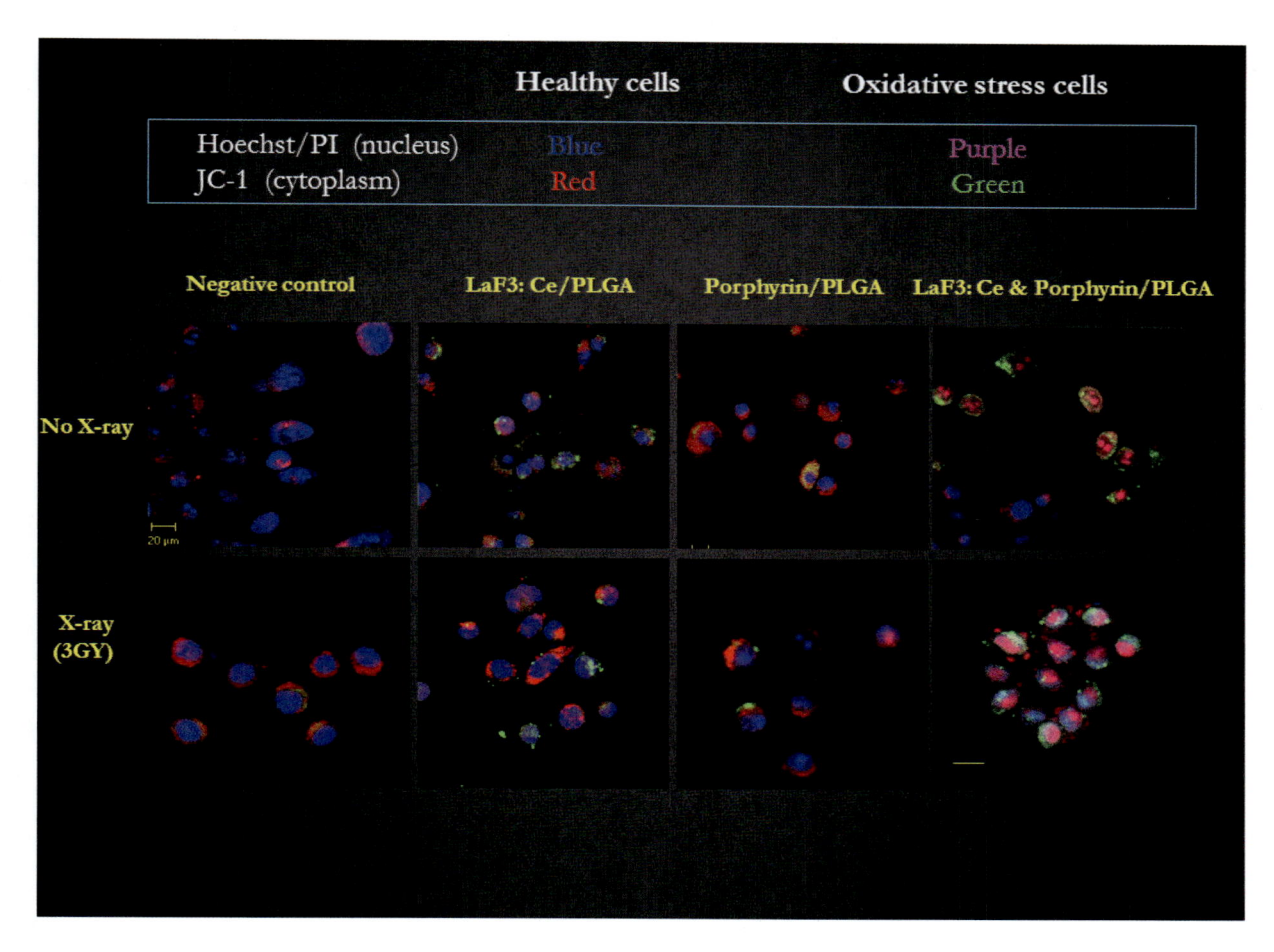

Figure 3-14. Confocal microscope images of the PC3 cells treated with the LaF$_3$:Ce/DMSO/PLGA, PPIX/PLGA and LaF$_3$:Ce^{3+}/DMSO/PPIX/PLGA microspheres. At the same dose of X-ray treatment (3 Gy), the percentage of the cells with mitochondrial perturbation was highest in the cells treated with the LaF$_3$:Ce^{3+}/DMSO/PPIX/PLGA microspheres. Treatment with the LaF$_3$:Ce^{3+}/DMSO/PLGA microspheres also resulted in a small population of the cells with unhealthy mitochondria, while exposure of the cells to PBS only (negative control) showed no sign of mitochondrial toxicity. The scale bar is 20 μm for all images. Adopted from ref. 5 with permission

The Bottom line

PDT is an effective treatment modality and has been widely used for the treatment of skin cancer. However, due to limited tissue penetration of light, PDT has been rarely applied for the therapy of solid and bulk cancers. The utilization of scintillating nanoparticles as an intracellular light source for photodynamic activation is a novel strategy to enable PDT of deep cancers. Here we report the application of LaF$_3$:Ce^{3+}/DMSO nanoparticles for photodynamic activation in prostate cancer cells *in vitro*. The results show that the encapsulation into PLGA microspheres facilitates energy transfer from the LaF$_3$:Ce^{3+}/DMSO nanoparticles to the PPIX molecules and consequently production of singlet oxygen. The LaF$_3$:Ce^{3+}/DMSO/PLGA and LaF$_3$:Ce^{3+}/DMSO/PPIX/PLGA microspheres induce sublethal damage to the cancer cells *in vitro*. Upon irradiation with X-rays the LaF$_3$:Ce^{3+}/DMSO/PPIX/PLGA microspheres induced cell killing while the microspheres without PPIX did not enhance the radiation effects. The described results indicate that X-rays can activate the LaF$_3$:Ce/DMSO/PPIX/PLGA microspheres for cancer treatment.

Executive Summary

- Experiments have been designed and conducted to prove the concept of X-ray induced photodynamic therapy for cancer treatment.
- LaF$_3$:Ce nanoparticles were synthesized by a wet-chemistry method in dimethyl sulfoxide (DMSO) and their application as an intracellular light source for photodynamic activation was investigated.
- The LaF$_3$:Ce^{3+}/DMSO nanoparticles have a strong green emission with a peak at around 520 nm which is effectively overlapped with the absorption of protoporphyrin IX (PPIX).
- The LaF$_3$:Ce^{3+}/DMSO nanoparticles were encapsulated into poly (D,L-lactide-co-glycolide (PLGA) microspheres along with PPIX.
- Upon irradiation with X-rays (90 kV), energy transfer from the LaF$_3$:Ce/DMSO nanoparticles to PPIX occurs and singlet oxygen is generated for cancer cell damage.
- Upon X-ray irradiation, the LaF$_3$:Ce/DMSO/PPIX/PLGA microspheres induced oxidative stress, mitochondrial damage and DNA fragmentation on prostate cancer cells (PC3).
- X-rays can activate LaF$_3$:Ce^{3+} and PPIX nanocomposites for cancer destruction.
- X-ray induced photodynamic therapy has a good potential for deep cancer treatment.

B. Copper Cysteamine – New Generation of Sensitizers for X-PDT

Here we introduce the structure and optical properties of a new Cu-Cyteamine complex (Cu-Cy) with formula of $Cu_3Cl(SR)_2$ (R = $CH_2CH_2NH_2$). This Cu-Cy has different structure from previous Cu-Cy in which both thio and amine groups from cysteamine bond with copper ions. Single-crystal X-ray diffraction and the solid-state nuclear magnetic resonance results show that the oxidation state of copper in the $Cu_3Cl(SR)_2$ is +1, rather than +2. Further, the $Cu_3Cl(SR)_2$ has been found with intense photoluminescence and X-ray excited luminescence. More interesting is that the $Cu_3Cl(SR)_2$ particles can produce singlet oxygen under irradiation by light or X-ray. This indicates that the $Cu_3Cl(SR)_2$ is a new photosensitizer that can be used for deep cancer treatment as X-ray can deeply penetrate soft tissues. All these mean that the $Cu_3Cl(SR)_2$ is a new material with potential applications for lighting, radiation detection and cancer treatment.

Cancer possesses the highest rate of mortality worldwide and is the second leading cause of death after heart disease, in the United State which is responsible for 25% of deaths overall. A total of 1,658,370 new cancer cases and 589,430 deaths from cancer were projected to occur in the United States in 2015. **To have a safe and effective treatment is always a good hope for cancer patients.** Photodynamic therapy (PDT) uses non-toxic photosensitizers and harmless visible light in combination with oxygen to produce reactive oxygen species (ROS), including peroxides, superoxide, hydroxyl radical, and **singlet oxygen,** that can kill malignant cells by apoptosis and/or necrosis, shut down the tumor microvasculature, and stimulate the host immune system. Preclinical studies have shown that local PDT enhances systemic antitumor immunity. In addition, PDT has a duality for targeting – the targeting of the drug and the light for activation. In case some photosensitizers distribute to the healthy tissue, if light is not exposed to the healthy tissue, it will not damage it. This duality for targeting is a big beauty of PDT as it can largely reduce the side-effects. Therefore, as a potential alternative to conventional cancer treatment methods, PDT has attracted ever-growing attention and is used with increasing frequency. **One of the limitations with PDT, however, is the need for direct light delivery for PDT activation.** Light delivery is challenging for the treatment of many tumors, such as those that are deeply located anatomically, and this is one reason that PDT use for deep tumors has been challenging.

There are three possible solutions to the light delivery of deep tumor treatment. The first prospect is to develop photosensitizers activated at near-infrared light, which can penetrate deeper into tissue than ultraviolet (UV) and visible light. Even though some research has been done toward developing NIR photosensitizers, there has been little success in this area. For near-infrared (NIR)-activated materials, the energy gaps are too narrow for singlet oxygen production. The second solution is to use upconversion nanoparticles that can be excited at NIR, such as 980 nm, which then emit light in the UV-Visible range for PDT activation. Several studies have reported that these upconversion nanoparticles can be used for PDT. However, NIR light can penetrate only 5 mm in tissue while retaining enough energy to activate photosensitizers. Therefore, this NIR light is not practically applicable for deep cancer treatment.

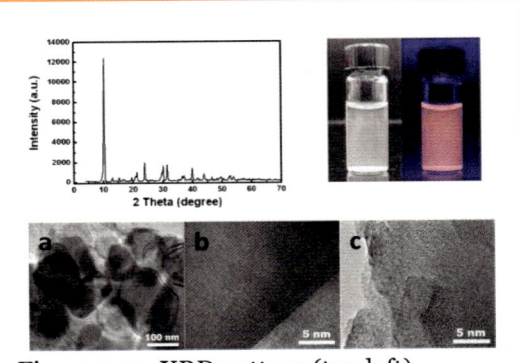

Figure 3-15. XRD pattern (top left), picture of solution sample (top right, under room and UV lighting) and HRTEM images (bottom a, b and c) of Cu-Cy particles. Adopted from ref.6 with permission

Although the above methods can solve the PDT light delivery to deep tumors at certain levels, they either have the limitation of light penetration or have additional energy transfer steps to perform, which result in complicated experimental procedures and may even decrease PDT treatment efficacy. It would be the best to develop a photosensitizer directly activated by X-ray to produce singlet oxygen. The possibility of using X-ray for photosensitizer activation has been reported in literature; however, the results are ambiguous. For some studies high enhancement was observed, while most studies found that the efficiency of photosensitizers for radiation enhancement is very low. In some cases, photosensitizers even decrease the efficiency of accompanying radiation treatments. One possible reason is that photosensitizers like porphyrin have very low stopping power and cannot effectively absorb X-rays for activation. We believe that the use of serendipitously invented Cu-Cy nanoparticles is a good solution for these issues and show great promise for breast cancer treatment as illustrated below.

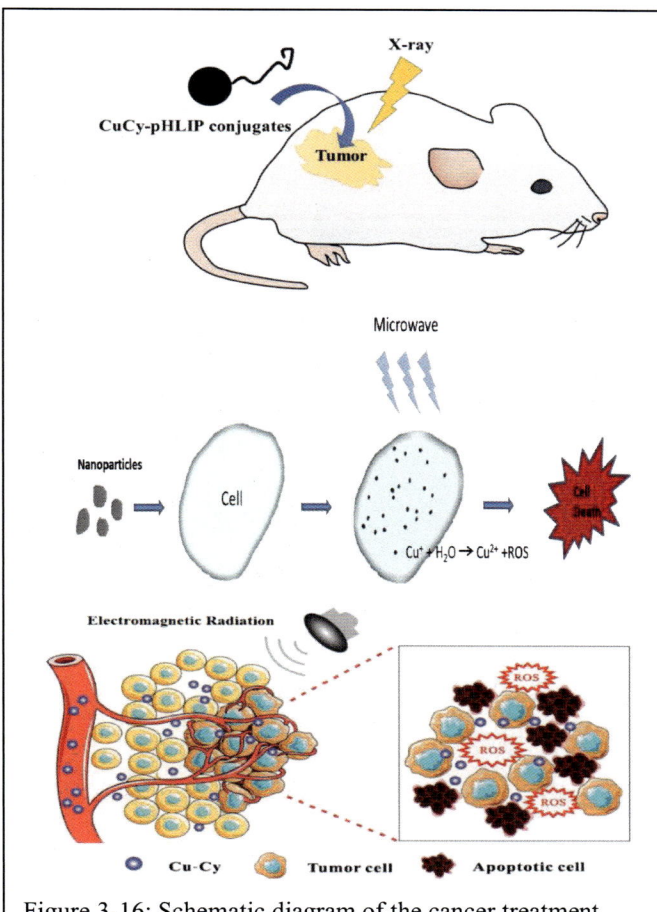

Figure 3-16: Schematic diagram of the cancer treatment principle of copper cysteamine photosensitizer under the activation of X-ray, microwave or ultrasound Adopted from refs. 9, 10 and 12 with permission

Cu-Cy, $Cu_3Cl(SR)_2$ (R= $CH_2CH_2NH_2$), as a new type of sensitizers we invented that have strong luminescence[22,23] and can produce ROS under UV light, X-rays, microwave radiation, and ultrasound. All these observations suggest that the Cu-Cy NPs are a new type of sensitizers with potential applications for infection inactivation and antitumor therapies. In addition, Copper-cysteamine (Cu-Cy) as a new type of materials also can be used for luminescence, solid state lighting, chemical sensing, radiation detection and plant cultivation lights. The crystal structure, optical properties and potential applications are described below.

Cu-Cy Crystal Structure

Figure 3-15 shows the X-ray diffraction (XRD) pattern, a photograph of the sample aqueous solution and the high resolution transmission electron microscopy (HRTEM) images of Cu-Cy particles. Their electron diffraction pattern (Figure 3-15 b and c) suggests that these small crystals are single crystals. Further HRTEM images display their continuous uniform lattice fringes. The HRTEM images demonstrate that these small crystals are highly crystalline and about 70 to 200 nm in size. The lattice spacing measured from the images are $d_1 = 0.347$ nm (Figure 3-15b) and $d_2 = 0.227$ nm (Figure 3-15c), respectively.

The powder XRD pattern of Cu-Cy displays very sharp and intense peaks. This is consistent with the HRTEM observations that the particles are highly crystalline and relatively large. However, the XRD pattern of Cu-Cy cannot be fitted with any known Cu-compounds in the present XRD database and this indicates that the Cu-Cy is a new compound that has never been reported before our publication.

Cu-Cy for Cancer treatment

With the development of nanotechnology, photodynamic therapy (PDT) has gradually become a cancer treatment method with many advantages. However, light-induced PDT, including ultraviolet, visible and near-infrared light bands, has poor penetration and significant energy attenuation in human tissue. Therefore, there have been great difficulties in the treatment of deep tumors.

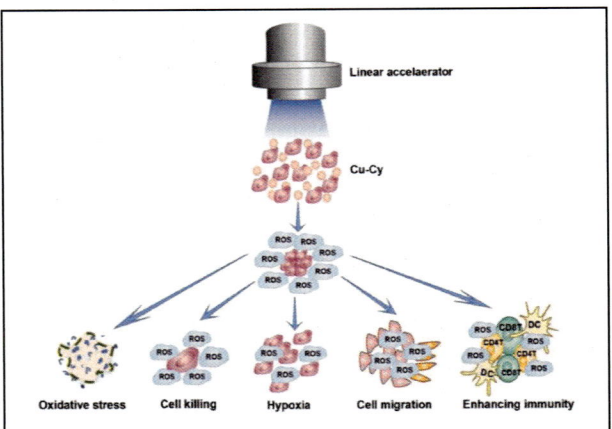

Figure 3-17: Schematic diagram of treatment and possible functions of copper cysteamine stimulated by clinic X rays Adopted from ref.17 with permission

Copper cysteine Cu-Cy photosensitizer we invented is a versatile new generation photosensitizer. The advantage of this photosensitizer over conventional photosensitizer is that Cu-Cy not only produces reactive oxygen (ROS) under the excitation of general light (e.g. ultraviolet light), but also ultrasound, X-rays or microwaves (Figure 3-16). So it can be used not only to treat superficial cancers but also to treat deep cancers, which have been evidenced in our sereies of publications.

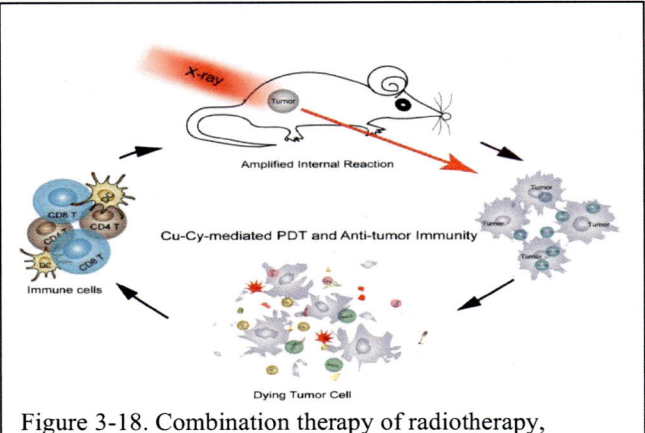

Figure 3-18. Combination therapy of radiotherapy, photodynamic and immune enhancement based on copper cysteamine Adopted from ref.16 with permission

The greatest advantage of this new generation of photosensitizer is that they can produce reactive oxygen with activation by X-rays, ultrasound or microwave to kill cancer cells or viruses. Applications that can be activated by X-rays have obvious advantages because they can be combined with modern radiotherapy techniques to improve treatment effectiveness and reduce harmful radioactive doses and side effects. A key question for this application is whether these new photosensitizer can be effectively used for treatment under the activation of X-rays used in clinical medicine. To this end, we have demonstrated for the first time that these photosensitizer can work effectively under the activation of clinical X-rays and the results show that Cu-Cy-mediated X-PDT can not only inhibit tumor growth, but also show good safety in animal experiments. It was verified from multiple cell levels (including HepG2, Li-7, SK-HEP-1, 4T1) how Cu-Cy-mediated X-PDT inhibited tumor proliferation and migration. The experimental results all show that Cu-Cy has a significant anti-cancer effect, and Cu-Cy has good safety under non-intervention conditions. The experimental results of body core magnetic resonance (MRI) showed that tumors with significantly restricted growth could be found in the Cu-Cy-mediated X-PDT treatment group, and no new metastases were found in the results of the whole body scan. During the whole treatment process, the mice did not show obvious toxic reactions and abnormal behavior changes. In addition, by constructing a large animal model of VX2 liver tumor in situ in rabbits, the effectiveness and safety of Cu-Cy-mediated X-PDT treatment were further verified from the experiments of multiple animal models.

In order to gain a deeper understanding of the potential molecular mechanisms behind the tumor inhibiting phenotypes by Cu-Cy-mediated X-PDT therapy, we used cell biology techniques to detect the expression of specific molecules corresponding to each phenotype. The results showed that in the X-PDT treatment group, the expression of PCNA molecules corresponding to the proliferation phenotype was the lowest, while the expression of E-cad molecules corresponding to the cell migration phenotype was the highest. It shows that X-PDT treatment has an inhibitory effect on tumor proliferation and metastasis compared with other groups. As a new type of photosensitizer, copper cysteamine Cu-Cy will become a promising tumor treatment method by combining with clinical linear accelerator. It has the dual effects of improving the efficiency of radiotherapy and inhibiting tumor growth and metastasis. This research has deepened our understanding of the treatment mechanism. And by simulating the clinical environment, it has been proved that Cu-Cy has the potential for clinical transformation, providing a new strategy for the clinical application of nanomaterials (Figure 3-17).

In addition, we found that this new photosensitizer can also activate the immunity of animals under X-ray excitation, which laid the foundation for the combination of radiotherapy, photodynamics and immunotherapy as desrcibed in our recent publication. (Figure 3-18)

In addition to cancer, **Cu-Cy NPs based PDT is also effective for Bacteria or virus Neutralization.** Diseases caused by Bacteria and virus have always been a big threat to human being. Excessive consumption and reliance upon antibiotics increase the chance of antibiotic resistance in different bacterial species. This understanding has led several researchers to talk about 'the end of the antibiotic epidemic. Bacterial resistance to antibiotics is a public health problem. Finding more effective antibacterial therapies to combat resistant strains is an ongoing subject of pertinence that can help stave epidemic. Our previous study revealed that Cu-Cy NPs alone can effectively kill gram-positive bacteria MRSA but not on gram-negative bacteria *E. coli* under UV light. Lately, We discovered that when KI is added to the Cu-Cy NPs, they can significantly inactivate both Gram-positive MRSA and Gram-negative *E.coli*. To uncover the mystery of killing, the interaction of KI with Cu-Cy NPs was investigated systematically, and

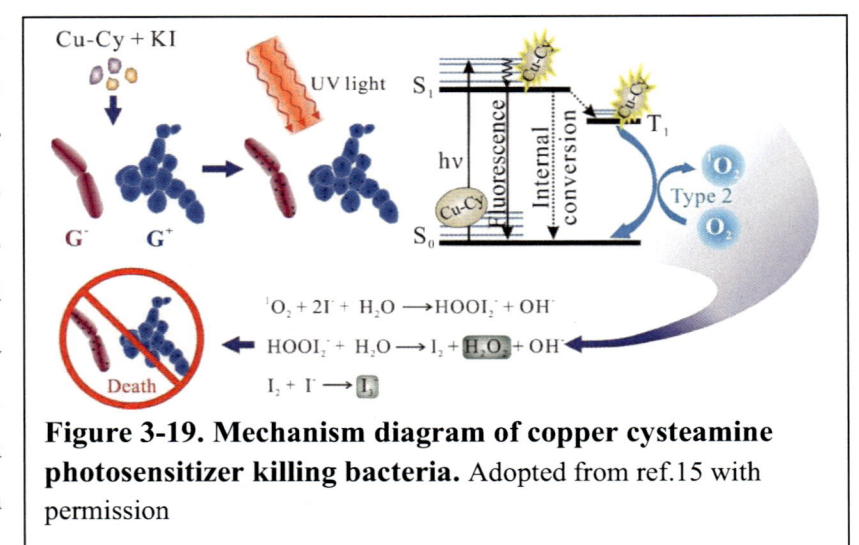

Figure 3-19. Mechanism diagram of copper cysteamine photosensitizer killing bacteria. Adopted from ref.15 with permission

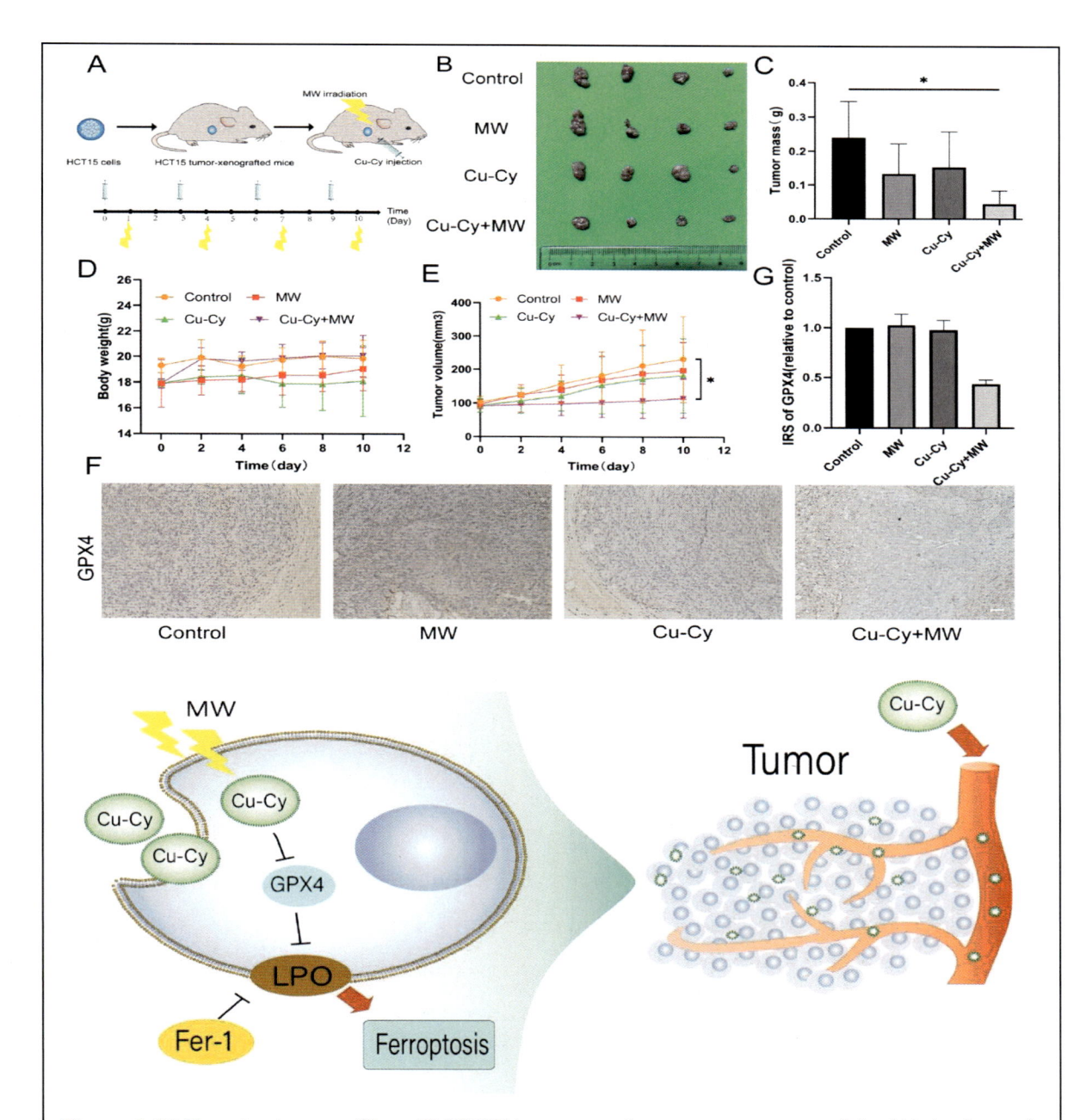

Figure 3-20 Top: Antitumor effect of MWDT in mouse subcutaneous tumor models. (A) A schematic diagram of MWDT scheme for animal experiments. HCT15 tumor-bearing mice were treated with three injections of Cu-Cy on 0th, 3rd, 6th, and 9th day. MW irradiation was performed on 1st, 4th, 7th, and 10th day. The tumor size and body weight were measured daily. (B) Images of each group at the end of the xenograft model experiment. (C) Tumor mass changes. (D) Body weight changes. (E) Tumor volume changes. (F) Histological observation of the tumor tissues with GPX4 staining. Scale bar: 50 μm. *p < 0.05. (G) Immunoreactive scores (IRSs) were calculated and compared among groups.

the products from their interaction were identified. No copper ions were released after adding KI to Cu-Cy NPs in cell-free medium and, therefore, it is reasonable to conclude that the Fenton reaction induced by copper ions is not responsible for the bacterial killing. Based on the observations, we propose that the major killing mechanism involves the generation of toxic species, such as hydrogen peroxide (H_2O_2), iodine tri-ions, iodide ions, singlet oxygen, and iodine molecules. This powerful combination of Cu-Cy NPs and KI has a good potential as an independent treatment or a complementary antibiotic treatment to infection diseases as reported in our recent publication (Fig. 3-19).

Most lately, we demonstrated that Cu-Cy nanoparticle-mediated microwave dynamic therapy, ferroptosis can be induced as a cancer treatment option. We used RNO-ID and SOSG to verify that ROS could be produced after MW irradiation of Cu-Cy, and the results showed that singlet oxygen increased with the increase of MW irradiation time and Cu-Cy concentration (Fig 3-20.A and B and C). In vitro experiments, Human CRC cells HCT15 can be inhibited by Cu-Cy nanoparticles activated with MW . Cu-Cy at 40 µg/mL almost killed all cells after microwave activation (Fig 3-20.D). A significant inhibition of cell colony formation was observed in Figs. 5.E and F when MW activated Cu-Cy nanoparticles were compared to other groups. In vivo experiments, compared to control group or MW group, Cu-Cy group, the Cu-Cy +MW group obviously inhibited the tumor mass and tumor growth (Fig 3-20). At the same time, by inducing ferroptotic death with microwave PDT using Cu-Cy nanoparticles, Zhou found that microwave PDT can effectively destroy colorectal cells. Western blot assay showed that GPX4 in HCT15 treated with MWDT was under expressed compared to other groups (Blank, MW alone or Cu-Cy alone group). However, when ferroptosis inhibitor Fer-1 were added, this change was reversed. Ferroptosis was generally considered to be characterized by lipid peroxidation (LPO) inside cells. C11-BODIPY fluorescent probe measurements showed that when HCT15 cells were treated with Cu-Cy + MW, the LPO was higher than when cells were treated with MW alone or Cu-Cy alone. As a result, human CRC cells were shown to undergo ferroptosis via MW activated Cu-Cy as illustrated in Figure 3-20 (bottom).

References for this chapter

1. **Wei Chen** and Jun Zhang, Using Nanoparticles to Enable Simultaneous Radiation and Photodynamic Therapies for Cancer Treatment, *J. Nanosci. Nanotechnol.* 2006, 6(4): 1159-1166

2. **Wei Chen**, Nanoparticle Self-Lighting Photodynamic Therapy For Cancer Treatment, J. Biomed. *Nanotechnol.* 2008, 4(4): 369-376 (cover story)

3. Wenjing Sun, Zijian Zhou, Guillem Pratx, Xiaoyuan Chen, Hongmin Chen, Nanoscintillator-Mediated X-Ray Induced Photodynamic Therapy for Deep-Seated Tumors: From Concept to Biomedical Applications, *Theranostics* 2020, 10(3): 1296-1318

4. Lun Ma, **Wei Chen**, ZnS:Cu,Co Water Soluble Afterglow Nanoparticles – Synthesis, Luminescence and Potential Applications, *Nanotechnology* 2010, 21: 385604

5. X. Zou, M. Yao, L. Ma, M. Hossu, W. Chen, X. Han, P. Juzenas, X-ray Induced Nanoparticles Based Photodynamic Therapy of Cancer, Future Nanomedicine 9 (15) (2014) 2339-2351.

6. L. Ma, W. Chen, G. Schatte, W. Wang, A.G. Joly, Y. Huang, R. Sammynaiken, M. Hossu, A new Cu–cysteamine complex: structure and optical properties, J. Mater. Chem. C 2(21) (2014) 4239-4246.

7. L. Ma, X. Zou, W. Chen, A New X-ray Induced Nanoparticle Photosensitizers For Cancer Treatment, J. Biomed. Nanotechnol. 10 (2014) 1501-1508.

8. Z. Liu, L. Xiong, G. Ouyang, L. Ma, S. Sahi, K. Wang, L. Lin, H. Huang, X. Miao, W. Chen, Y. Wen, The Investigation of Copper Cysteamine Nanoparticles as a new type of radiosenstizers for Colorectal Carcinoma, Scientific Reports 7 (2017) 9290.

9. S. Shrestha, J. Wu, B. Sah, A. Vanasse, L.N. Cooper, L. Ma, G. Li, H. Zhen, W. Chen, M.P. Antosh, X-ray Induced Photodynamic Therapy with pH-Low Insertion Peptide Targeted Copper-Cysteamine Nanoparticles in Mice, PNAS 116 (34) (2019 (accepted)) 16823–16828.

10. M. Yao, L. Ma, L. Li, J. Zhang, R.X. Lim, W. Chen, Y. Zhang, A New Modality for Cancer Treatment—Nanoparticle Mediated Microwave Induced Photodynamic Therapy, J. Biomed. Nanotechnol. 12 (2016) 1835–1851.

11. N.K. Pandey, L. Chudal, J. Phan, L. Lin, O. Johnson, M. Xing, P. Liu, H. Li, X. Huang, Y. Shu, W. Chen, A facile method for synthesis of copper-cysteamine nanoparticles and study of ROS production for cancer treatment, J. Mater. Chem. B (in press) (2019).

12. P. Wang, X. Wang, L. Ma, S. Sahi, L. Li, X. Wang, Q. Wang, Y. Chen, W. Chen, Q. Liu, Nanosonosensitization by Using Copper–Cysteamine Nanoparticles Augmented Sonodynamic Cancer Treatment, Part. Part. Syst. Charact. 35(4) (2018) 1700378 (1-10).

13. L. Huang, L. Ma, W. Xuan, X. Zhen, H. Zheng, W. Chen, M.R. Hamblin, Exploration of Copper-Cysteamine nanoparticles as a new type of agents for Antimicrobial photodynamic inactivation, J. Biomed. Nanotechnol. 15 (2019) 2142–2148.

14. L. Shi, P. Liu, J. Wu, L. Ma, H. Zheng, M.P. Antosh, H. Zhang, B. Wang, W. Chen, X. Wang, The effectiveness and safety of copper-cysteamine nanoparticle mediated X-PDT for cutaneous squamous cell carcinoma and melanoma Nanomedicine (London) 14(15) (2019) 2027-2043.

15. X. M. Zhen, L. Chudal, N.K. Pandey, J. Phan, X. Ran, E. Amador, X. Huang, O. Johnson, Y. Ran, W. Chen, M.R. Hamblin, L. Huang, A Powerful Combination of Copper-Cysteamine Nanoparticles with Potassium Iodide for Bacterial Destruction, Mater. Sci. Eng. C 110 (2020) 110659 1-8.

16. Qi Zhang, Xiangdong Guo, Yingnan Cheng, Lalit Chudal, Nil Kanatha Pandey, Jieyou Zhang, Lun Ma, Qing Xi, Guangze Yang, Ying Chen, Xin Ran, Chengzhi Wang, Jingyi Zhao, Yan Li, Li Liu, Zhi Yao, **Wei Chen**, Yuping Ran, and Rongxin Zhang, Use of copper-cysteamine nanoparticles to simultaneously enable radiotherapy, oxidative therapy and immunotherapy for melanoma treatment, *Signal Transduction and Targeted Therapy* (Nature), 2020, 5:58

17. Xiangyu Chen, Jiayi Liu, Ya Li, Nil Kanatha Pandey, Taili Chen, Lingyun Wang, Eric Horacio Amador, Weijun Chen, Feiyue Liu, Enhua Xiao, **Wei Chen**, Study of copper-cysteamine based X-ray induced photodynamic therapy and its effects on cancer cell proliferation and migration in a clinical mimic setting, Bioactive Materials, 2022, 7:504-514

18. Hui Zhou, Zhongtao Liu, Zijian Zhang, Nil Kanatha Pandey, Eric Amador, William Nguyen,

Lalit Chudal, Li Xiong, **Wei Chen**, and Yu Wen, Copper-cysteamine nanoparticle-mediated microwave dynamic therapy improves cancer treatment with induction of ferroptosis, *Bioactive Materials*, 2023, 24: 322–330

Chapter 4

Microwave induced photodynamic therapy

4.1 A Novel Cancer Treatment Modality—Microwave-Induced Photodynamic Therapy through Nanoparticles

Photodynamic therapy (PDT) is a type of phototherapy and photochemotherapy in which photosensitizers (PSs) are used to generate extremely reactive oxygen species (ROS) such as hydroxyl radicals (OH), singlet oxygen ($^1O_2$), and peroxides (R—O—O) that cause irreversible cell damage. However, one of the constraints of the existing PDT is the requirement for direct light supply to activate the PDT. Light delivery is tough for many cancers, particularly those that are anatomically distant, which is one reason PDT usage for deep cancer has proved difficult. Numerous solutions to the light delivery challenge have been researched for the treatment of deep cancer. The first possibility is to produce photosensitizers that are activated by near-infrared (NIR) light, which penetrates tissues deeper than ultraviolet (UV) or visible light. NIR light, on the other hand, cannot penetrate deeper than 10 mm into tissue while still having sufficient energy to activate PSs. The second method is to activate PDT using upconversion nanoparticles that can be energized in the near infrared and emit light in the UV-visible region. However, NIR-upconversion nanoparticles for PDT activation suffer from the same light penetration limitation. Thirdly, scintillation or afterglow nanoparticles can be used to activate PDT, allowing for treatment of deeper cancers. Cerenkov light was recently reported to be effective for PDT activation.

The purpose of this article is to introduce microwave-induced photodynamic therapy (MIPDT) as a novel idea in cancer therapy and to discuss its potential uses in cancer treatment. Microwave Ablation (MWA) is a relatively safe and non-invasive method of treating cancer. MWA utilizes electromagnetic radiation in the microwave energy spectrum to induce tissue necrosis within solid tumours. Microwave energy is unique among thermal treatment energies in a number of ways. The most significant of them is that microwaves penetrate all sorts of tissues and non-metallic materials, including water vapour and dried, burned, and desiccated tissues formed during the ablative process.

As a result, the combination of microwaves and PDT may result in the development of a novel therapeutic for deep cancer treatment.

Components and Procedures

Cu-Cy Particle Synthesis

$CuCl_2$ $2H_2O$ (0.460 g, 2.698 mmol) was dissolved in DI water and then cysteamine was added (0.636 g, 8.244 mmol). After adjusting the pH to 8, the solution was agitated for approximately 2 hours at room temperature and then heated to its boiling temperature for 30 minutes. The crude product was centrifuged and washed three times with a solution of DI water and ethanol (v/v = 5:4) followed by adequate sonication to yield Cu-Cy particles. Finally, the particles were thoroughly dried overnight in a vacuum oven set to room temperature.

Measurement of Photoluminescence and X-ray Excited Luminescence

The photoluminescence spectrum was acquired using a Shimadzu RF-5301PC fluorescence spectrophotometer after scattering 0.1 mg Cu-Cy particles in 3 mL DI water (Kyoto, Japan). The X-ray luminescence was determined in a light-proof X-ray cabinet connected to an external detector through an optic fibre. At 90 kV, a Faxitron RX-650 (Faxitron X-ray Corp., IL, USA) was used to irradiate the samples. The luminescence spectra were acquired using a QE65000 spectrometer (Ocean Optics Inc., FL, USA) connected to the X-ray chamber via a 0.6 mm core diameter optic fibre (P600-2-UV-Vis, Ocean Optics Inc., FL, USA) with a probe head extended inside the X-ray chamber and positioned 45° and 5 mm from the sample surface. A FLS920 spectrofluorometer was used to determine the luminescence decay and time-gated emission spectra (Edinburgh Instruments).

Observations on Cell Culture and Nanoparticle Uptake

The ATCC CRL-1661 rat osteosarcoma UMR-106 cells were grown in Dulbecco's Modified Eagle's Medium (DMEM, Gibco, USA) supplemented with 10% fetal bovine serum (FBS, Sciencell, USA) and containing 100 U/mL penicillin and 100 µg/mL streptomycin. UMR-106 cells were seeded at a density of 1×10^6 cells/mL into a 6-well plate and incubated for 24 hours at 37 C in a humidified environment containing 5% v/v CO2. After draining the culture medium, different doses of Cu-cysteamine (Cu-Cy) nanoparticle solution (0, 25 and 100 µg/mL) were applied to the 6-well plate at a concentration of 2 mL per well. After 24 hours, cells were separated using trypsinization (0.25 percent trypsin in Ethylenediaminetetraacetic acid (EDTA)) and concentrated using 1,000 rpm centrifugation for 5 minutes. The cell sample was then fixed in 3% glutaraldehyde for 24 hours, washed three times with phosphate-buffered saline (PBS), and fixed again in 1% osmium tetroxide for 2 hours. The cells were dehydrated sequentially with 30 percent, 50 percent, 70 percent, 80 percent, 90 percent, and 100 percent ethyl alcohol for ten minutes each. Epon812 was used to embed the fixed cells, and tiny blocks of cells within the Epon812 were sliced using an ultramicrotome (Leica Ultracut, Germany). Following that, positive staining with uranylacetate and lead citrate was performed on the ultrathin slices. A transmission electron microscope was used to study the nanoparticles' absorption into cells (H-7650, HITACHI, Japan).

The cell suspension (100 L) was seeded at a density of 2×10^4 cells/mL into a 96-well cell culture plate. After 24 hours, the culture media was withdrawn and different concentrations of Cu-Cy nanoparticle solutions (0, 6.25, 12.5, 25, 50, 100, 200, and 400 µg/mL) were introduced to the plate at a rate of 100 L per well. The Cell Counting Kit-8 (CCK-8, Dojindo, Japan) was used to determine the cytotoxicity of cells. When performing the CCK-8 experiment, the culture media was removed at each of the required time intervals (24, 48, and 72 h), 10 L of CCK-8 solution and 90 L DMEM were added to each well of the plate, and the cytotoxicity was determined after 4 hours of cell incubation. The optical density of the formazan solution was determined using a microplate reader (Thermo, Multiskn Go) set to 450 nm for all samples.

Microwave-Induced Photodynamic Therapy in In Vitro Cells

UMR-106 cells were seeded at a density of 2×10^4 cells/mL into a 6-well plate and incubated for 24 hours at 37°C in a humidified environment containing 5% v/v CO_2. The plate was then filled with various concentrations (0, 6.25, and 25 µg/mL) of Cu-Cy nanoparticle solutions at a rate of 400 L per well, and the microwave was given to the cells via a radiator probe (frequency of 2450 MHz). The microwave was created by a Xuzhou Baoxing Medical Equipment Co. Ltd. WB-3100A I medical microwave generator. The viability of the cells was assessed using live/dead staining following 24 h incubation with Cu-Cy nanoparticles via MW at 20 W for 5 min. The cells were gently washed with PBS before being incubated with 100 L solutions of calcein AM and ethidium homodimer (Sigma, USA). After staining the cells for 30 minutes at 37°C, they were visualized using a fluorescence microscope.

Microwave-Induced Photodynamic Therapy in Vivo Animal Studies

To produce the UMR-106 tumour xenografts, we used six- to eight-week-old female naked mice (C57BL/6, Medical Experimental Animal Center of Guangdong Province, China). Subcutaneous injections of a suspension of 1 106 UMR-106 cells were made into the shoulder and leg of naked mice. Microwave treatment involves delivering microwaves directly to tumours using a radiator probe, as described before in in vitro research. Daily tumour growth was observed in mice. When the tumours attained a diameter of about mm, the mice were sedated with 1% chloral hydrate solution and randomly assigned to one of three groups: Cu-Cy, MW, or Cu-Cy+MW (n = 6 for each group). Cu-Cy and Cu-Cy +MW nanoparticles (concentration: 1 mg/mL) were administered intratumorally into anaesthetized mice in the Cu-Cy and Cu-Cy +MW groups. The MW group received 30, 50, or 100 μL of normal saline (NS). After 30 minutes, the tumours on mice in the MW and Cu-Cy +MW groups were irradiated directly with MW at 20 W for 5 minutes. Every day following the initiation of radiation treatment, the tumour size was determined using a digital caliper. The volume of the tumour was calculated using the following formula: /6 greater diameter (smaller diameter)2. Each group's animals assigned to day 14 were used to generate a tumour growth curve. On the fourteenth day, mice were euthanized. The tumours were dissected surgically and their volumes (cubic millimetres) were determined. The tumours were fixed in 4% paraformaldehyde solution and then dried and embedded in paraffin using standard techniques. Finally, the frozen specimens were cut into cryosections, and two adjacent 5 μm thick cryosections were utilized to examine tumour proliferation using Ki-67 immunohistochemistry (IHC) and immunofluorescent (IF) staining. To observe the morphological changes in the cells and tissues, one of the adjacent 5 μm thick slices was stained with hematoxylin and eosin (H&E). A fluorescence microscope was used to view tumour slices stained with anti-Ki-67 antibody and H&E.

Measurement of Singlet Oxygen in Aqueous Solution

The RNO-ID (p-nitrosodimethylaniline (RNO)-imidazole (ID)) method was used to determine singlet oxygen in aqueous solutions, as stated in the literature. 0.225 mg RNO (Sigma, USA) and 16.34 mg ID (Sigma, USA) were added to 30 mL de-ionized (DI) water that had been sufficiently bobbled to achieve air saturation. 1.5 mg of the testing sample (Cu-Cy) was added to 3 mL of the aforesaid RNO-ID solution to create the sample solution. Then, using a microwave treatment apparatus, the RNO-ID solution and sample solutions were subjected to microwaves (MW) for 5 minutes at varied output powers (0—30 W) (WB-3100A1, BXING, China). Meanwhile, the other set of RNO-ID solutions and sample solutions were exposed to MW at a power level of 20 W for varying durations (0—30 min). The intensity of the RNO absorption peak at 440 nm was used to determine the singlet oxygen content using a microplate reader (Thermo, Multiskn Go). Singlet oxygen emission spectra were obtained using a home-built spectrometer equipped with a Hamamtsu In/InGaAsP detector (H10330A-45) excited at 447 nm at room temperature.

Detection of Reactive Oxygen Species in UMR-106 Cells

2′,7′-dichlorodihydrofluorescin diacetate was used to determine the intracellular ROS (DCFH-DA, Sigma, USA). DCFH-DA enters the cell in a passive manner and interacts with singlet oxygen to create the highly fluorescent dichlorofluorescein (DCF). 0.1 M MDCFH-DA stock solution (in methanol) was diluted 5,000-fold in DMEM without serum or other additives to obtain a working solution of 20 μM. The UMR-106 cell suspension (400 L) was seeded at a density of 2104 cells/mL into three 24-well cell culture plates (A, B, and C). The cell suspensions were then incubated for 24 hours at 37°C in a humidified 5% CO_2 environment. At 400 L per well, different concentrations of Cu-Cy nanoparticle solution (0, 6.25, and 25 μg/mL) were applied to the plates. After 24 hours, the cells in the 24-well plates were washed twice with PBS, incubated for 30 minutes at 37 C in a 400 L solution of DCFH-DA, and gently rinsed three times with PBS. The plates were then filled with 400 L of DMEM. For 5 minutes, culture plate A was exposed to MW at a dosage of 20 W. For 30 minutes, culture plate B was exposed to UV radiation at a dosage of 10 mW/cm^2. Plate C served as an untreated control. The fluorescence intensity of the cells was then quantified using a fluorescent microscope (Olympus BX51, Japan).

Intracellular ROS Quantitative Detection

The intracellular singlet oxygen was quantified using an oxidation-sensitive fluorescence sensor (DCFH-DA). Cells on culture plates A and B were co-cultured for 24 hours with varied concentrations of Cu-Cy nanoparticles (0, 6.25, and 25 μg/mL), washed three times with PBS, and incubated for 30 minutes at 37°C in a 400 L DCFH-DA solution. Three times with DMEM, the cells were gently washed, and 400 L of DMEM was added to the plate. Plate A cells were exposed to MW at a power level of 20 W for 5 minutes, whereas plate B cells were utilized as a control. The fluorescence was measured using a Guava Easy Cyte 5HT flow cytometer (Millipore, USA) with a 488 nm excitation and a 525 nm DCF detection filter. Each sample was measured using 6,000 cells.

Cell Death Observation

The UMR-106 cell suspension (400 L) was planted at a density of 5104 cells/mL into a 24-well cell culture plate. After 24 hours of incubation, the plate was filled with varied concentrations (0, 6.15, and 25 g/mL) of Cu-Cy nanoparticle solution at a rate of 400 L per well. After 24 hours of incubation with Cu-Cy nanoparticles, cells in the plate were radiated for 5 minutes with MW at 20 W. Guava Nexin Reagent was used to visualize changes in the nucleus morphology of UMR-106 cells (Millipore, USA). To summarize, UMR-106 cells were gently washed with PBS and centrifuged at 1,000 rpm for 5 minutes. The pelleted cells were resuspended in 100 μL DMEM supplemented with 1% FBS and then treated for 20 minutes at room temperature with 100 L of Annexin V-PE and 7-AAD labelling solution. Finally, cells were examined using a Guava EasyCyte 5HT flow cytometer (Millipore, USA) at 488 nm with a 575 nm band-pass filter for Annexin V-PE detection and at 546 nm with a 647 nm band-pass filter for 7-AAD detection. Guava Nexin Software v2.2.2 was used to evaluate 6,000 cells.

Following rehydration and antigen retrieval, endogenous peroxidase activity in IHC and IF was inhibited by incubation in methanol containing 0.3 percent hydrogen peroxide. Following that, slices were treated overnight with Ki-67 antibody and subsequently with a secondary Anti-Rabbit IgG antibody (Alexa Fluor 488, Beyotime, China). Counterstained the slides with 4′,6-diamidino-2-phenylindole (DAPI) (C1002, Beyotime, China). A fluorescent microscope was used to acquire images of tumour slices stained with the anti-Ki-67 antibody (Olympus BX51, Japan).

Outcomes

Copper cysteamine (Cu-Cy) is a novel type of photosensitizer that may be activated by light or X-rays to generate singlet oxygen for cancer killing. The particle size is around 250 nm, as determined by transmission electron microscopy (TEM), and the microanalysis, which includes particle size, crystal structure, optical and copper valence, is reported in our earlier paper. The size determined by dynamic light scattering (DLS) is around 230 nm, which is comparable to the size determined by transmission electron microscopy (TEM). The photoluminescence excitation (PLE), emission (PL), and X-ray excited luminescence (XL) spectra of Cu-Cy nanoparticles are depicted in Figure 1(A). The insets in Figure 1(A) show images of the Cu-Cy aqueous solution under ambient light (a) and when activated by a UV lamp (b).

We discovered that microwaves may also be used to activate Cu-Cy, resulting in the production of singlet oxygen. This discovery establishes a new modality for cancer treatment known as MIPDT. For PDT to work, reactive oxygen species (ROS) such as singlet oxygen are required. We employed the p-nitrosodimethyl-aniline (RNO)-imidazole (ID) technique to measure the singlet oxygen generated by Cu-Cy after exposure to various MW dosages. RNO is a water-soluble molecule whose absorption can be irreversibly stopped in the presence of ID by singlet oxygen. We found singlet oxygen created by the Cu-Cy nanoparticles at various MW dosages by comparing the relative quenching of RNO absorption with and without Cu-Cy nanoparticles. As illustrated in Figure 1(B), MW irradiation did not cause any singlet oxygen to quench the RNO absorption in the control of RNO-ID. However, when Cu-Cy particles were used, the RNO absorption was quenched constantly as a function of the MW dose, showing that singlet oxygen was generated continually. Additionally, we determined the formation of singlet oxygen when Cu-Cy nanoparticles were irradiated with MW at a power of 20 W for various time durations, as shown in Figure 1. (C). The results indicated that as the microwave irradiation time grew, the RNO absorption was quenched constantly, implying that more singlet oxygen was created.

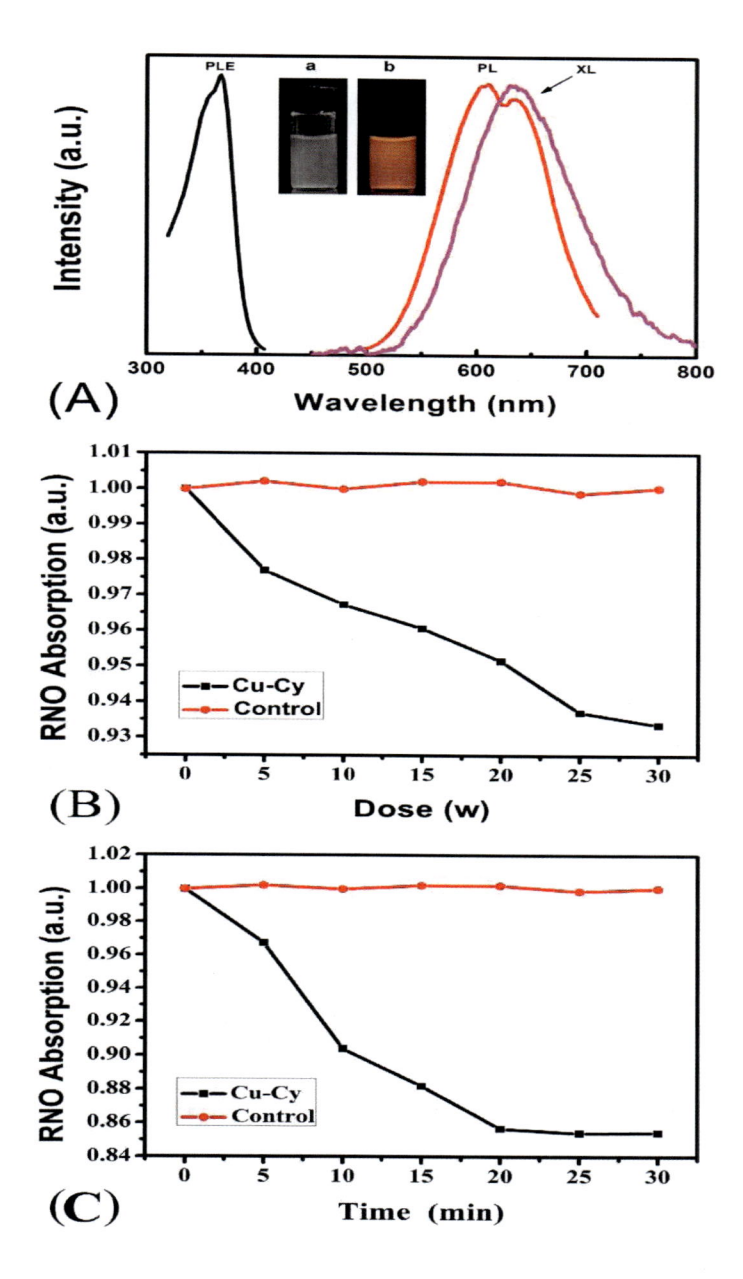

Figure 4-1 **Optical properties of Cu-Cy nanoparticles**. A: The photoluminescence excitation (PLE, emission at 650 nm), emission (PL, excitation at 360 nm) and X-ray excited luminescence (XL) spectra of Cu-Cy nanoparticles. The inset are photos of the Cu-Cy aqueous solution at room light (a) and excited by a UV lamp (b). B: RNO absorption quenched by singlet oxygen produced in Cu-Cy aqueous solution (0.5 mg/ml) irradiated by MW for 5 min at different outputs. (C): RNO absorption quenched by singlet oxygen produced in Cu-Cy aqueous solution (0.5 mg/ml) irradiated by MW at 20 W for various time durations. Adopted from ref. 1 with permission

The anti-tumor effects of various concentrations of Cu-Cy nanoparticles produced by microwaves were assessed by live/dead staining, as illustrated in Figure 4-2. When UMR-106 cells were cultivated with Cu-Cy nanoparticles at concentrations ranging from 0 µg/ml to 25 µg/ml for 24 hours, only a few cells died (red, Figs. 4-2(d and g)). However, within 5 minutes of exposure to MW at 20 W, some UMR-106 cells became hazy and died (red, Figs. 4-2(e and h)). The results shown in Figure 4-2 indicate that increasing the Cu-Cy nanoparticle concentration or/and the MW irradiation period resulted in a greater number of UMR-106 cancer cells being destroyed. At a Cu-Cy concentration of 25 µg/ml, combined with ten minutes of MW irradiation at a power of twenty watts, nearly 100% of cancer cells were destroyed. The green and red cells (in Fig. 4-2) in five random scopes were counted for quantification, and the results are given in Figure 4-3.

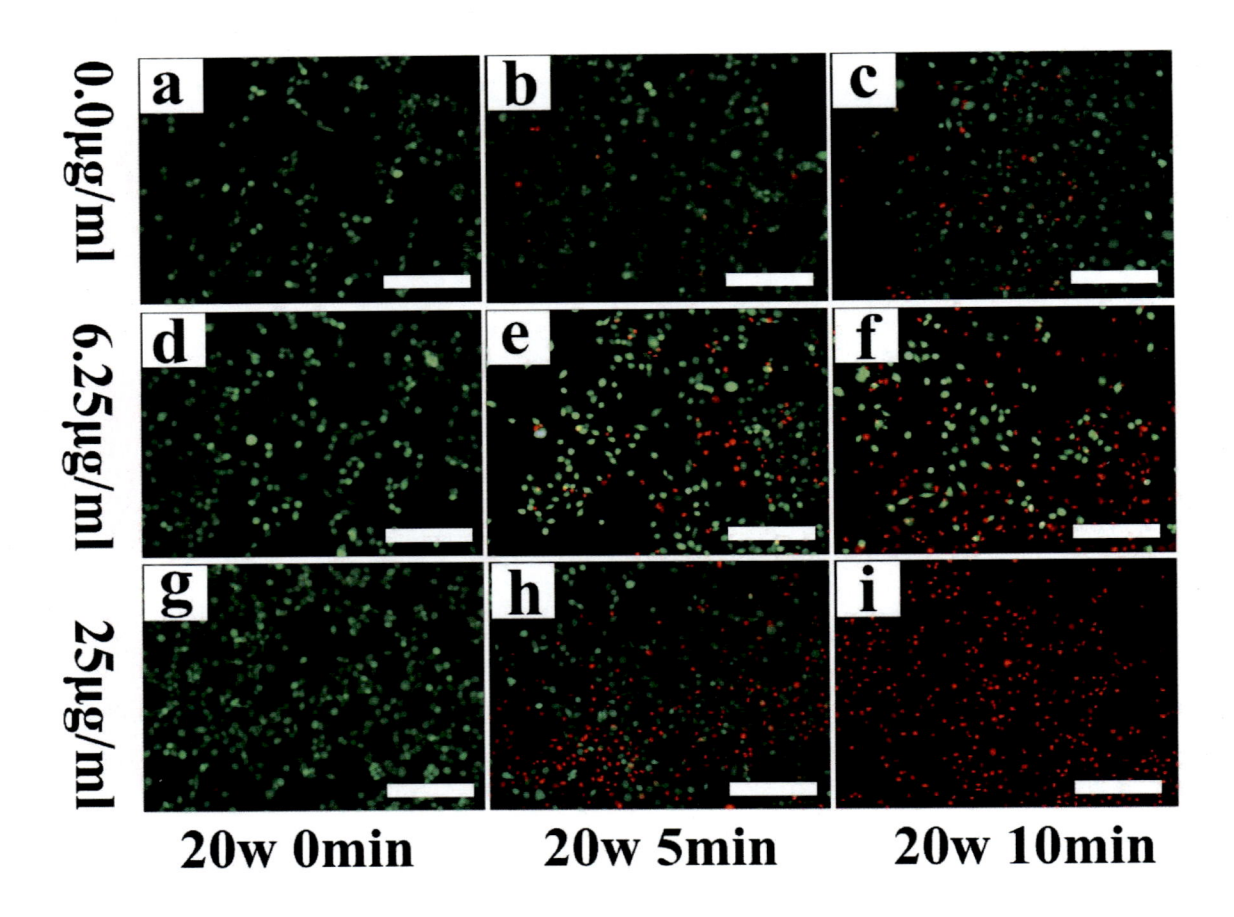

Figure 4-2. *In vitro* **cell study of MIPDT.** The live/dead staining images of UMR-106 cells with Cu-Cy nanoparticles and MW. a, control group; b, control + 5 min MW at 20 W; c, control + 10

min MW at 20 W; d, 6.25μg/ml Cu-Cy; e, 6.25μg/ml Cu-Cy + 5 min MW at 20 W; f, 25μg/ml Cu-Cy +10 min MW at 20 W; g, 25.0μg/ml Cu-Cy; h, 25.0μg/ml Cu-Cy + 5 min MW at 20 W; i, 25.0μg/ml Cu-Cy +10min MW at 20 W. Adopted from ref. 1 with permission

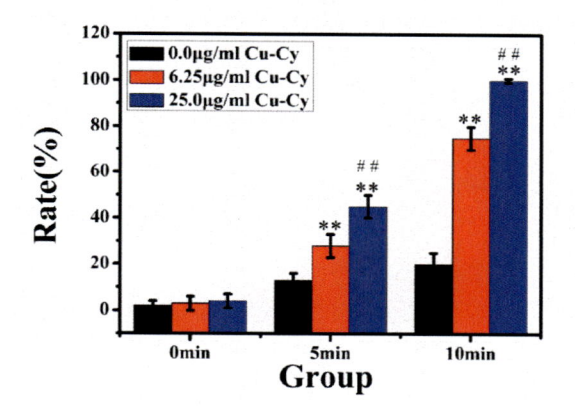

Fig. 4-3. The death cell rates in cells treated with different concentrations of Cu-Cy for 1, 5 and 10 minutes of microwave irradiation. Adopted from ref. 1 with permission

MIPDT was also tested in vivo on animals. As illustrated in Figure 4-4 (top left), tumours in the MW treatment group (top row) and the Cu-Cy treatment group (middle row) expanded over time, with no obvious difference in tumour growth between Cu-Cy and normal saline (NS, 100 L 0.9 percent NaCl, as a control) at dosages of 20, 50, and 100 l. Meanwhile, tumours treated with Cu-Cy alone were much smaller than tumours treated with NS alone, notably in the Cu-Cy group (100 l Cu-Cy dosage). However, no statistically significant difference between the MW and Cu-Cy groups was identified. This data implies that the Cu-Cy particles are slightly toxic in vivo; nevertheless, this does not result in a significant reduction in tumour size or growth inhibition. With MW radiation (bottom row), tumour development was significantly slowed at 50 and 100 l Cu-Cy doses. Each group's tumour growth curve was determined from the animals allocated to day 14 (Figure 4-4 (Bottom A—D). Tumors on various body areas of mice in the MW and Cu-Cy groups were comparable in size, and no statistically significant difference was seen between them (See Fig.4- 4, Bottom (A and B)). The tumour volume decreased as the Cu-Cy dose was raised in the Cu-Cy+MW group. On day 3, there was a significant difference in tumour volume between the left leg (LL) and the left shoulder (LS) (#$P < 0.05$, ##$P < 0.01$) and the right leg (RL) and the left shoulder (LS) ($P < 0.05$, $P < 0.01$) (Fig. 4, Bottom (C)). On day 3, a significant difference in tumour volume was found between the Cu-Cy+MW group and the Cu-Cy group (##P 001) and the Cu-Cy+MW group and the MW group (P 001). Between the MW and Cu-Cy groups, no statistically significant change was seen (Fig. 4-4, Bottom (D)).

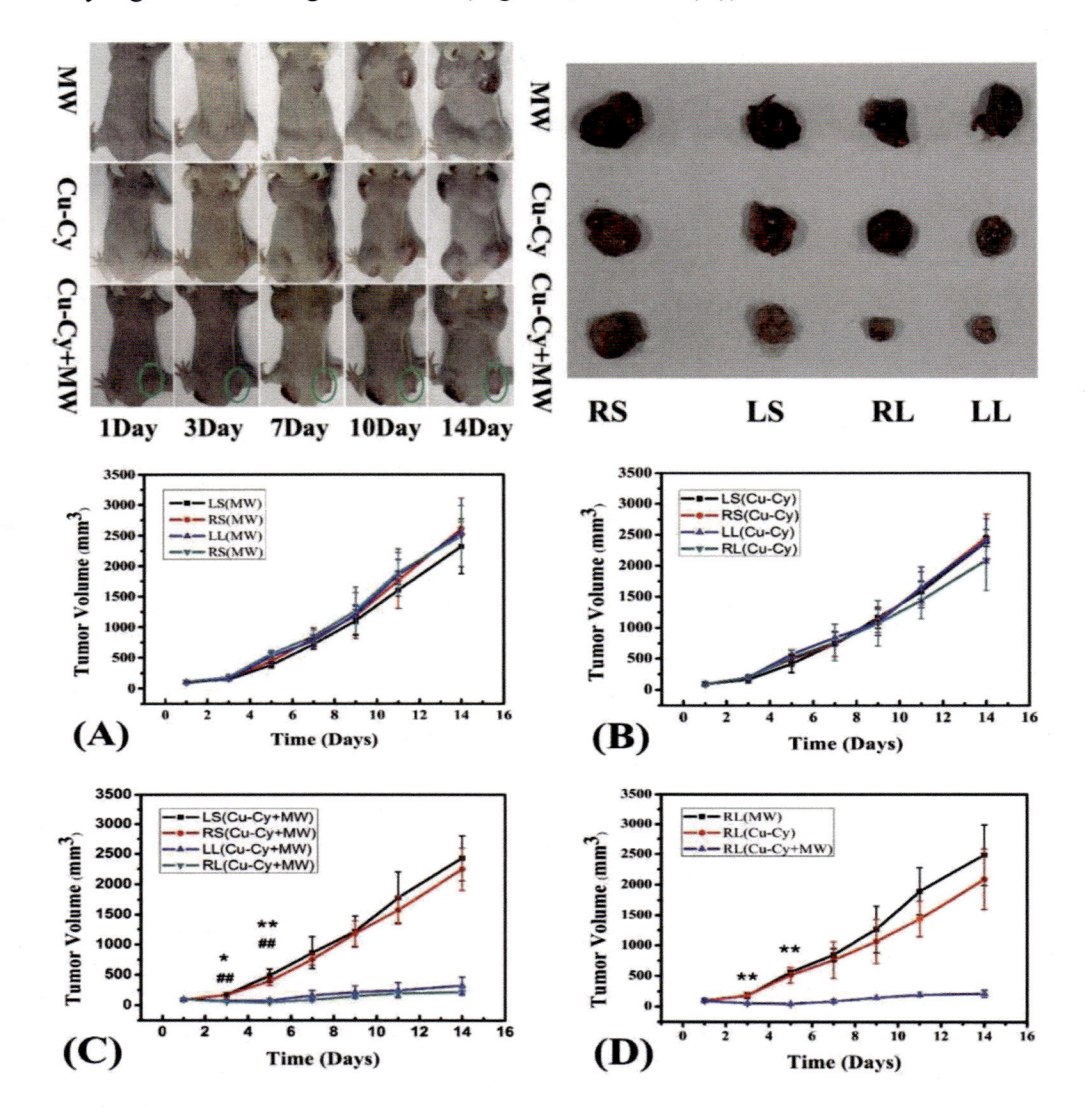

Figure 4-4 **in vivo animal study of MIPDT. Top Left:** Time-dependent in vivo images of mice with differently sized UMR-106 tumors after treatment at 1, 3, 7, 10 and 14 days. MW group: left shoulder, 100 μl normal saline (NS); right shoulder 20 μl NS; left leg, 50 μl NS; right leg, 100 μl NS. Cu-Cy group and Cu-Cy + MW group: left shoulder, 100 μl NS; right shoulder 20 μl Cu-Cy solution (concentration: 1mg/ml); left leg, 50 μl Cu-Cy solution; right leg, 100 μl Cu-Cy solution. At 30 minutes post-injection, the tumors in MW and Cu-Cy + MW groups were irradiated with MW at 20 W for 5 min directly to the tumors. **Top Right**: The tumor collected after UMR-106 tumor-bearing mice were sacrificed on the 14th day of treatment. **Bottom:** The tumor growth curves. (A): MW group. (B):Cu-Cy group; (C):Cu-Cy + MW group; (D):Tumor volume in the left leg of MW, Cu-Cy, Cu-Cy + MW groups. Adopted from ref. 1 with permission

On the fourteenth day, the mice were euthanized and decapitated. The tumours were surgically dissected and are depicted in Figure 4 at the top right. Clearly, tumours treated exclusively with NS or Cu-Cy (top and middle rows) developed to a little higher volume than those treated exclusively with Cu-Cy +MW. The identical size of tumours treated with 20, 50, or 100 μl of Cu-Cy particles demonstrates that these Cu-Cy dosages have a minimal influence on tumour growth. However, when triggered with MW, Cu-Cy nanoparticles (at concentrations of 50 and 100 μl) can significantly reduce tumour volume (the bottom row of the top right in Fig. 4-4). These observations corroborate the results depicted in the top left corner of Figure 4-4. The preliminary results indicate that MW can activate Cu-Cy particles to generate singlet oxygen for tumour cell killing, and that Cu-Cy is a promising photosensitizer for cancer treatment.

Staining with hematoxylin and eosin (H&E) on tumour tissues20 (Fig. 4-5, left) demonstrates that tumour tissues treated with Cu-Cy nanoparticles or MW alone exhibit no evidence of cell damage or injury, and that these tumours are formed primarily of malignant cells (Fig. 4-5, left top and middle rows). This demonstrates that MW or Cu-Cy therapy alone is incapable of successfully destroying or suppressing malignancies. When Cu-Cy nanoparticles are irradiated with MW, they can significantly destroy tumour cells. Nuclear pyknosis, cytoplasmic edoema, and some leaky patches of eosinophils are observed in the Cu-Cy + MW group, indicating tumour necrosis (Fig.4-5 left bottom row).

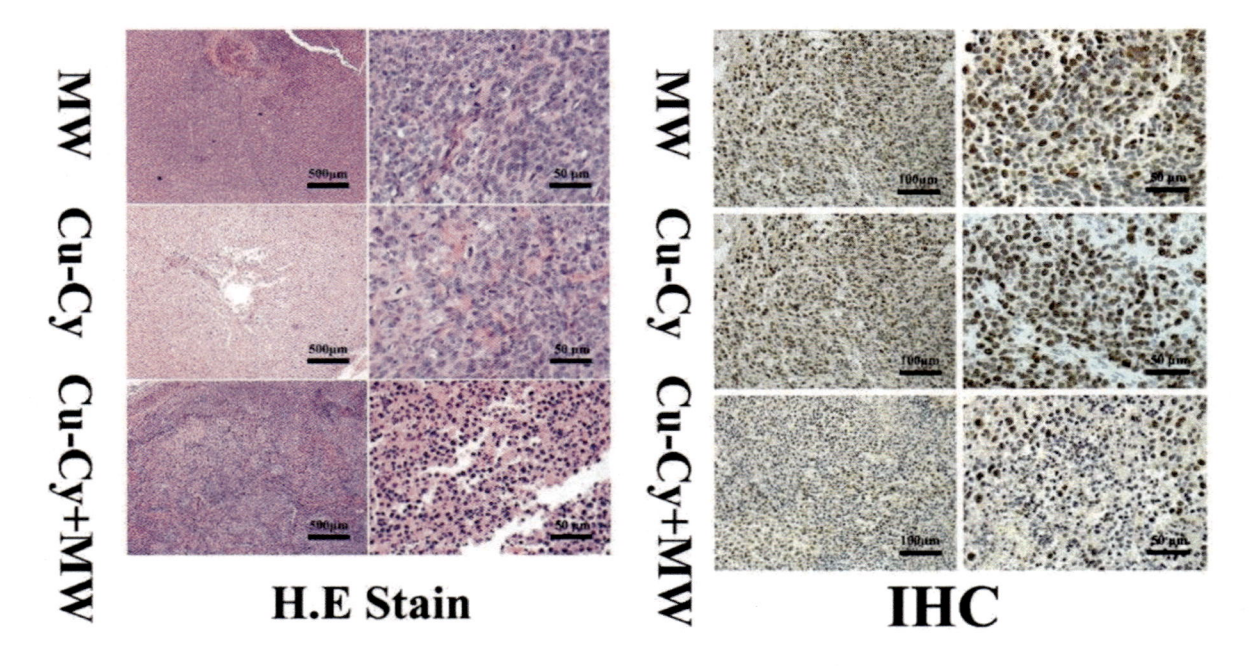

Figure 4-5. **Staining imaging for the effects of MIPDT on tumor tissues.** Left: Hematoxylin and eosin (H&E) staining. Top row, the tumor at RL after MW treatment; middle row, the tumor at RL after Cu-Cy treatment; bottom row, the tumor at RL by Cu-Cy + MW treatment. Right: IF and IHC staining with Ki-67. Top row, the tumor at RL after MW treatment; middle row, the tumor at RL by Cu-Cy treatment; bottom row, the tumor at RL after Cu-Cy + MW treatment. The MW treatment was conducted at 20 W for 5 min. Adopted from ref. 1 with permission

Ki-67 is a non-histone nuclear protein that is present at low levels in quiescent cells but is upregulated in proliferating cells, particularly in the G2, M, and late S phases. Thus, Ki-67 reactivity, defined as the proportion of positive tumour cells as determined by immunohistochemistry (IHC) labelling, is a particular nuclear marker for cell proliferation. Overexpression is frequently observed in a number of malignant tissues and is associated with a poor prognosis for cancer patients. A staining procedure can be used to determine the percentage of tumour cells positive for Ki-67. The greater the number of positive cells, the more rapidly they divide and generate new cells. The application of Ki-67 labelling to tumour cells treated with Cu-Cy, MW, and Cu-Cy + MW is illustrated in detail in Figures 4-5 and 4-6. Only the combination of Cu-Cy and MW has been shown to be effective in inhibiting tumour growth. Overexpression of Ki67 is observed in tumours treated with Cu-Cy nanoparticles or MW at 20 W alone. This suggests that treatment with Cu-Cy or MW alone is ineffective at destroying or suppressing cancer cells.

However, when Cu-Cy and MW were combined (at the same dose as MW alone), the majority of tumour cells were destroyed and the expression of Ki67 was significantly reduced (Fig. 4-6). All of these findings suggest that the combination of Cu-Cy and MW is an effective strategy for cancer treatment and cell proliferation reduction.

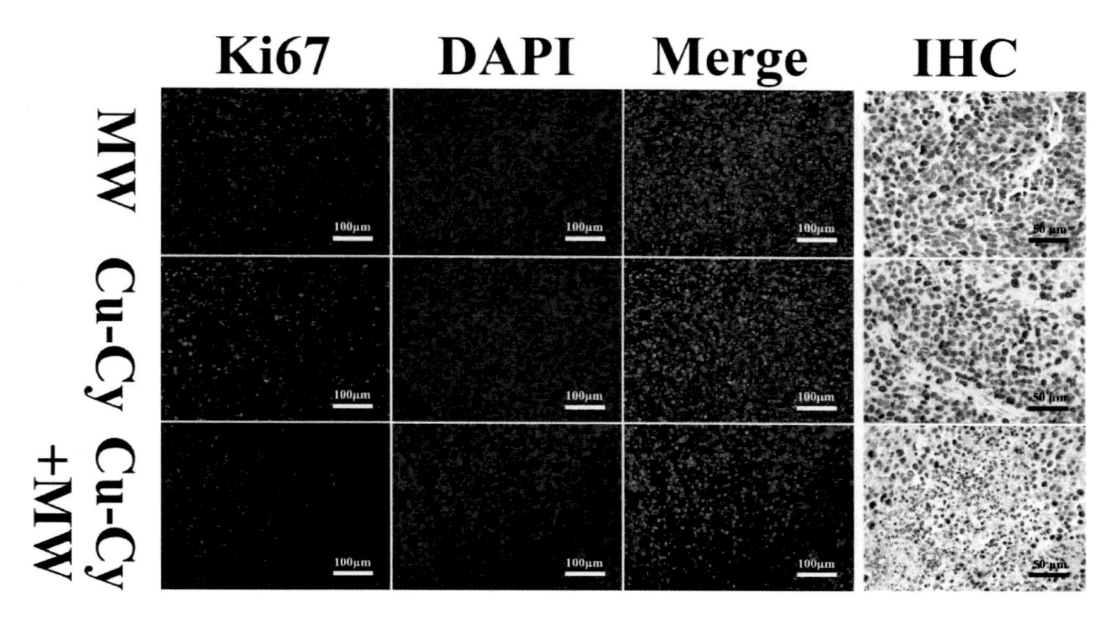

Fig.4-6 IHC staining. Top row, RL of MW treatment group; middle row, RL of Cu-Cy treatment group; bottom row, RL of Cu-Cy+MW treatment group. Adopted from ref. 1 with permission

Cu-Cy nanoparticles are readily taken up by UMR-106 tumour cells, and their uptake increases with increasing Cu-Cy nanoparticle concentration, as shown in Figure 4-7. As can be shown, UMR-106 cells took in a large number of Cu-Cy nanoparticles at a concentration of 100 μg/ml. To elucidate the mechanism of tumour elimination, the DCFH-DA technique was used to quantify intracellular ROS generation. The cells were seen using a fluorescent microscope (Fig. 4-8(a)) following 24 h incubation with Cu-Cy nanoparticle concentrations of 25 (a, d, g), 6.25 (b, e, h), and 0 μg/ml (c, f, I with UV (d—f) and MW (a—c), respectively. UMR-106 cells treated with 25 g/ml Cu-Cy nanoparticles triggered with UV or MW show green fluorescence (a, d), indicating that the cells produce reactive oxygen species (ROS). There was no fluorescence observed in control or UMR-106 cells treated with 6.25 μg/ml Cu-Cy nanoparticles triggered with UV or MW (b, c, e, f), indicating that no ROS were generated in these cells. Flow cytometry was used to quantify the fluorescence intensity within cells (see Fig. 4-8(b)). The mean fluorescence intensity (MFI) of UMR-106 cells represents intracellular oxidative stress. The results indicate that the MFI is always greater in UMR-106 cells treated with Cu-Cy + MW (Figs. 4-8(b(D—F)) than in untreated cells (Figs. 4-8(b(A—C)). The MFI increases as the Cu-Cy concentration increases. The MFI of cells treated with MW and 25 µg/ml Cu-Cy is twofold that of cells treated with MW alone (Fig. 8(b(D)) and threefold that of the control (Fig. 4-8(b(A)). By comparing Figures 4-8(b (A and D)), it is possible to see that the level of intracellular singlet oxygen is slightly enhanced in UMR-106 cells activated with low doses of microwaves (20 W for 5 min).

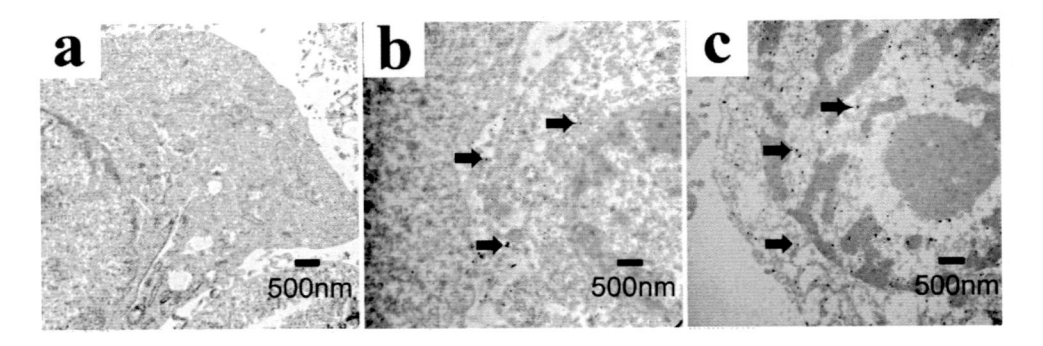

Figure 4-7. TEM images of different concentrations of Cu-Cy nanoparticles in UMR-106 cells (a: control, b: 25µg/ml Cu-Cy, c: 100µg/ml Cu-Cy). Adopted from ref. 1 with permission

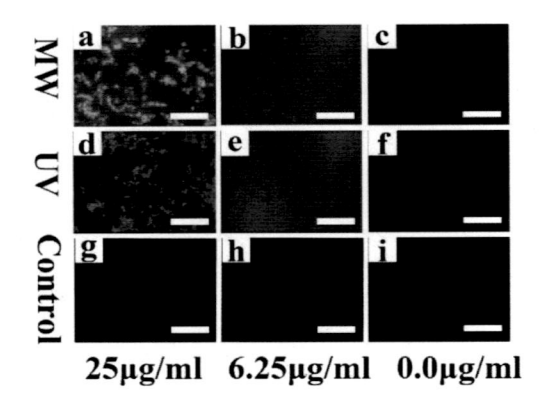

Figure 4-8a. Fluorescence images of singlet Oxygen in UMR-106 cells. The microwave irradiation is at 20 W for 5 min and the ultraviolet (UV) irradition is conducted by a UV lamp for 5 min. Adopted from ref. 1 with permission

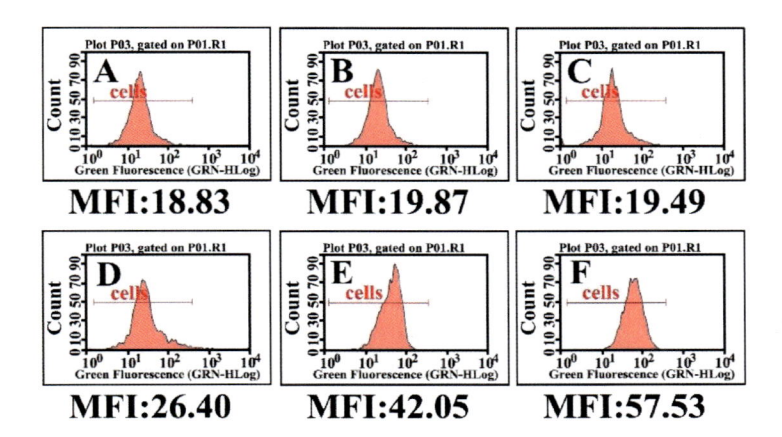

A MFI:18.83	B MFI:19.87	C MFI:19.49
D MFI:26.40	E MFI:42.05	F MFI:57.53

Figure 4-8b. **The quantitative detection of intracellular singlet oxygen.** The quantitative detection was conducted by means of oxidation-sensitive fluorescent probe (DCFH-DA) using flow cytometry. The mean fluorescence intensity (MFI) reflects the intracellular singlet oxygen concentration and oxidative stress in the UMR-106 cells. The MFI is shown for: (A) 0.0 µg/mL Cu-Cy; (B) 6.25 µg/mL Cu-Cy; (C) 25.0 µg/mL Cu-Cy; (D) 0.0 µg/mL Cu-Cy + MW at 20 W for 5 min; (E) 6.25 µg/mL Cu-Cy + MW at 20 W for 5 min; and (F) 25.0 µg/mL Cu-Cy + MW at 20 W for 5 min. Adopted from ref. 1 with permission

Apoptosis and necrosis are two distinct cell death mechanisms that may be evaluated using flow cytometry. As illustrated in Figure 4-9, no discernible difference in the number of cells undergoing apoptosis or necrosis is found ($p_{apoptosis} < 0.01$, $P_{necrosis} < 0.05$ for 6.25 µg/ml) or ($P_{apoptosis} < 0.01$, $P_{necrosis} < 0.01$ for 0 µg/ml). However, after 24 hours of treatment with 25 µg/ml Cu-Cy nanoparticles, the overall number of cells undergoing apoptosis or necrosis rose, with no discernible difference between apoptosis and necrosis. When Cu-Cy nanoparticles with and without MW were used, apoptosis rose from 4% (without MW) to 8% (with MW) (Fig. 9 bottom). There is essentially little difference between the treatments at 0, 6.25, and 25 g/ml. For necrosis, the MW therapy significantly increases cell death. Necrosis cell death is over 50% for Cu-Cy triggered with MW at 25 µg/ml, and for each concentration, MW-induced necrosis cell death is much greater than apoptotic cell death. All of these results indicate that the combination of Cu-Cy nanoparticle photosensitizers with MW is a successful approach for cancer treatment that falls under the category of MIPDT.

Biocompatibility and Pharmacokinetics

Cu-Cy nanoparticles are a novel class of photosensitizers that can be triggered using UV-visible light, X-rays, or microwaves, as explained in this article for PDT. Their biocompatibility, toxicity, and pharmacokinetics have all been well investigated. The hemocompatibility of the nanomaterials is determined using the hemolysis ratio, and the results indicate that they are extremely blood compatible.

Biodistribution

As illustrated in Figure 4-10, the biodistribution of Cu-Cy nanoparticles in the major organs (heart, liver, spleen, lung, kidney, brain, and intestines was determined, and it was discovered that the nanoparticles were primarily distributed in the lung and liver, which is consistent with the H&E results. After 72 hours, both the high dosage and low dose groups returned to normal levels completely.

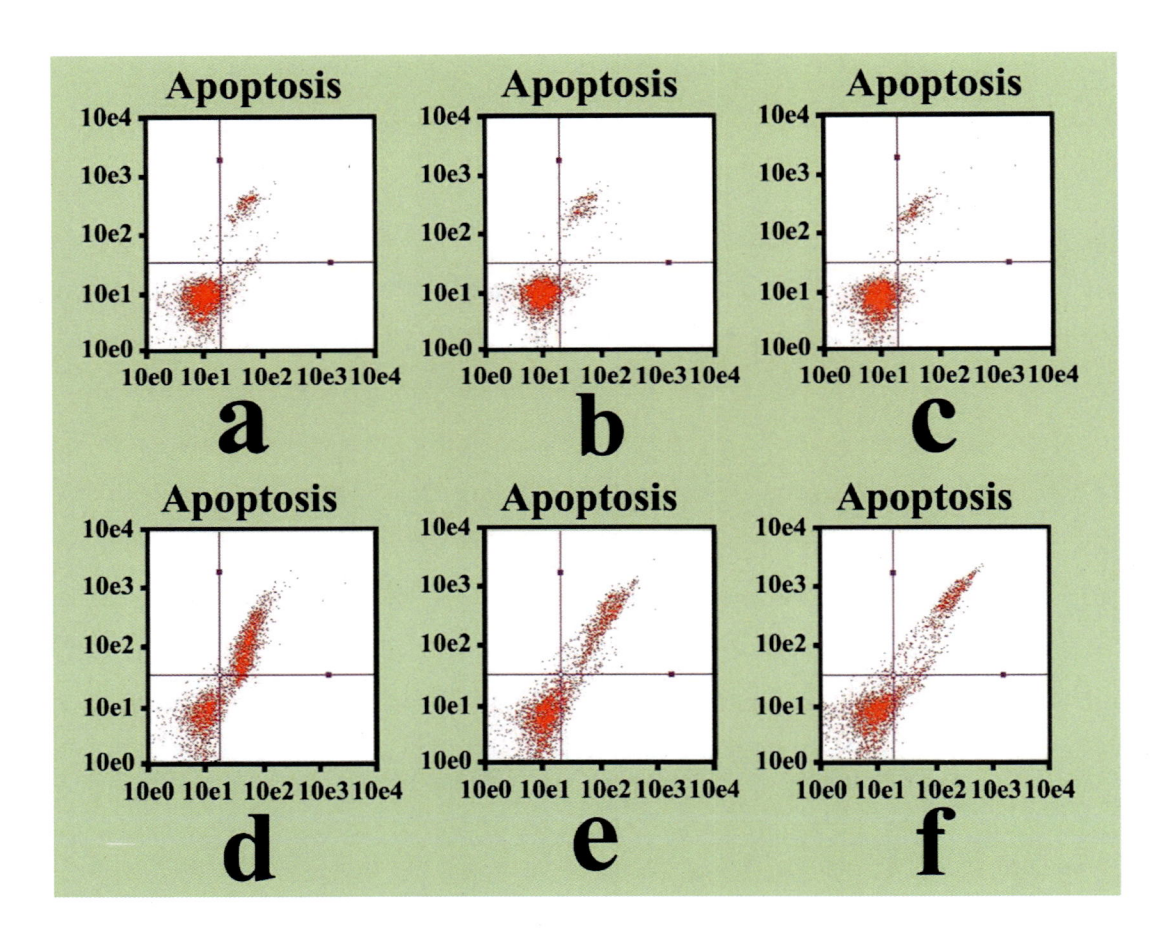

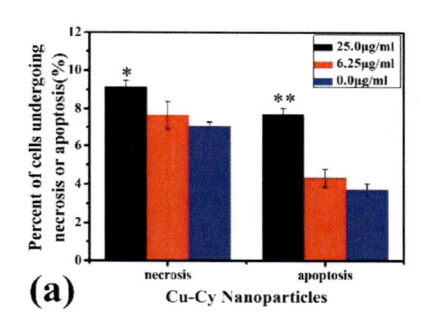

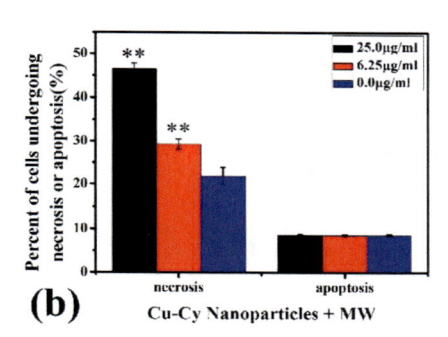

Figure 4-9. **Top:** Apoptosis and necrosis of UMR-106 cells analyzed by Flow Cytometry. a, 25.0μg/ml Cu-Cy; b, 6.25μg/ml Cu-Cy; c: 0.0μg/ml Cu-Cy; d, 25.0μg/ml Cu-Cy + MW; e, 6.25μg/ml Cu-Cy + MW; f, 0.0μg/ml Cu-Cy + MW. **Bottom:** Percentage of cells undergoing apoptosis and necrosis. Adopted from ref. 1 with permission

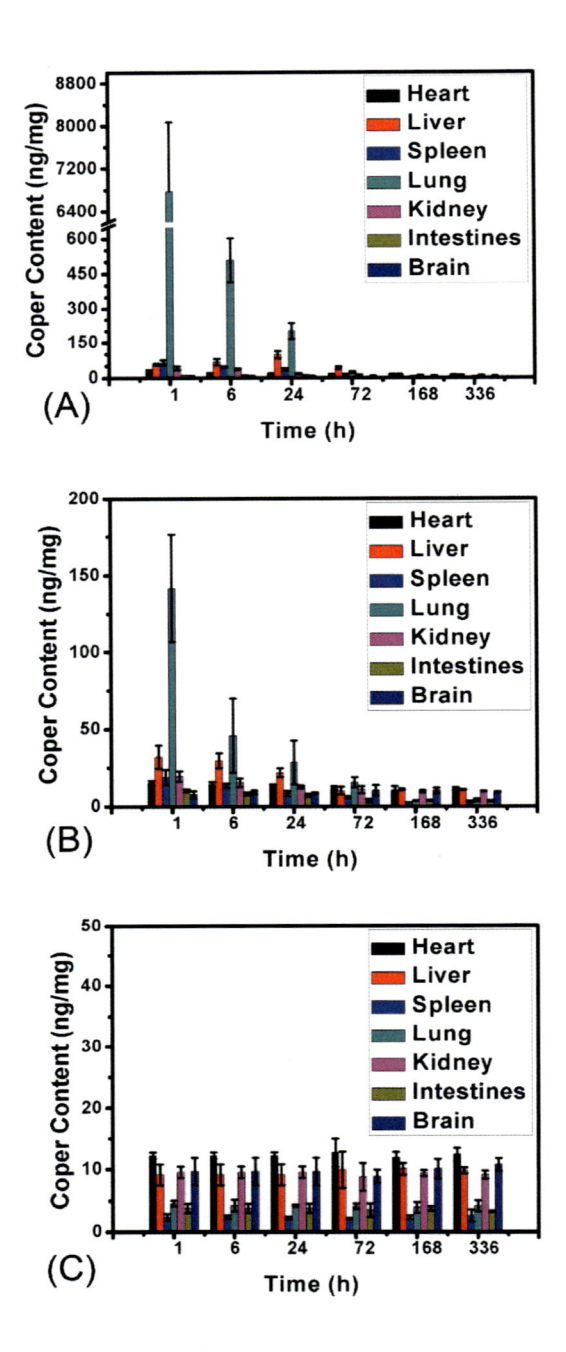

Figure 4-10. Biodistribution of Cu-Cy particles in Balb/c mice. Adopted from ref. 1 with permission

Clearance of Particles

120 female Balb/c mice (20—25 g, 5 weeks) were randomly assigned to one of three groups: high dose (100 mg/kg), which was 20 times the cure dose; low dose (5 mg/kg, the treat dose); or control

group. At various time points, the mice (n = 3) were euthanized (1 h, 6 h, 24 h, 72 h, 168 h, 336 h). Blood, urine, feces, and tissue samples from the major organs (brain, heart, liver, spleen, lung, and kidney) were collected and dissolved in 2 ml HNO$_3$ and HCl (v/v = 1:3), followed by 5 minutes at 70 C to create clear solutions. After centrifuging the solutions at 3000 rpm for 10 minutes, the supernatants were retained for subsequent inductively coupled plasma mass spectrometry (ICP-MS) analysis. Dehydration of main organs (heart, liver, spleen, lung, kidney, and brain intestines) was performed using buffered formalin, various doses of ethanol, and xylene. Following that, they were imbedded in liquid paraffin. Organs were cut (3–5 mm) and stained with hematoxylin and eosin (H&E) before being examined under a microscope (Olympus, BX51). Figures 4-11 and 4-12 illustrate the results. The observations indicate that copper's metabolic activity was highest during the first three days via blood and urine. This indicates that the optimal metabolic approach may be to deliver copper nanoparticles into the bloodstream via the liver or kidney. Copper was found to be eliminated from the body through the urine.

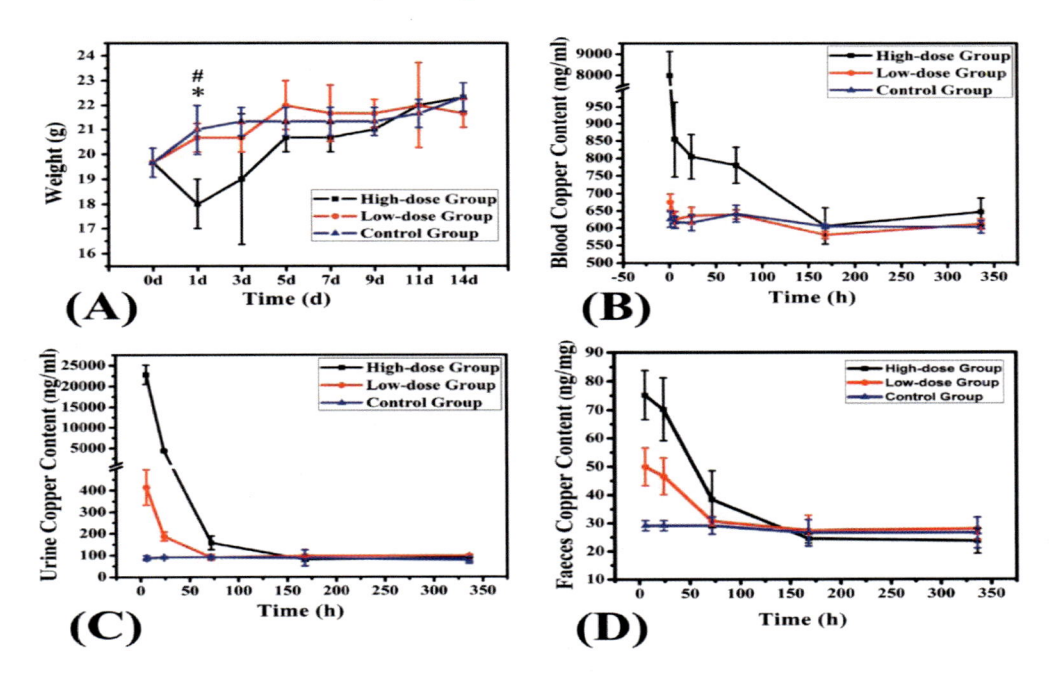

Figure 4-11. **The change of weight and copper concentration in blood, urine, and feces in 14 days**. (A) Body weight curve of Balb/c mice in different groups with time. (B) Blood copper content; (C) Urine copper content and (D) Feces copper content in different groups with time. Adopted from ref. 1 with permission

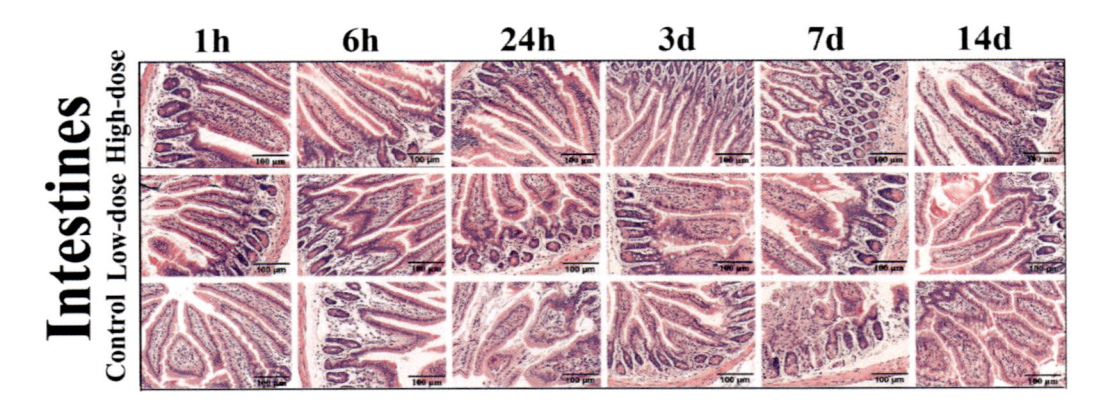

Figure 4-12. The H&E stained images of Lung, Liver and Intestines in different groups for different times. Adopted from ref. 1 with permission

Toxicity in Vivo

We assessed weight changes as well as changes in the copper concentration of blood, urine, and faeces. Weight is a critical component in determining acute and prospective toxicity. Weight variations were recorded throughout a 14-day period, as illustrated in Figure 4-11. (A). The mice treated with a high dose lost weight within the first three days (P < 0.01). The high dose group mice gradually regained their weight over time, eventually returning to normal in 14 days. Thus, we investigated the cause of this alteration and discovered that the mice in the high dosage groups were in a lower activity and diet condition during the first two days following drug administration, which may have been caused by the single big dose of Cu-Cy nanoparticles. Additionally, no difference was observed between the low-dose and control groups, indicating that there was no clear toxicity associated with the treatment levels.

Copper levels in blood, urine, and feces are markers to examine while examining the metabolic pathway of Cu-Cy nanoparticles. We examined the changes in copper concentrations in blood, urine, and feces for various groups and time periods (Figs. 4-11(B—D)). Copper levels in blood and urine fluctuate, as illustrated in Figures 4-11(B and C). At first, the high dose group exhibits very comparable symptoms to the low dose group, following a rapid spike in copper levels following the injection. The copper level in the blood then reduced significantly after 6 hours and reached 800 μg/ml at 24 hours, which was comparable to the low dose and normal groups. The copper content in urine initially reached 25,000 ng/ml, approximately three times that of blood, but subsequently fell substantially and returned to normal after 72 hours. However, the copper concentration in feces is proportionate to the quantity injected. Copper levels in feces have been reported to decrease over time. At 72 hours, both the high and low dose groups had copper levels that were consistent with normal rates.

The lung, liver, and intestines are stained with H&E in Figure 4-12. Mild pulmonary congestion was present, as were moderate ingested particles in the lung. This behaviour subsided after 24 hours, and there was no difference between the three groups after 72 hours. There was no difference between the low dose and control groups, indicating that Cu-Cy is safe at therapeutic doses.

As illustrated in Figure 4-12, there was a modest enlargement of hepatocyte cells at 1 and 6 hours. After 24 hours, the hepatocyte cells became normoxic and showed no difference between the low dosage and control groups. No swelling cells were observed in the low dosage group, and no significant differences were observed between the low dose and control groups. Additionally, none of the groups had fragmented or necrotic cells. The results indicated that high dosage treatments can cause hepatocyte cell swelling for a brief period, after which the hepatocyte cells recover.

Additionally, we examined H&E pictures of the heart, spleen, kidney, intestines, and brain and found no difference between the high dose, low dosage, and control groups. All of these tissues' cells were normal in structure and exhibited no evident toxicity.

These findings suggest that Cu-Cy is a relatively safe medication with a favourable biocompatibility and minimal toxicity. Copper's metabolic activity was greatly concentrated in the first three days via blood and urine. The most effective metabolic pathway may be to inject the copper nanoparticles straight into the bloodstream, where they will pass via the liver and kidneys before being eliminated in the urine.

Analysis

Cu-Cy is a good photosensitizer that may be activated with light or X-rays to treat cancer. Cu-Cy nanoparticles have two appropriately long decay times—one of 7.399 microseconds and another of 0.363 milliseconds. These extended decays are comparable to the luminescence decay lifetimes of photosensitizer triplet states. This suggests that Cu-Cy nanoparticles possess long-lived triplet states, which are necessary for energy transfer to ground state triplet oxygen in order to generate singlet oxygen. However, the MW energy is insufficient to excite Cu-Cy nanoparticles for the formation of singlet oxygen. There must be another mechanism for the microwave-induced ROS generation involving Cu-Cy.

Indeed, ROS production by microwaves is a common occurrence that has been raised as a concern for the effect of cell phones on human health. According to Huang et al., 900 MHz mobile phone radiation can trigger the generation of reactive oxygen species (ROS) and apoptosis in human peripheral blood mononuclear cells. Shahin et al. investigated the effect of oxidative stress on implantation and pregnancy in mice induced by 2.45 GHz microwave irradiation. They concluded that a low level of MW irradiation-induced oxidative stress not only inhibits implantation, but may also result in embryo deformity if pregnancy continues. All of these studies established that microwaves can generate reactive oxygen species.

Microwave Heating and the Production of Reactive Oxygen Species

Heating is the primary impact of microwaves' interaction with cells, tissues, and nanomaterials. Microwave energy absorption accelerates the travel of charged particles and the rotation of water molecules, hence increasing the temperature. To determine the effect of the Cu-Cy nanoparticles on microwave heating, we compared the microwave-induced heating temperature in the Cu-Cy particle solutions to the temperatures in DI water, as shown in Figure 4-13. After microwave irradiation, we discovered that the temperatures in Cu-Cy aqueous solutions were nearly identical to those in DI water. As illustrated in Figure 4-3, heating has a significant effect and can destroy tumour cells. However, the primary effect identified here is the destruction of cancer cells. This may also be seen in the change in the shape of the cell prior to and during microwave-induced photodynamic therapy. If heating kills the cells, the cells will have a more rounded form, probably due to the condensation of skeletal proteins. As illustrated in Figure 4-2, the shape of the cells is nearly same before and after treatment. This suggests that with the current treatment, hyperthermia caused by heating is not a significant factor in cell death. However, heating may aid in the generation of ROS. It has been reported that heat can result in the creation of reactive oxygen species (ROS) and 8-oxoguanine. Temperature elevation to 37—50°C was found to result in increased ROS production. The formation of reactive oxygen species (ROS) was increased following a temperature increase to 37°C. These findings demonstrate that heat can activate dissolved oxygen, resulting in the production of reactive oxygen species (ROS) (singlet oxygen, superoxide radicals, hydrogen peroxide, and hydroxyl radicals). The production of hydrogen peroxide (H_2O_2) is initiated by thermal activation of dissolved oxygen to the singlet state.

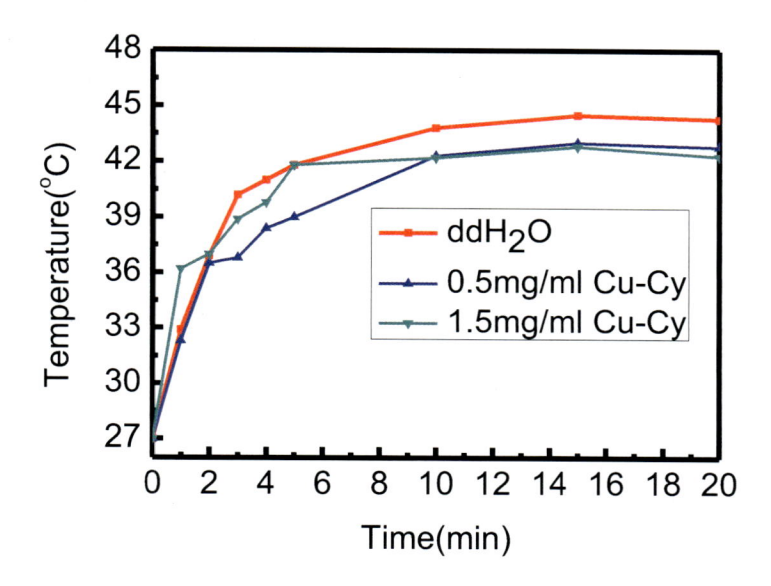

Figure 4-13. **Microwave induced heating in water and Cu-Cy aqueous solutions.** Adopted from ref. 1 with permission

It has been demonstrated that mitochondria are a significant generator of reactive oxygen species (ROS) in response to hyperthermia. Superoxide is the primary ROS produced by mitochondria as a result of unpaired electrons lost from the electron transport chain reacting with oxygen molecules. By superoxide dismutase, superoxide produced as the principal ROS is reduced to H_2O_2 (SOD). This process is particularly sensitive to the potential of the mitochondrial membrane. Heat exposure has been shown to increase mitochondrial potential, and elevated temperatures in plants resulted in increased ROS production. Heat-induced reactive oxygen species (ROS) can damage and/or inhibit proteins in a variety of ways, one of which is through the direct oxidation of amino acids by ROS. We use the reactive oxygen species (ROS) generated by Cu-Cy microwave heating to cure cancer in this study.

Effects of Copper

Cu-Cy may emit copper ions as the pH of the surrounding environment decreases. This is a significant contributor to ROS creation, as copper ions can significantly increase ROS production in biological systems. Three observations demonstrate the decomposition of Cu-Cy and the subsequent release of Cu ions in the tumor's acidic environment. To begin, the original Cu-Cy particles are 250 nm in diameter, but following uptake by cancer cells, their size is decreased to 15-20 nm, as illustrated in Figure 4-14 by transmission electron microscopy (TEM) photos. This results in the dissolution of Cu-Cy particles in acidic solutions, resulting in their reduction in size. Second, when the original Cu-Cy particles were treated with HCl acid aqueous solution, as illustrated in Figure 4-15, the luminescence of Cu-Cy was quenched. Third, in acidic solutions, Cu^+ in Cu-Cy is oxidized to Cu^{2+}, as demonstrated by electron spin resonance (ESR) and depicted in Figure 4-16. All of these studies demonstrate that the release of copper ions from Cu-Cy particles in acidic environments can expedite the generation of reactive oxygen species (ROS). It is generally established that the pH of tumours is lower than that of normal tissue. Tumors typically have a pH of 3 to 5, however some have a pH as low as 0. As a result, when Cu-Cy is administered to tumours, a portion of the Cu-Cy nanoparticles degrades and copper ions are liberated. Copper ions can be either monovalent (Cu^+) or divalent (Cu^{2+}, indicating that copper is a redox active transition metal capable of accelerating ROS formation in biological systems, as has been extensively researched. For instance, amounts of soluble copper have been shown to catalyze the transition of a superoxide radical anion ($^{\cdot}O_2^-$) to the highly reactive hydroxyl radical (OH) via the metal-catalyzed Haber-Weiss reaction. Cu^{2+} is quickly transformed to the potent and reactive Cu^+ ion in reducing cell-free circumstances, where it is capable of producing tissue-damaging reactive oxygen species (ROS), such as H_2O_2.

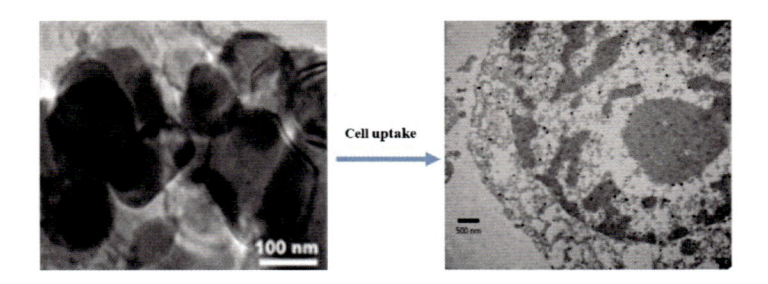

Figure 4-14. **TEM images of Cu-Cy particles** for the original particles (left) and particles after uptake by osteosarcoma cells (right). Adopted from ref. 1 with permission

Cu must cycle between the Cu+ and Cu^{2+} redox states in order to accelerate the generation of ROS. Mitochondria are constantly metabolizing oxygen, resulting in the production of reactive oxygen species (ROS). Typically, a single electron is transferred to oxygen to generate superoxide (O$_2^-$), which then dismutase (either spontaneously or by superoxide dismutase) to form H2O2. Although superoxide is insoluble in membranes and has a limited half-life and a local effect, superoxide dismutase transforms superoxide to the longer-lasting and membrane-diffusible H2O2. Peroxidases catalyze hydrogen peroxide reactions, culminating in the formation of hypochlorous acid (HOCl) and singlet oxygen (^{1}O$_2$). Finally, the Haber-Weiss reaction generates hydroxyl radicals from superoxide and hydrogen peroxide via an iron or copper ion catalyst. Copper ions generated from Cu-Cy in the acidic environment of the tumour upon MW activation may enhance ROS generation via the Fenton and Haber-Weiss reactions, as follows:

Cu+ + H$_2$O → CU^{2+} + OH. + -OH (Fenton Reaction) (1)

O2- + H$_2$O$_2$ → O$_2$ + ·OH +⁻OH (Haberweiss Reaction) (2)

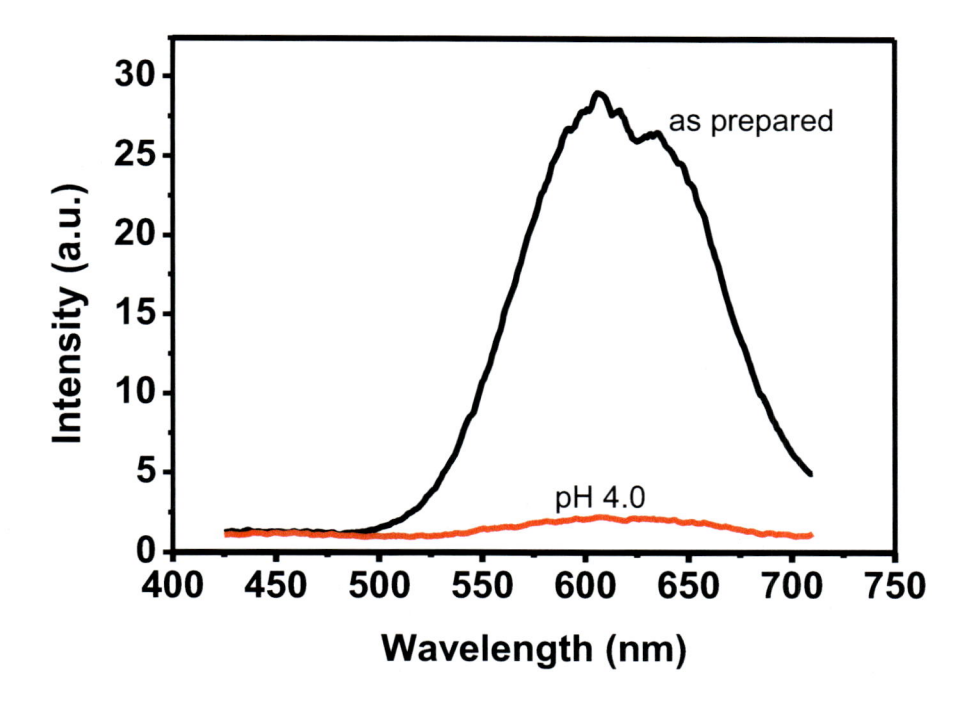

Figure 4-15. **The luminescence spectra of Cu-Cy particles** for the original particles as prepared and after acid (HCl, volume 10 % in DI water, pH = 4) treatment at for 5 hours. The excitation is at 360 nm. Adopted from ref. 1 with permission

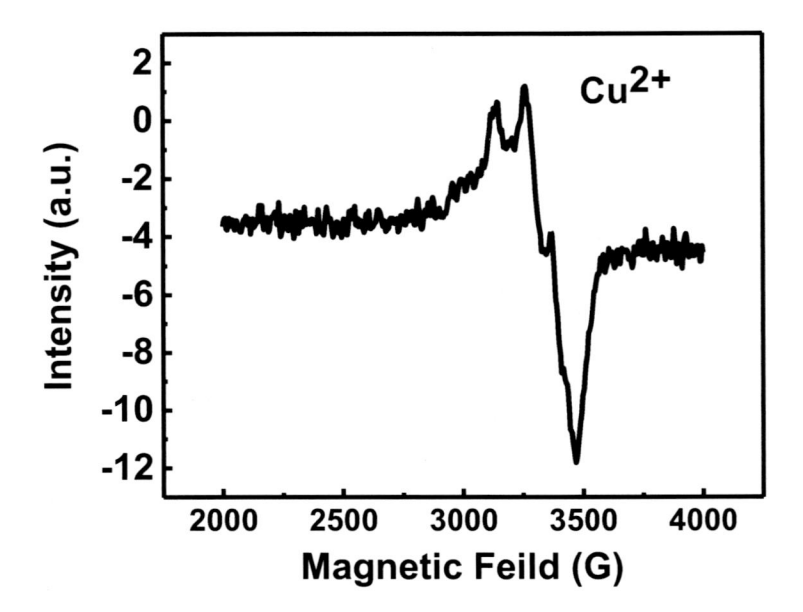

Figure 4-16. The ESR spectrum of Cu-Cy in acidic solution at pH of 4.0 indicating the conversion of Cu^+ to Cu^{2+}. Adopted from ref. 1 with permission

Because the copper in Cu-Cy is recognized as Cu^+ during decomposition, the copper ions liberated are Cu^+ ions. This lends substantial support to the copper-based Fenton reaction discussed previously. Additionally, in an acidic environment, such as that found in cancer cells or tumours, Cu^+ may convert oxygen to hydrogen peroxide by the following mechanism:

$$Cu^+ + O_2 + 2H^+ \rightarrow Cu^{2+} + H_2O_2 \qquad (3)$$

H_2O_2 is a significant ROS because it reacts with a wide variety of biological species and acts as a precursor to or product of events involving other ROS. On the other hand, free redox metal ions such as Cu^{2+} can produce hydroxyl radicals (OH) via the Haber-Weiss and Fenton reactions with H_2O_2:

$$H_2O_2 + Cu^{2+} \rightarrow Cu^{+\cdot}O_2H^{\cdot} + H^+ \qquad (4)$$
$$Cu^{+\cdot}O_2H^{\cdot} + H_2O_2 \rightarrow Cu^+ + O^2 + OH^{\cdot} + H_2O \qquad (5)$$
$$Cu^+ + H^+ + H_2O_2 \rightarrow Cu^{2+} + OH^{\cdot} + H_2O \qquad (6)$$

Additionally, singlet oxygen can be generated by disproportioning hydrogen peroxide into water and singlet oxygen ($2H_2O_2 \rightarrow 2H_2O + {}^1O_2$) using metal catalysts such as copper. These findings support the concept that ROS are created in tumour cells when Cu-Cy is microwave activated. The generation of singlet oxygen, superoxide, hydrogen peroxide, and hydroxyl radicals as a result of microwave heating and the copper free ions released from Cu-Cy in an acidic environment upon MW activation may provide the groundwork for microwave-induced PDT using Cu-Cy.

The Bottom Line

ROS can be created naturally within a biological system as a consequence of oxygen metabolism. Cells overcome ROS levels in typical physiological conditions by balancing ROS creation with ROS removal via a scavenging system. On the other hand, when cells are subjected to oxidative stress, excessive ROS disrupt the actin cytoskeleton's dynamics and can damage cellular proteins and DNA, finally resulting in cell death. Tumor cells generate far more reactive oxygen species (ROS) than normal cells. As a result, cancer cells are more susceptible to oxidative stress caused by anticancer drugs. Over the last few decades, medical researchers have made significant progress in developing a variety of antitumor physical and chemical agents, including ionizing radiation, novel chemical molecules, and other systems that exhibit anticancer activity via a ROS-dependent activated apoptotic cell death pathway, implying the possibility of using ROS as an antitumor strategy to treat human cancers. Nevertheless, numerous disadvantages remain linked with these medicines as a result of resistance and systematic toxicity toward normal cells. The specific ROS types implicated in cell death remain unknown. Numerous techniques based on oxidative stress have been developed, including the injection of reactive oxygen species (ROS) such as hydrogen peroxide (H_2O_2, hydroxyl radicals (HO), or other ROS-generating compounds to cancer cells. Nonetheless, no successful outcomes were obtained, possibly because the ROS components generated by tumour cells lacked selectivity and specificity, leading in the production of adverse effects. As schematically indicated in Figure 4-17, we believe that directing Cu-Cy nanoparticles to tumour cells and microwave activation for copper ion release within the tumour cells is a viable solution to the above-mentioned problematic issues. Controlling the processes that generate ROS within tumour cells and using microwave to release the copper and generate heat to enhance ROS development constitutes a novel technique for cancer treatment that we refer to as microwave-induced photodynamic therapy (MIPDT) (Fig. 4-17).

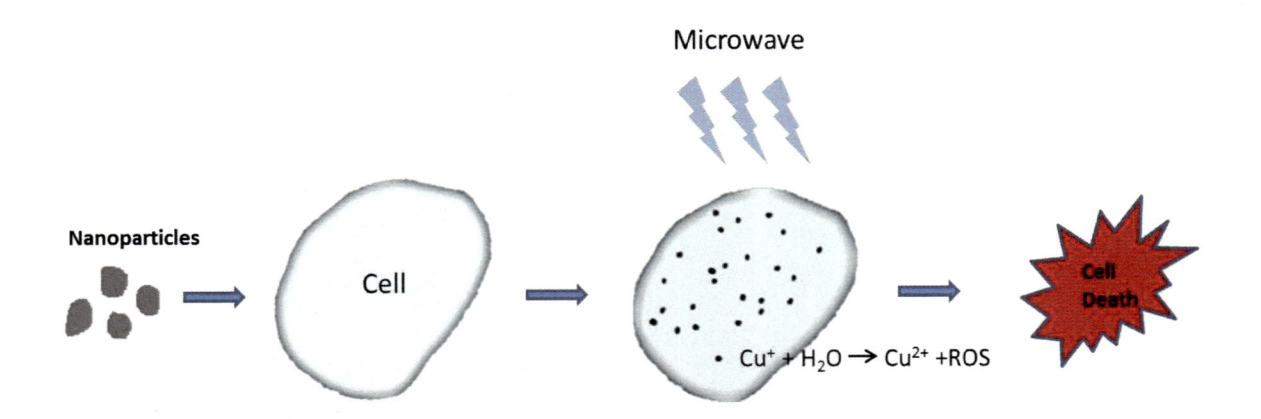

Figure 4-17. **A schematic illustration for microwave induced photodynamic therapy for cancer treatment**. Adopted from ref. 1 with permission

MIPDT is a cutting-edge form of cancer treatment. To begin, the Cu-Cy is a novel sort of photosensitizer that can be triggered not only by light and X-rays but also by microwaves to generate singlet oxygen. Additionally, Cu-Cy nanoparticles exhibit strong fluorescence, allowing for their usage as a diagnostic imaging agent. Additionally, they can be synthesized on the nanoscale, labelled with functional groups for targeted administration, and modified to improve water solubility, circulation time, and cellular uptake. Cu-Cy nanoparticles are extremely cytotoxic. Additionally, they are simple to create and inexpensive. MIPDT using Cu-Cy particles can be utilized to treat cancers that are deep in the body, beyond the limitations of conventional PDT, which is limited to superficial tumours. This also enables the simultaneous use of PDT and MWA in the treatment of osteosarcoma. Due to the fact that hyperthermia or heating can increase the efficacy of PDT, combining MWA and PDT allows for a lower microwave dosage while minimizing side effects. The heating effects and the release of copper ions from Cu-Cy are the primary mechanisms by which ROS are generated for cancer killing when MW is stimulated. MIPDT, in general, will pave the way for the treatment of cancer and other disorders.

4.2 For highly effective microwave dynamic treatment with aggregation-induced emission luminogens

Photodynamic therapy (PDT), a promising cancer treatment modality with low invasiveness, low drug resistance, and few side effects, utilizes a photosensitizer (PS) that is excited by light of a suitable wavelength to form reactive oxygen species (ROS) that can induce apoptosis and/or necrosis in treated cells. Additionally, PDT may be utilized alone or in conjunction with other therapeutic modalities, including surgery, chemotherapy, radiation, or immunotherapy. While PDT has enormous clinical promise, traditional PSs often exhibit fluorescence quenching and a large reduction in ROS generation in aqueous conditions. Fortunately, aggregation-induced emission luminogens (AIEgens) may provide a way around this constraint. AIEgens are a class of compounds that are slightly emissive when molecularly dissolved but emit strong fluorescence when aggregated due to intramolecular motion restriction. Interestingly, numerous AIEgens exhibit efficient photosensitizing capacity and distinctive light-up properties when aggregated, which is advantageous for developing image-guided PDT for cancer treatment. However, the low penetration depth of light continues to limit the practical applicability of AIE PSs as a primary or supplementary therapy. Additionally, because PDT is oxygen-dependent, both types of PSs (conventional and AIE) are less effective at treating hypoxic tumours, thus restricting their clinical utility.

Thermal ablation has been intensively studied in the therapeutic context as an alternate mode of tumour destruction. It is one of the most successful therapies in combination oncotherapy because it increases tumour sensitivity to PDT, chemotherapy, immunotherapy, or radiation by increasing blood flow to the tumour. When tissues are heated, the blood arteries widen, increasing the flow of blood. Due to the fact that haemoglobin carries oxygen, tissue heating increases the amount of oxygen in the blood, hence increasing the efficacy of the therapies. MW technology has several advantages over other thermal therapies, including mobility, shorter ablation time, deeper tissue penetration, greater tumour ablation volumes, less procedure discomfort, consistently higher intertumoral temperature, and negligible adverse effects. Notably, MWs are capable of spreading easily across a wide variety of tissues and nonmetallic materials, including burned or desiccated tissues formed during the ablation process. Despite these advantages, the inability of MWs to selectively target tumours may result in substantial harm to adjacent normal tissues during therapy. As a result, additional research and development of a more robust system are necessary to avoid nonspecific heating of healthy tissues.

Recently, microwave dynamic therapy (MWDT) has gained widespread interest, in which MW sensitizers can generate reactive oxygen species (ROS) in response to MW irradiation, thereby destroying tumour cells. Numerous MW-responsive agents have been reported to generate ROS in response to MW radiation, including copper-cysteamine (Cu-Cy) nanoparticles, g-C_3N_4 quantum dots, TiO_2 nanoparticles, Fe-metal organic framework nanoparticles, liquid metal super nanoparticles, Cu₂ZnSnS₄ nanocrystals, Mn-doped zirconium metal-organic framework nanocubes, and While all of these sensitizers are sensitive to MWs and hence interesting for applications involving MWs, the poisonous nature of certain of these metal ions and/or excessive sensitizer concentrations may result in serious adverse effects. Thus, the development of more efficient sensitizers capable of circumventing the aforementioned constraints is critical for optimizing the therapeutic efficacy of MWDT.

In prior work, we demonstrated that pyridinium-substituted tetraphenylethylene salt-based AIEgens (TPEPy-I and TPEPy-PF6, Figure 4-18) had a PDT effect on cancer cells and bacterial inactivation when exposed to white light. To our knowledge, however, there is no study on AIEgen-mediated ROS generation in response to MW irradiation. The reason for this could be because MW has an energy of just 10^{-3} eV, which is insufficient to rupture chemical bonds and generate ROS. Given that these two AIEgens are composed of a TPE segment (donor), a thiophene vinyl fragment (bridge), and a cationic pyridinium moiety (acceptor) with a strong charge-transfer property and effective ISC channels with a low ΔE_{S-T} (S1→T3: -0.22 eV), they can be activated via MW irradiation to generate ROS.

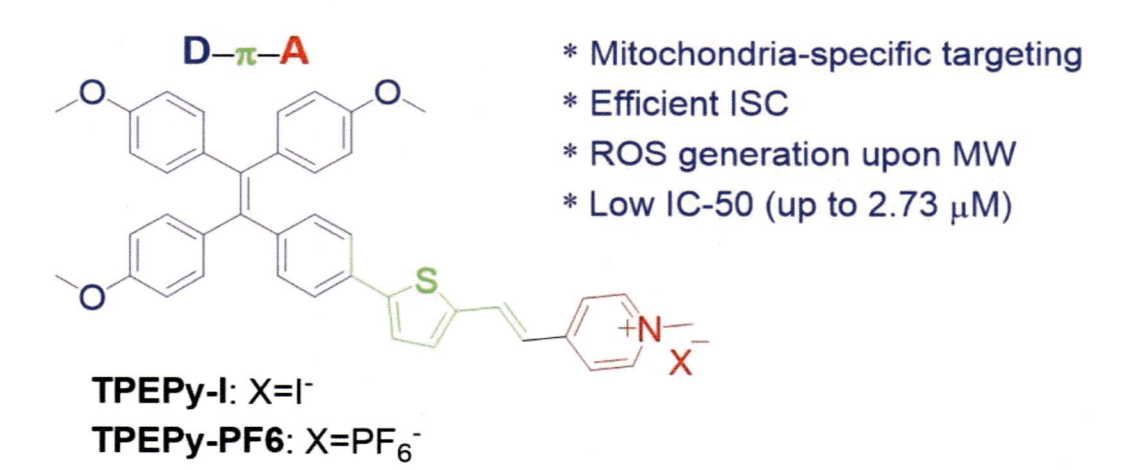

Figure 4-18. The chemical structures of two MW sensitizers (**TPEPy-I** and **TPEPy-PF6**). Adopted from ref. 2 with permission

The two AIEgens (TPEPy-I and TPEPy-PF6) are described in this contribution for the first time as MW sensitizers with efficient ROS production and cancer cell killing properties when exposed to MW irradiation. In summary, this work paves the way for the treatment of tumours with AIEgens under MW irradiation and enables the use of conventional PDT for deep cancer treatment, even in hypoxic conditions.

Components and Procedures

Components

Sigma-Aldrich, USA, provided p-nitrosodimethylaniline (RNO), imidazole, 1,4-benzoquinone (BQ), sodium azide (NaN3), 2′,7′-dichlorodihydrofluorescein diacetate (DCFH-DA), 9,10-anthracenediyl-bis(methylene)dimalonic acid (ABDA), 2,2,6,6-tetramethyl Thermo Fisher Scientific, USA, provided the 3-(4,5-dimethylthiazol-2-yl)-2,5-diphenyltetrazolium bromide (MTT). All compounds were utilized in their unpurified state.

Spectroscopy of ultraviolet–visible absorption and fluorescence

The UV–vis optical absorption and photoluminescence spectra of TPEPy-I and TPEPy-PF6 (stock solutions in DMF) were obtained using a Shimadzu UV–Vis spectrophotometer (UV-2450) and a Shimadzu spectrofluorophotometer (RF-5301PC), respectively.

SEM and fluorescence microscopy imaging

The SEM pictures were acquired with the help of a Hitachi S-4800 FE-SEM. To obtain dried samples for SEM measurements, samples were dropped on the surface of the silicon substrate and subsequently dried. To obtain fluorescence microscopy images, TPEPy-I or TPEPy-PF6 was added to an imaging plate and viewed using an OLYMPUS IX71 fluorescence microscope.

Detection of reactive oxygen species in a cell-free system using the RNO bleaching method

We used the RNO bleaching method to determine the amount of extracellular ROS produced in response to MW excitation. At various time intervals during MW exposure, the intensity of RNO absorption was determined spectrophotometrically (2450 MHz). The MW was supplied in complete darkness using a radiator probe equipped with a microwave therapy device (WB-3100AI, BXING, China). Specifically, 0.45 mg of RNO and 32.68 mg of imidazole were dissolved separately in 30 mL of DI water and then air saturated for 15 minutes through air bubbling.

Following that, a 3 mL solution of RNO and imidazole was created in a cuvette (10 mm path length) under dark conditions by combining 1 mL of RNO, 1 mL of imidazole, and 1 mL of the testing sample. Meanwhile, a control experiment was conducted using the same approach but with DI water as the testing sample to determine the influence of MW irradiation on RNO's absorption.

Utilization of an ABDA probe and electron spin resonance (ESR) spectroscopy to detect singlet oxygen ($^1O_2$) in aqueous solution

To further validate the $^1O_2$ production under MW activation, we assessed the $^1O_2$ produced by the TPEPy-I and TPEPy-PF6 nanoaggregates using the commercially available $^1O_2$ indicator ABDA. To summarize, a stock solution of ABDA (1.5 mM) in DMF was prepared. The working solution (3 mL final volume) was produced in DI water by dissolving 30 M ABDA and 15 M TPEPy-I or TPEPy-PF6 in a 10 mm path length cuvette in the dark. The solution was then subjected in the dark to MW (2450 MHz), and the absorbance of ABDA at 379 nm was evaluated using a spectrophotometer. To assess the influence of MW on the absorbance of ABDA, a control experiment was conducted using DI water alone in place of the testing sample under the identical conditions.

The ESR measurements were carried out at the University of Texas at Dallas's Nanotech Institute utilizing a Bruker EMX Xband ESR spectrometer (Bruker Biospin, Billerica, MA). Each sample was aliquoted in 0.5mm ID heparinized hematocrit capillary tubes and then transferred to 4mm thin wall quartz ESR tubes (Wilmad LabGlass, Vineland, NJ). At room temperature, field swept continuous wave ESR spectra were acquired.

Detection of extracellular ROS using the DCFH-DA probe

The ROS generated by the TPEPy-I and TPEPy-PF6 nanoaggregates in aqueous solution upon MW stimulation were further examined using the photoluminescence (PL) method in conjunction with DCFH-DA as a ROS probing agent. DCFH-DA (1.8 mM) stock solution was prepared in DMF. Following that, the working solution (final volume 3 mL) was produced in a cuvette (10 mm path length) using DCFH-DA (30 M) and TPEPy-I or TPEPy-PF6 (10 M). The solution was then subjected in the dark to MW (2450 MHz), and the PL intensity was measured at 523 nm using a spectrofluorophotometer equipped with a 505 nm excitation wavelength. Under the same conditions, a control experiment was conducted using DI water instead of TPEPy-I and TPEPy-PF6.

Intracellular ROS generation detection

We investigated the intracellular production of reactive oxygen species (ROS) utilizing DCFH-DA as a fluorescent detection probe. 1 x 10^5 HeLa cells were seeded into nine separate imaging plates and cultured for 24 hours at 37 °C in a humidified cell incubator containing 5% CO_2. Following that, the cells were cultured for 4 hours in fresh culture media with or without TPEPy-I and TPEPy-PF6 (5 μM) (3 mL). Cells were then washed twice with PBS and incubated for another 45 minutes at 37 °C in the dark with 20 M DCFH-DA in DMEM (500 L). Following that, the cells were washed three times with PBS to remove the unloaded probe. The specified cells were then subjected to 10 W (2450 MHz) of MW irradiation in the dark for 1 or 1.5 minutes after adding 3 mL of DMEM. Finally, the cells were resuspended in PBS (500 μL) and immediately viewed under the same instrumental circumstances using the OLYMPUS IX71 fluorescent microscope.

A study of microwave dynamic treatment (MWDT) utilizing the MTT assay

The cytotoxicity of TPEPy-I and TPEPy-PF6 nanoaggregates was determined using the MTT test following MW irradiation. HeLa cells were planted at a density of 2 x 10^4 cells per well in 24-well plates. After 24 hours, the old medium was removed from each well and replaced with 2.4 mL of fresh culture media (DMF-culture medium containing 99.92 percent culture medium) containing various concentrations of TPEPy-I or TPEPy-PF6 (0–10 μM). After an additional 4 hours of incubation, the cells were treated with or without 10 W of MW radiation (2450 MHz) for 1.5 minutes in the dark (by putting the MW probe into the culture medium without touching the plate surface) and then incubated for an additional 20 hours. After removing the old medium, 400 μL of fresh culture media containing 40 μL of MTT solution (5 mg/mL MTT reagent in PBS) was added to each well and cultured in the dark for an additional 4 hours. The formazan product was then dissolved in DMSO, and the formazan crystal's absorbance at 540 nm was measured using a microplate reader (Multiskan FC). Finally, the vitality of cells was measured using the equation:

$$\text{Cell viability} = \frac{\text{The absorbance of the treated group}}{\text{The absorbance of the untreated group}} \times 100\%$$

The effect of MWDT was investigated using a live/dead experiment

The viability of cells exposed to MW irradiation was further investigated using a live/dead test. HeLa cells were cultivated at a density of 1 x 10^5 cells/well and then incubated for 24 hours at 37

°C in a humidified 5% v/v CO_2 environment. Following incubation, the old medium was removed and 3 mL of fresh media (DMF-culture medium with 99.92 percent culture medium content) was added to each well, either with or without 10 M TPEPy-I and TPEPy-PF6. There were nine groups: control, TPEPy-I, TPEPy-PF6, 1.5-minute MW, 2 minute MW, TPEPy-I + 1.5 minute MW, TPEPy-I + 2 minute MW, TPEPy-PF6 + 1.5 minute MW, TPEPy-PF6 + 2 minute MW, TPEPy-PF6 + 1.5 minute MW, and TPEPy-PF6 + 2 minute MW. After 4 hours of incubation, the MW, TPEPy-I + MW, and TPEPy-PF6 + MW groups were irradiated with 1.5 or 2 minutes of MW (10 W; 2450 MHz) in the dark using the radiator probe (inserting the probe into the medium without touching the plate surface). Following that, the cells were placed in an incubator for 20 hours. On the day of the experiment, the old medium was replaced with 500 litres of fresh media containing calcein-AM and propidium iodide (PI) and incubated for an additional 45 minutes at 37 °C in the dark. Finally, the marked cells were examined using a fluorescent microscope, the OLYMPUS IX71.

Imaging in broad daylight

To investigate the morphological changes in the cells following MW treatment, bright-field pictures of HeLa cells were acquired using the OLYMPUS IX71 fluorescent microscope.

Analyses statistical

At least three times, the data were given as mean standard deviation. To establish the statistical significance of the control and experimental groups, one-way analysis of variance (ANOVA) was used followed by the Tukey test. Statistical significance was defined as a p-value of <0.05.

Outcomes and Analysis

TPEPy-I and TPEPy-PF6 synthesis and characterization

Our recent paper describes the synthesis and comprehensive characterization of the two AIEgens TPEPy-I and TPEPy-PF6 (Figure 4-18). The absorption spectra of TPEPy-I and TPEPy-PF6 nanoaggregates in a DMF-water mixture (99.75 percent water) are shown in Fig. 4-19a, with the absorption maxima located at around 440 and 450 nm, respectively. The PLE and PL spectra of TPEPy-I and TPEPy-PF6 nanoaggregates in a DMF-water mixture (99.75 percent water) are shown in Fig. 4-19b, with emission peaks at around 652 and 663 nm, respectively, when stimulated at 467 nm. Additionally, their PL spectra remained nearly identical after 4 months of storage, indicating their high stability. The mean hydrodynamic diameters of the nanoaggregates generated in the DMF-water combination (99.67 percent water) were (119 ± 32) and (152 ± 48) nm for TPEPy-I and TPEPy-PF6 nanoaggregates, respectively (Fig. 4-19c and d).

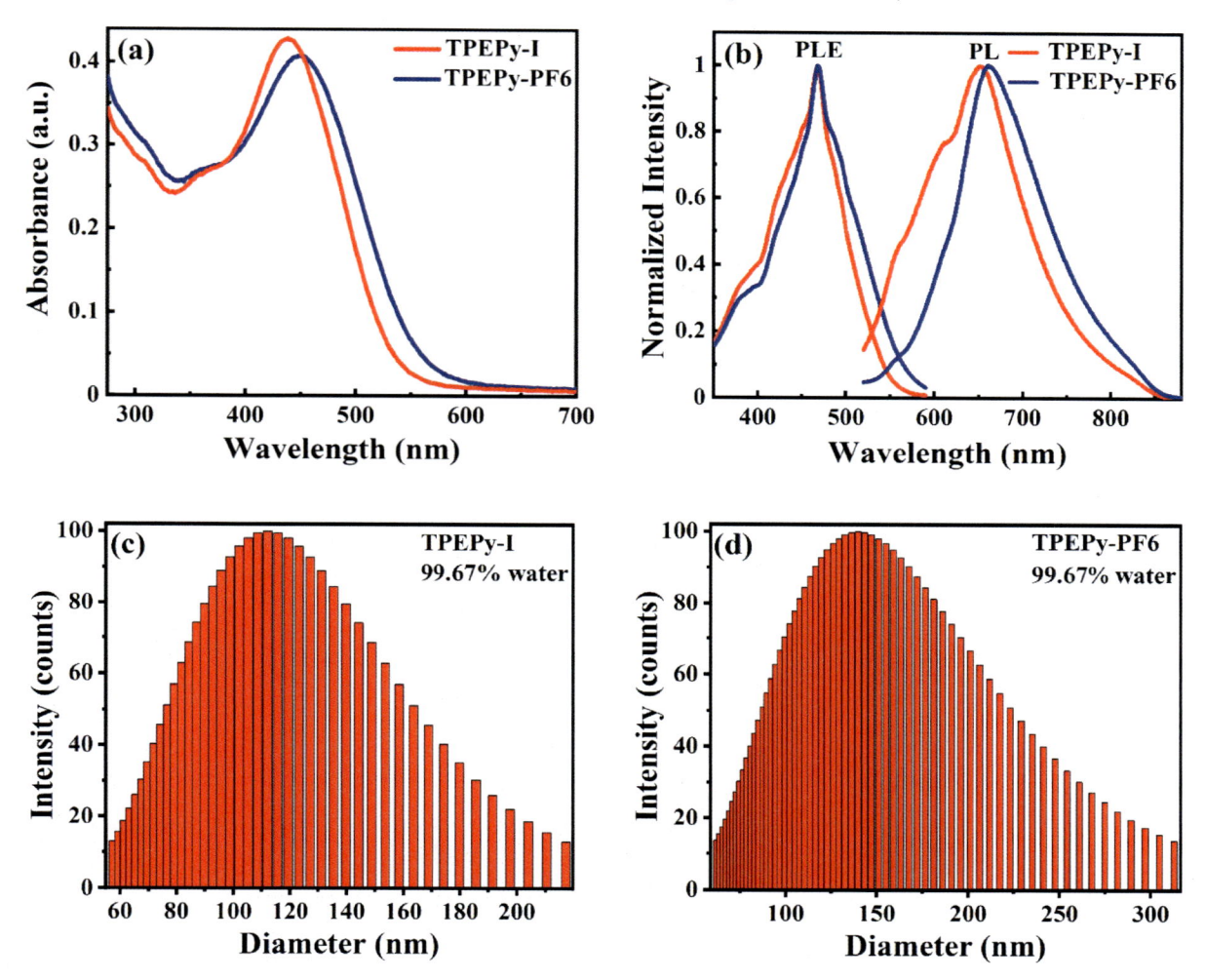

Fig. 4-19. (a) UV-vis absorption spectra of **TPEPy-I** and **TPEPy-PF6** nanoaggregates in the DMF-water mixture with 99.75% water content. (b) Normalized photoluminescence excitation (PLE) spectra at 467 nm (left) and PL emission spectra at 652 and 663 nm (right) of the **TPEPy-I** and **TPEPy-PF6** nanoaggregates, respectively, in DMF-water mixture with 99.75% water content. Emission wavelengths of **TPEPy-I** and **TPEPy-PF6** nanoaggregates were 652 and 663 nm, respectively. The excitation wavelength was 467 nm for both cases. (c and d) Particle size distribution of (c) **TPEPy-I** and (d) **TPEPy-PF6** nanoaggregates in DMF-water mixture with 99.67% water content measured by DLS. Adopted from ref. 2 with permission

SEM and fluorescence microscopy images

The morphology and self-assembly behaviours of both AIEgens were investigated using SEM. When no water was applied, both AIEgens self-assembled into nano/micro-architectures (Fig. 4-20 (a–f). Additionally, we performed SEM measurements when the water content of both AIEgens was 90% and 99.67%. As illustrated in Fig. 4-20 (g-o), molecules self-assembled into micro/nanostructures as a result of water evaporation. Due to the fact that the solvent must be evaporated prior to doing SEM observations, just a tiny change was seen between circumstances. Due to the fact that the properties of these AIEgens are largely dependent on their water content and all water content was evaporated prior to SEM observations, SEM results revealed a larger range of sizes than DLS measurements. SEM studies indicate that both AIEgens were assembled into distinct shapes, as AIEgens have a difficult time self-assembling into well-defined structures due to their nonpolar topology. In essence, the aggregation behaviour of AIEgens is a self-assembly process facilitated by the molecules' solvophobic properties.

169

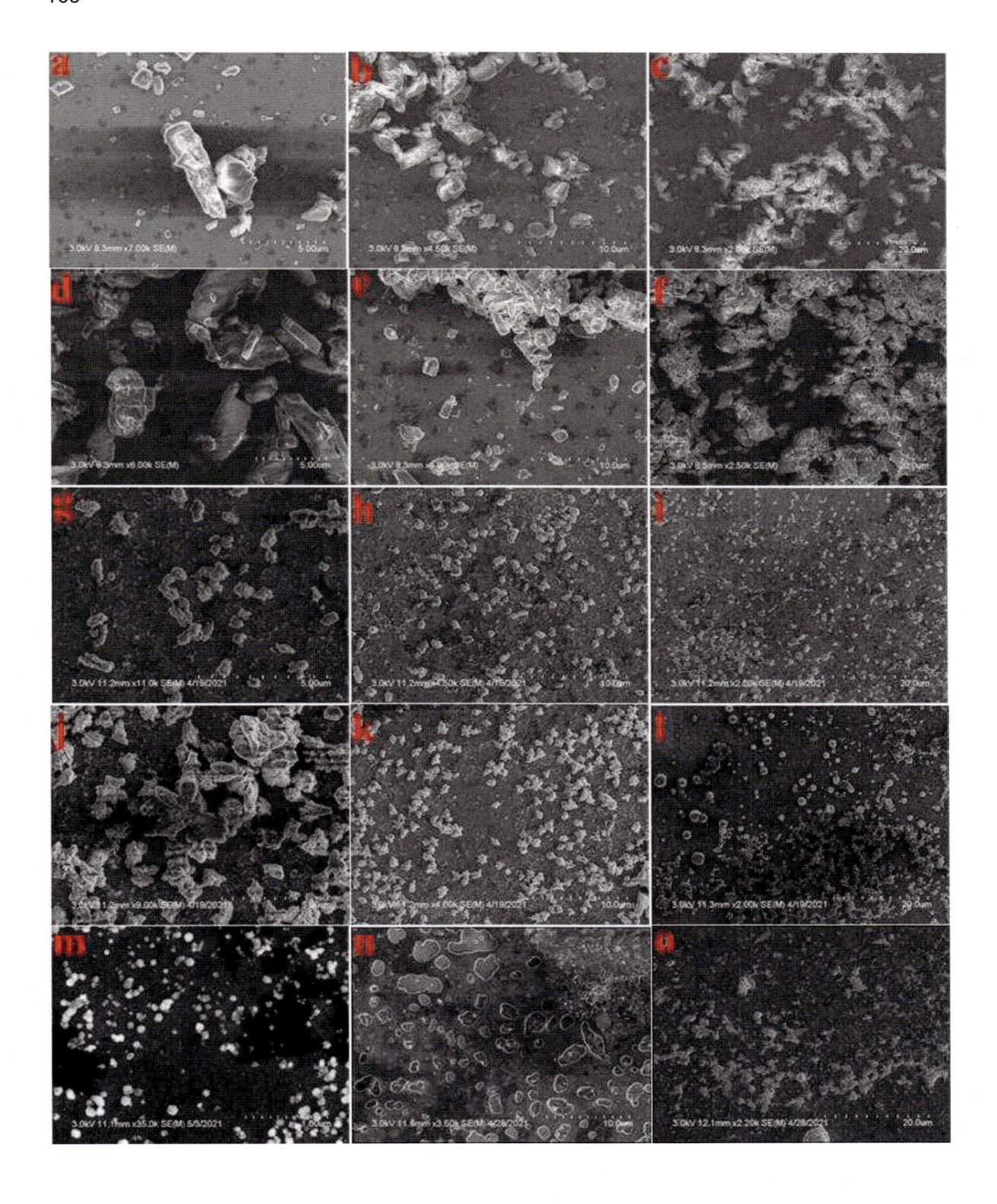

Fig. 4-20. Representative SEM images of (a-c) **TPEPy-I** with no water (powder sample), (d-f) **TPEPy-PF6** with no water (powder sample), (g-i) **TPEPy-I** with 90% water content, (j-l) **TPEPy-PF6** with 90% water content, (m-n) **TPEPy-I** with 99.67% water content, and (o) **TPEPy-PF6** with 99.67% water content. Adopted from ref. 2 with permission

It is intriguing that TPEPy-I caused a higher level of ROS, which could be attributable to the beneficial action of iodide anions as stated in our recent work. Another possibility is that the nanoaggregates of TPEPy-I are smaller in size, as smaller particles have bigger surface areas, which aids in regulating the amount of reactive sites on the particles' surface. However, the precise reason for the variation in ROS generating capability between the two samples is unknown at the moment.

As noted previously, TPEPy-I nanoaggregates produce more ROS than TPEPy-PF6, compelling us to conduct more tests on TPEPy-I nanoaggregates. The comparison of ROS generated by TPEPy-I nanoaggregates (10 µM) at 2 and 10 W of MW irradiation. As a result, a larger MW dose generates more ROS. Additionally, ROS generation is concentration-dependent. Interestingly, 5M of TPEPy-I nanoaggregates exposed to 10 W of MW generated nearly the same amount of ROS as 10M exposed to 2 W of MW. Taken together, irradiation time, MW dose, and sample concentration were identified as significant determinants of ROS production.

To determine whether the ROS detected in the RNO bleaching assay was $^1O_2$, we treated TPEPy-I nanoaggregates with sodium azide (NaN$_3$), a physical quencher of $^1O_2$. The bleaching of RNO was significantly reduced in the presence of NaN$_3$ (40 mM), indicating that $^1O_2$ was the major component of the produced ROS.

We are all aware that $^1O_2$ is typically formed as a result of energy transfer from the excited state of photosensitive substances to molecular oxygen ($^3O_2$). However, several researchers have demonstrated that 1O2 can be generated under certain conditions by the oxidation of superoxide radicals ($^•O_2^-$). To test this theory, we added 1,4-benzoquinone (BQ), a well-known quencher of $^•O_2^-$, to TPEPy-I nanoaggregates solution. Interestingly, adding BQ (340 M) to the solution of TPEPy-I nanoaggregates significantly prevented RNO bleaching, showing that $^•O_2^-$ was created concurrently in the reaction system. On the basis of this discovery, it is fair to assume that $^1O_2$ is produced during the oxidation of $^•O_2^-$, as indicated in Figure 4. According to the molecular orbital diagram (Fig. 4-21), the loss of an electron with the appropriate spin can produce either $^1O_2$ or $^3O_2$.

The odds of producing $^1O_2$ and $^3O_2$ via oxidation of $·O_2^-$ are determined to be 2/5 and 3/5, respectively. The confirmation of the synthesis of $·O_2^-$ implies the possibility of the generation of other forms of ROS, as $·O_2^-$ is the precursor to the majority of ROS and acts as a mediator in oxidative chain reactions. It is worth noting that the rise in RNO absorbance at 440 nm observed in the DI water + BQ +10 W group (black curve in Fig. 3d) is due to imidazole-BQ interaction. As shown in Fig. S5a, the absorption of RNO at 440 nm was unaffected by BQ, showing that RNO does not interact with it. However, the absorption of RNO at 440 nm increased somewhat in the presence of imidazole and BQ (Fig. S5c), indicating that imidazole interacts with BQ, as previously indicated. Additionally, Fig. S5d demonstrates that the interaction becomes more pronounced with MW irradiation.

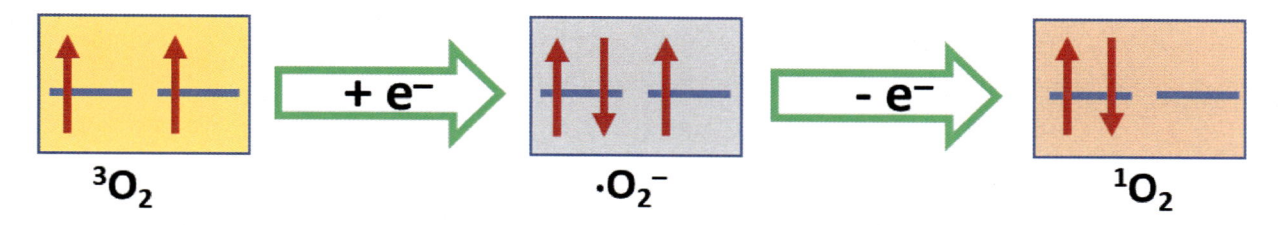

Fig. 4-21. The schematic molecular π* orbitals of molecular oxygen ($^3O_2$), superoxide radical ($·O_2^-$), and singlet oxygen ($^1O_2$). Adopted from ref. 2 with permission

Additionally, we used another scavenger of $·O_2^-$, chloroform, to demonstrate that the nanoaggregates may produce $·O_2^-$ in the presence of MW radiation. The bleaching of RNO was significantly reduced when chloroform (4.2 or 21 mM) was added to the TPEPy-I solution, showing that the nanoaggregates may generate $·O_2^-$ under MW irradiation.

Measurements of $^1O_2$ with electron spin resonance (ESR) spectroscopy

All of these observations suggest that MW can create $^1O_2$ only in the presence of compact nanoaggregates, as proven by DLS measurements (Fig. 4-22a and b). Fig. 4-22c illustrates the AIEgen-mediated MWDT schematically.

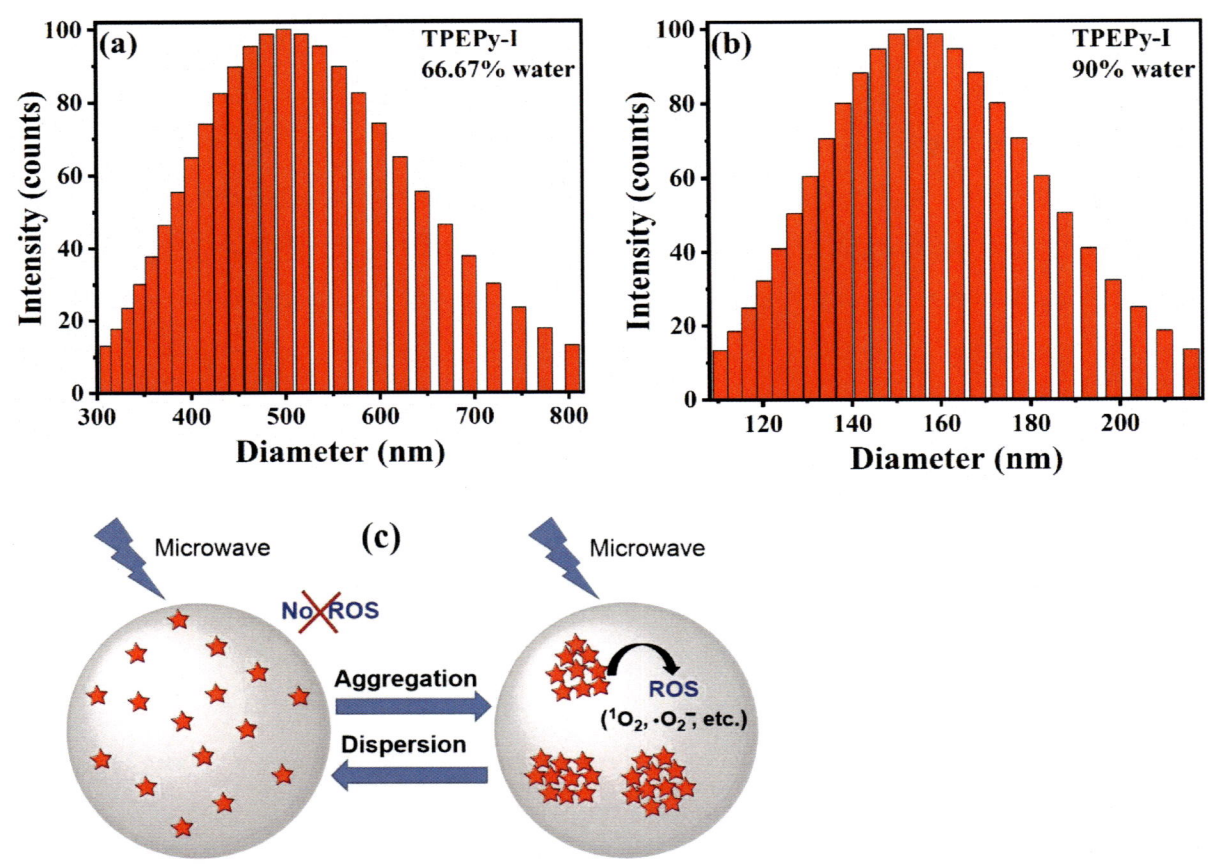

Fig. 4-22. The particle size distribution of nanoaggregates of **TPEPy-I** formed in DMF-water mixture with (a) 66.67% and (b) 90% water content measured by DLS. The average hydrodynamic diameters were found to be (517 ± 108) and (157 ± 24) nm, respectively. (c) Schematic diagram of the AIEgen-mediated microwave dynamic therapy (MWDT). Adopted from ref. 2 with permission

The ESR approach was utilized to confirm the creation of $^1O_2$ further by trapping it using 2,2,6,6-tetramethylpiperidine (TEMP), a well-known probe molecule for trapping $^1O_2$. When TEMP is oxidized with $^1O_2$, the stable free radical 2,2,6,6-tetramethyl-1-piperidinyloxy (TEMPO) is formed, which may be easily identified by ESR. As illustrated in Fig. 4-23, the distinct and characteristic 1:1:1 triplet signal (i.e., three lines of equal intensity) of the TEMPO was identified following MW irradiation of TPEPy-I nanoaggregates (10 M), hence providing direct evidence of $^1O_2$ production. However, without MW irradiation, such a distinct TEMPO characteristic signal could not be observed. Similarly, we conducted studies with TPEPy-PF6 nanoaggregates to determine whether they could yield $^1O_2$ when excited with MW (Fig. 7). Additionally, the amount of $^1O_2$ created by TPEPy-I nanoaggregates was greater than that produced by TPEPy-PF6, which was consistent with our previous findings.

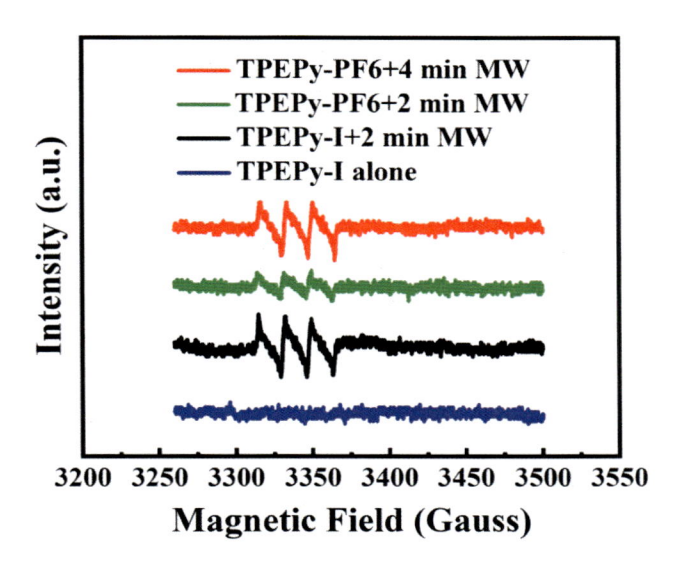

Fig. 4-23. ESR spectra of $^1O_2$ trapped by TEMP in the presence of **TPEPy-I** and **TPEPy-PF6** nanoaggregates (10 µM) under 10 W of MW irradiation. Concentration of TEMP was 20 mM. Adopted from ref. 2 with permission

Intracellular detection of reactive oxygen species

The results of our investigation into ROS production in a cell-free setup prompted us to investigate ROS detection in cells. The intracellular ROS generation was examined using DCFH-DA, an oxidation-sensitive probe. DCFH-DA is a nonpolar and cell permeant molecule that is converted to DCFH by intracellular esterase and then to the extremely fluorescent DCF upon oxidation by intracellular reactive oxygen species (ROS). The representative photos in Fig. 4-24 reveal that cells treated with MW (1 or 1.5 min, 10 W) exhibited no green fluorescence, whereas cells treated with TPEPy-I or TPEPy-PF6 nanoaggregates (5 M) exhibited faint green fluorescence. Meanwhile, the intensity of green fluorescence was significantly raised in cells treated with the TPEPy-I or TPEPy-PF6 nanoaggregates in combination with MW, demonstrating that the two nanoaggregates are capable of producing significant amounts of ROS when stimulated with MW. Additionally, by increasing the MW exposure duration from 1 to 1.5 minutes, the intensity of green fluorescence was increased. Additionally, these data demonstrate that the two AIEgens can generate ROS in the presence of MW and are hence promising sensitizers for MWDT.

Investigation of the MWDT impact using the MTT test

Using the MTT assay, we determined the MWDT effect of the two AIEgens. It is a quantitative colorimetric assay in which the yellow tetrazolium salt MTT is converted to purple formazan crystals by the metabolically active cells' mitochondrial dehydrogenase. The results shown in Figure 4-25 indicate that nanoaggregates treated with MW killed considerably more cells than their comparable controls (MW alone and nanoaggregates alone). Additionally, our data indicate that the mortality of TPEPy-I and TPEPy-PF6 nanoaggregates increased with increasing concentration, indicating a dose-dependent cytotoxic action. These findings further established that the combination of MW and TPEPy-I or TPEPy-PF6 nanoaggregates was lethal to HeLa cells. For instance, the average viability of HeLa cells was found to be 58.4 percent vs. 62.5 percent, 31.1 percent vs. 36.7 percent, and 9.3 percent vs. 14.2 percent at 2.5, 5, and 10 M of TPEPy-I and TPEPy-PF6 nanoaggregates, respectively, after 1.5 minutes of 10 W MW irradiation. While it is not entirely reasonable to compare our findings to previously published results due to methodological differences, the high MWDT effect of the two AIEgens at low concentrations indicates that the present AIEgen system is superior to the majority of MW sensitizers reported to date, which require high concentrations to achieve the desired cytotoxicity.

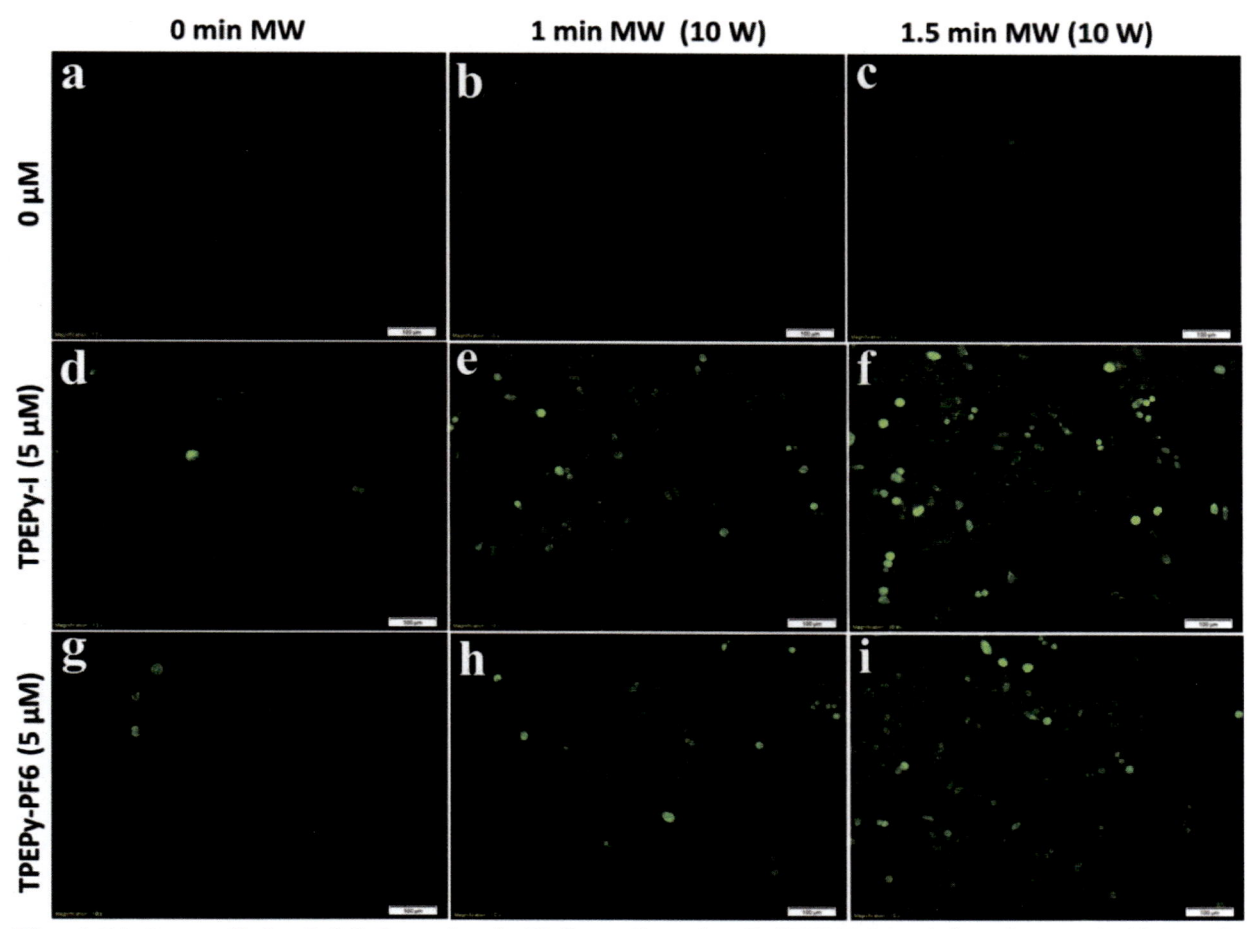

Fig. 4-24. Intracellular ROS detection in HeLa cells using DCFH-DA staining dye upon 10 W of MW irradiation. (a) Cells without any treatments. (b) Cells treated with MW for 1 min. (c) Cells treated with MW for 1.5 min. (d) Cells treated with **TPEPy-I**. (e) Cells treated with **TPEPy-I** upon MW for 1 min. (f) Cells treated with **TPEPy-I** upon MW for 1.5 min. (g) Cells treated with **TPEPy-PF6**. (h) Cells treated with **TPEPy-PF6** upon MW for 1 min, and (i) cells treated with **TPEPy-PF6** upon MW for 1.5 min. The increase in green fluorescence intensity shows ROS production. Scale bar = 100 μm; magnification = 10×. Adopted from ref. 2 with permission

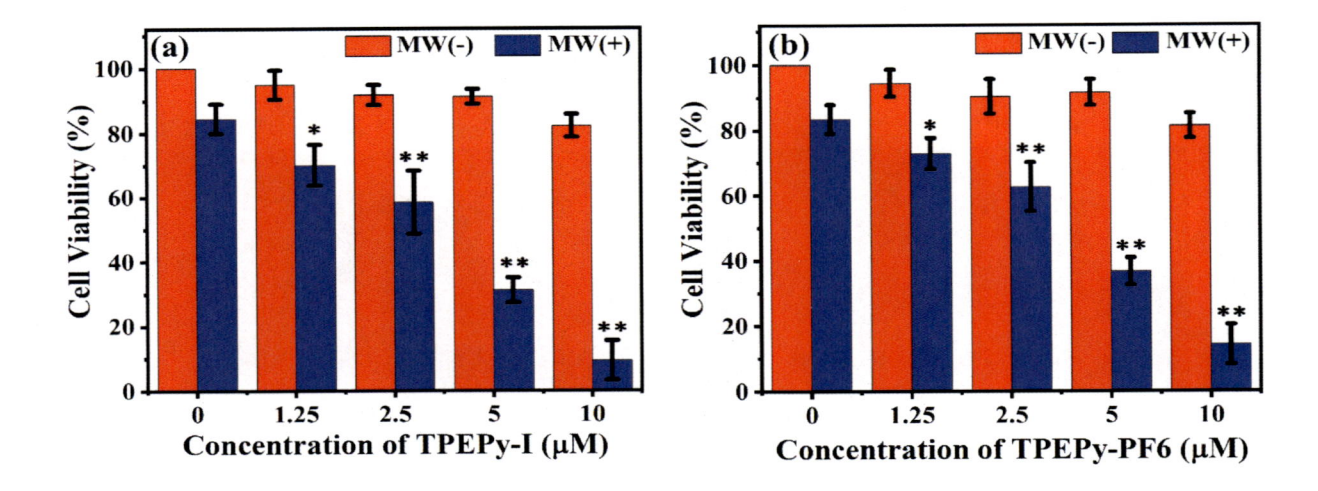

Fig. 4-25. Evaluation of MWDT effect of (a) **TPEPy-I** and (b) **TPEPy-PF6** nanoaggregates under MW irradiation (10 W) on HeLa cells for 1.5 min. Statistical analysis was performed with respect to MW alone and the corresponding concentration of the nanoaggregate alone (*$p < 0.05$ and **$p < 0.0001$). Adopted from ref. 2 with permission

The IC50 values for TPEPy-I and TPEPy-PF6 nanoaggregates were determined to be (2.73 ± 0.52) and (3.22 ± 0.55) M, respectively, upon MW (Fig. 11). This indicates that TPEPy-I nanoaggregates had a greater overall MWDT effect, which is consistent with the ROS generation and cytotoxicity investigations.

MWDT investigation using a live/dead test

The antitumor effect of TPEPy-I and TPEPy-PF6 nanoaggregates following MW exposure was also determined utilizing a live/dead cell viability assay. Calcine-AM was used to label viable HeLa cells and PI was used to stain nonviable cells. Calcein-AM is a cell-permeable dye that has been widely used to assess the viability and/or cytotoxicity of the majority of eukaryotic cells. Intracellular esterase convert the calcein-AM to a green luminous calcein in living cells. On the other hand, PI is excluded from live cells with intact plasma membranes but penetrates damaged cells, attaching to nucleic acids and identifying the presence of dead cells in a population.

The green (life) and red (dead) channels were combined for each group, and representative live/dead assay images are given in Fig. 4-26. When TPEPy-I or TPEPy-PF6 nanoaggregates were activated for 1.5 or 2 minutes with MW (10 W), their cytotoxicity was dramatically increased when compared to their respective controls (MW alone and nanoaggregates alone). Additionally, as shown in Fig. 4-26, more cells were eliminated when the MW exposure period was increased (from 1.5 to 2 minutes), indicating that TPEPy-I and TPEPy-PF6 nanoaggregates are viable options for noninvasive therapy of deep cancers and infectious disorders in MWDT. To quantify the cell viability, the number of live (green fluorescence) and dead (red fluorescence) cells was counted using ImageJ software, and the findings are shown in Fig. 4-27. The average cell viability of HeLa cells in the presence of TPEPy-I and TPEPy-PF6 nanoaggregates was found to be 23.8 percent and 29.1 percent for 1.5 minutes, and 4.7 percent and 7.5 percent for 2 minutes, respectively, when exposed to 10 W of MW (Fig. 4-27). Again, this indicates that TPEPy-I nanoaggregates outperformed TPEPy-PF6 nanoaggregates on average, which could be attributed to the action of iodide ions, as discussed in our recent work.

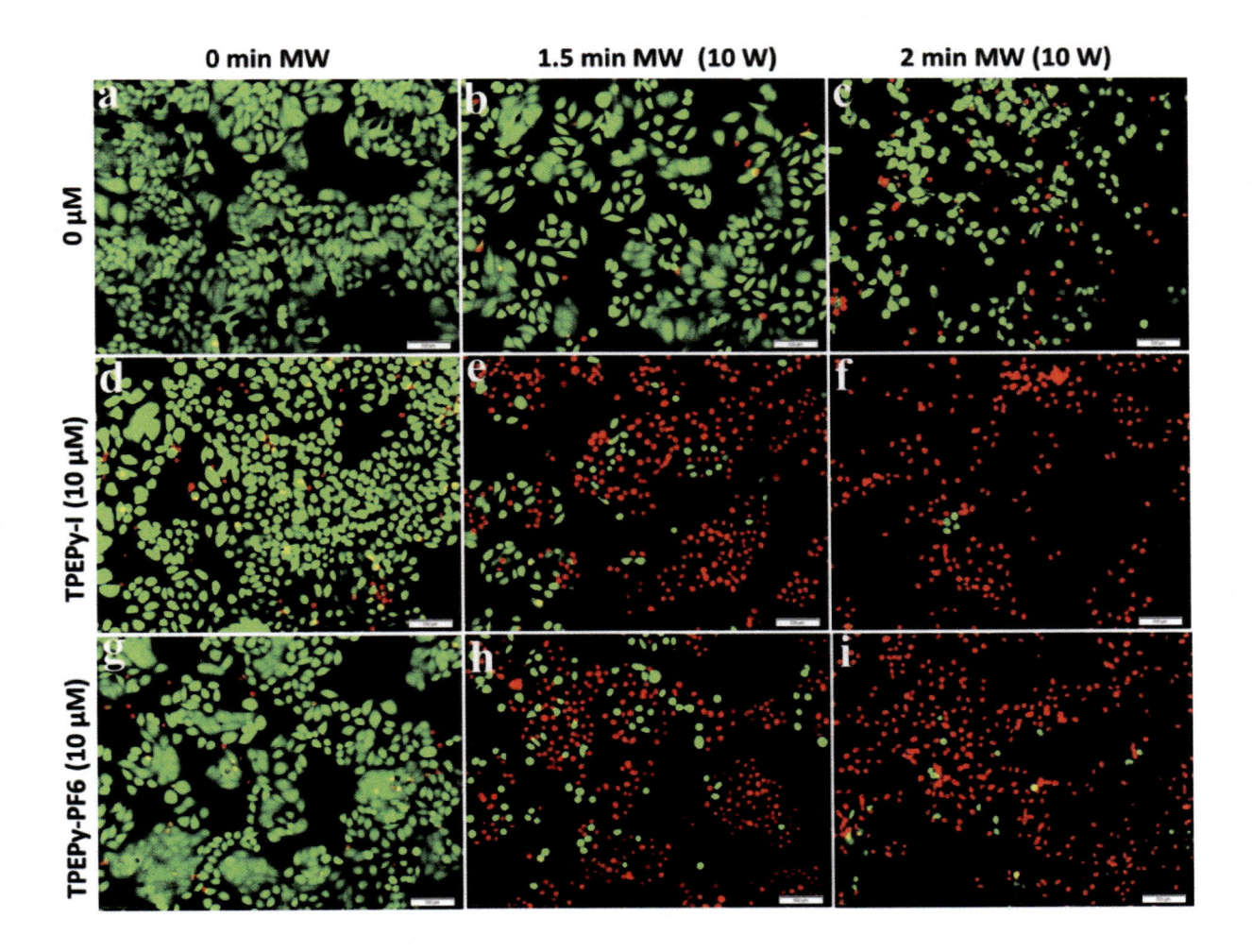

Fig. 4-26. The effect of **TPEPy-I** and **TPEPy-PF6** nanoaggregates (10 μM) in HeLa cells upon 10 W of MW irradiation. (a) Cells without any treatments. (b) Cells treated with MW for 1.5 min. (c) Cells treated with MW for 2 min. (d) Cells treated with **TPEPy-I**. (e) Cells treated with **TPEPy-I** upon MW for 1.5 min. (f) Cells treated with **TPEPy-I** upon MW for 2 min. (g) Cells treated with **TPEPy-PF6**. (h) Cells treated with **TPEPy-PF6** upon MW for 1.5 min, and (i) cells treated with **TPEPy-PF6** upon MW for 2 min. Green fluorescence represents viable cells, whereas red fluorescence represents dead cells. Scale bar = 100 μm; magnification = 10×. Adopted from ref. 2 with permission

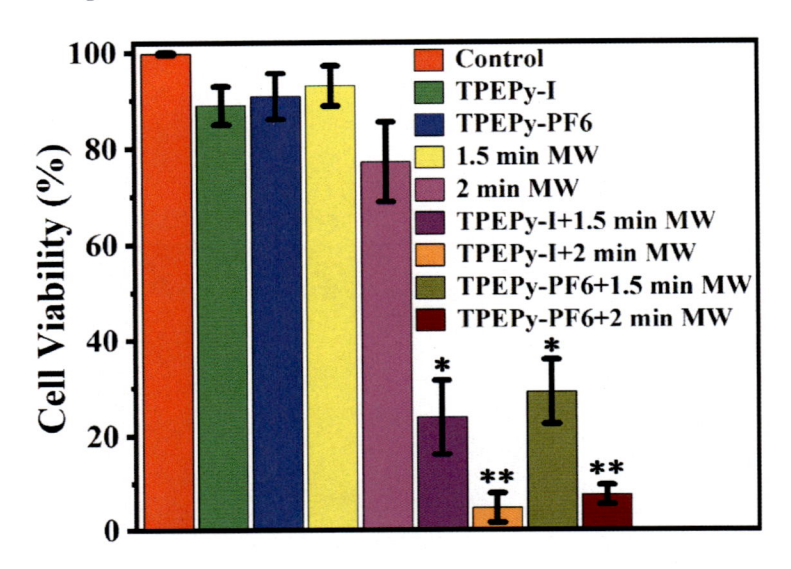

Fig. 4-27. The quantitative analysis of the live/dead cell assay using ImageJ software. *$p < 0.0001$ compared with 1.5 min MW alone and the corresponding nanoaggregate alone; **$p < 0.00001$ compared with 2 min MW alone and the corresponding nanoaggregate alone. Adopted from ref. 2 with permission

Images with a bright field

Additionally, we observed alterations in the shape of HeLa cells following MW treatment. As illustrated in Fig. 4-28, cells treated with TPEPy-I nanoaggregates alone maintained their regular and normal cell shape, demonstrating a minimal level of dark cytotoxicity against HeLa cells. By contrast, the combination of MW and nanoaggregates generated a substantial change in cell shape, indicating that the nanoaggregates and MW are highly hazardous to cancer cells. The results were consistent with those obtained using the MTT and live/dead tests.

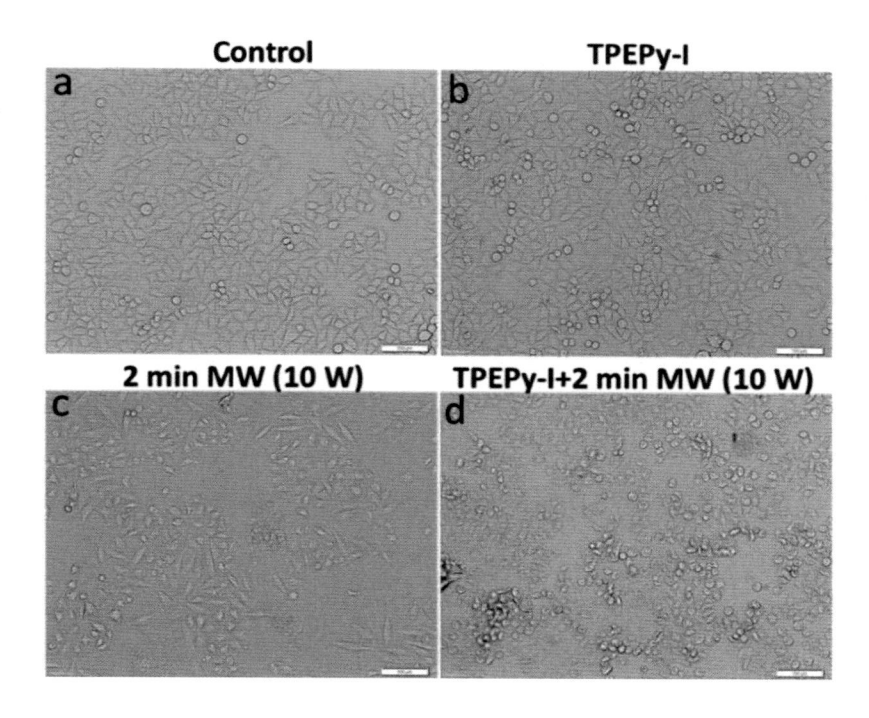

Fig. 4-28. Bright-field images of HeLa cells (a) without any treatments (control), (b) treated with **TPEPy-I** (10 µM), (c) treated with MW for 2 min, and (d) treated with **TPEPy-I** (10 µM) upon MW for 2 min. Scale bar = 100 µm; magnification = 10×. Adopted from ref. 2 with permission

Production of reactive oxygen species and MW heating

Despite significant attempts by numerous groups, including ours, to elucidate the processes of MW-induced ROS formation, the specific mechanism remains unknown because MW irradiation lacks the energy required to break chemical bonds or initiate any chemical reactions. One plausible explanation is that some of the MW energy may be condensed into hot areas, resulting in electron transfer from the nanoaggregates to the surrounding water and oxygen, thereby forming ROS. Another option is that the nanoaggregates have a catalytic function comparable to that of other materials such as copper-chromium nanoparticles, g-C_3N_4 quantum dots, gold nanoparticles, and activated carbon. Additionally, the non-thermal action of MW may lead the reactant molecules to be excited to higher vibrational and rotational energy levels. Shahin et al. hypothesized that the MW's non-thermal action may be responsible for the increased ROS generation. Although the precise method by which ROS are produced is still debated, it is widely accepted that MW irradiation causes polar molecules to constantly realign with the oscillating electric field, thereby increasing their kinetic energy and, consequently, heat. Tissues having a high-water content (for example, solid organs and tumours) are excellent candidates for this form of treatment. There is mounting evidence that heat can act as a catalyst for ROS formation, especially $^1O_2$.

To evaluate whether MW irradiation may generate $^1O_2$ by dismutation of hydrogen peroxide (H_2O_2), we used the singlet oxygen sensor green (SOSG) reagent, which reacts with $^1O_2$ and emits a brilliant green fluorescence with a peak at around 525 nm. When H_2O_2 (100 M) was stimulated with MW (2 and 10 W), the normalized PL intensity at 525 nm increased significantly in both time and dose-dependent fashions compared to H_2O_2 alone and MW alone (Fig. 16a), providing strong evidence that MW can create $^1O_2$ by decomposing H_2O_2. Indeed, ROS formation by MW is a typical occurrence, which has been cited as a major issue for the influence of mobile phones on human health as their use in daily life increases.

To characterize the heating effect of MW, temperatures of DI water with or without the two nanoaggregates were measured up to 6 minutes after 10 W of MW irradiation (2450 MHz). The temperature of the DI water was not significantly different in the presence of TPEPy-I or TPEPy-PF6 nanoaggregates (20 μM), indicating that the MW thermal effect is unlikely to be a significant factor in the killing of cancer cells and excluding the possibility that these nanoaggregates may increase the temperature of MW heating. Based on this observation and our findings, it is plausible to assume that the killing of cancer cells is predominantly caused by reactive oxygen species (ROS), and hence we classify microwave dynamic therapy as such (MWDT).

It is well established that photodynamic treatment (PDT) has a significant disadvantage due to its oxygen-dependent nature, which restricts its effectiveness against hypoxic malignancies. Numerous strategies have been investigated to address this issue, one of which is increasing blood flow in tumours. Because tumour hypoxia is primarily caused by changes in the tumour microenvironment and disordered blood flow, increasing blood flow has proven an effective strategy for increasing tumour oxygenation. It has been observed that modest heating can enhance blood flow in tumours and the oxygen level within the tumour. Thus, microwave-induced photodynamic therapy combined with ROS dynamic therapy is an excellent combination for cancer treatment, since it not only improves efficacy but also may provide a remedy for hypoxic difficulties.

The Bottom Line

We demonstrated for the first time that two AIEgens (TPEPy-I and TPEPy-PF6) may generate ROS and thereby kill cancer cells when exposed to MW irradiation. We used a variety of ways to demonstrate that the two AIEgens can generate ROS in response to MW exposure. The AIEgens exhibited considerable cytotoxicity toward HeLa cells when stimulated by MW, as determined by the MTT and live/dead assays. Given the NIR emission, stability, and efficacy of TPEPy-I or TPEPy-PF6 nanoaggregates in killing cancer cells even at low concentrations, we anticipate that these nanoaggregates will be worthy candidates for further investigation in the study of image-guided MWDT, either alone or in combination with other treatment modalities such as radiotherapy, chemotherapy, immunotherapy, or surgery. This groundbreaking finding paves the way for a new viewpoint on the molecular design of AIEgens with the goal of advancing clinical use and increasing the efficacy of cancer treatments.

References for this chapter

1. Mengyu Yao, Lun Ma, Lihua Li, Junying Zhang, Rebecca X. Lim, **Wei Chen**, and Yu Zhang, A New Modality for Cancer Treatment—Nanoparticle Mediated Microwave Induced Photodynamic Therapy, *J. Biomed. Nanotechnol.*, 2016, 12: 1835–1851
2. Nil Kanatha Pandey, Wei Xiong, Lingyun Wang, **Wei Chen**, Brian Bui, Jian Yang, Eric Amador, Mingli Chen, Christina Xing, Aseem Atul Athavale, Yaowu Hao, Wirya Feizi, Lloyd Lumata, Aggregation-induced emission luminogens for highly effective microwave dynamic therapy, Bioactive Materials, 2022, 7:112-125

Chapter 5

Sonodynamic Therapy

5.1 Basic Concept of Sonodynamic Therapy

Ultrasound is a type of sound that humans cannot hear, and it has a frequency higher than 20 kHz. It creates vibrations in the surrounding environment by compressing and expanding it. Scientists have found many ways to use ultrasound in medicine, both for diagnosis and treatment. (Figure 5-1)

For diagnostic purposes, ultrasound uses a wide range of frequencies from 2.0 to 28.0 MHz. On the other hand, for treatments like tissue repair and drug delivery, lower frequencies from 0.5 to 3.0 MHz are used. Diagnostic ultrasound uses low-energy waves to avoid harming cells, while therapeutic ultrasound requires higher energy to achieve the desired results. (Figure 5-1)

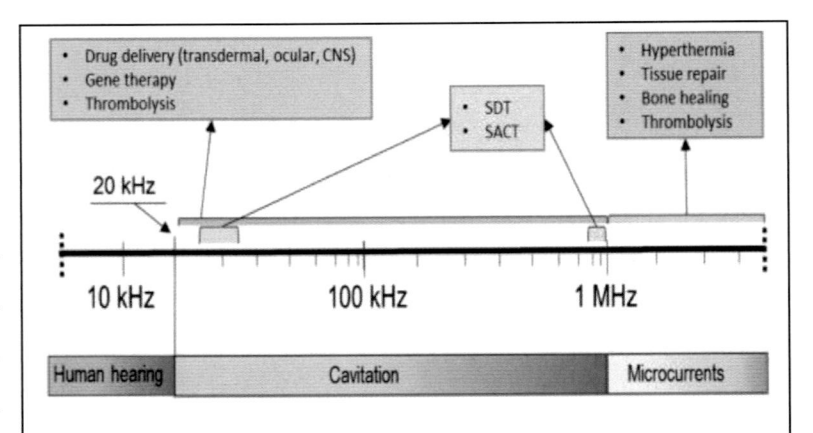

Fig. 5-1. Simplified diagram of the ultrasound frequencies used for therapeutic applications. Adopted from ref. 1 with permission

Ultrasound interacts with living systems through three main pathways: thermal (generating heat), chemical (forming radicals), and mechanical (causing shear stress and shock waves). These interactions lead to specific effects on cells and tissues. In therapeutic applications like high-intensity focused ultrasound (HIFU) therapy for cancer, the goal is to create a localized increase in temperature (hyperthermia) to destroy cancer cells.

The mechanical effects of ultrasound can temporarily increase the permeability of cell membranes, making it easier for cells to absorb drugs. This property is used in drug delivery, allowing targeted and controlled release of medications in various medical fields.

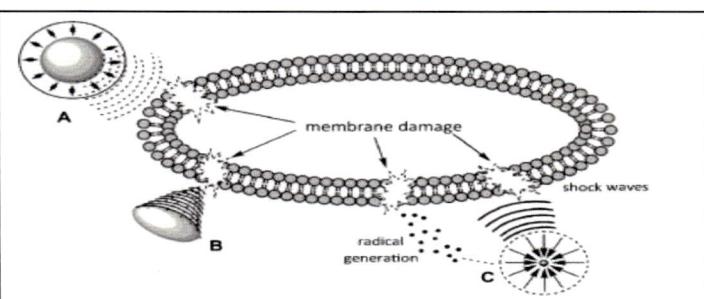

The chemical effects of ultrasound involve sonochemical reactions and the formation of free radicals. These processes have potential therapeutic applications, but their short lifetimes make them challenging to harness effectively.

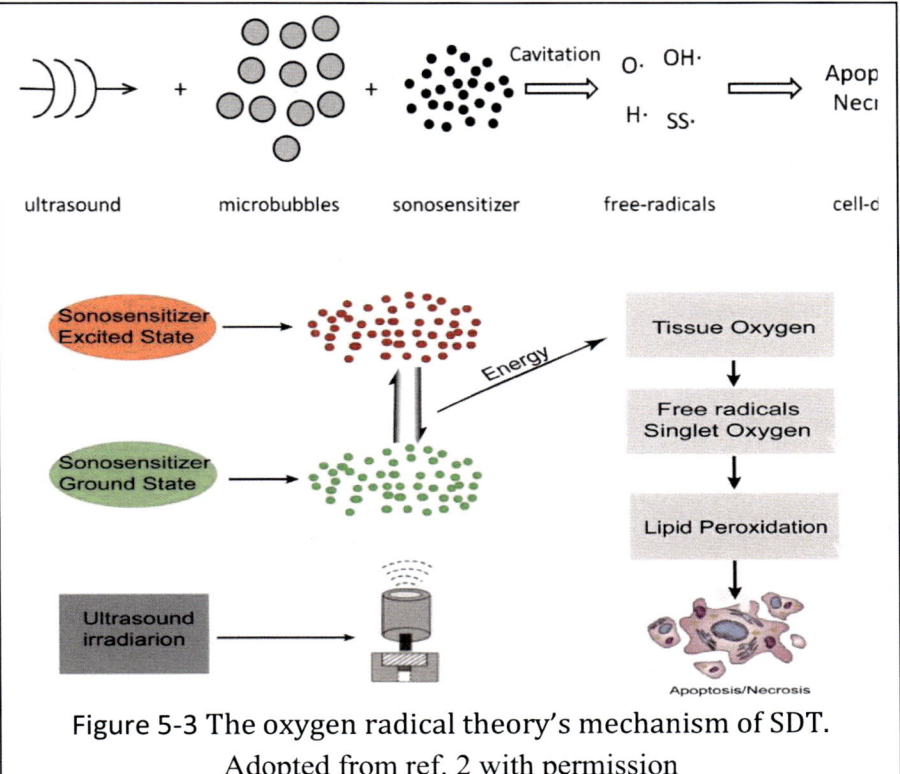

Fig. 5-2. Membrane damages following acoustic cavitation. Adopted from ref. 1 with permission

The primary phenomenon responsible for ultrasound's effects in tissues is called acoustic cavitation (Figure 5-2). Ultrasound waves in liquid create tiny bubbles (microbubbles) filled with gas or vapor. Depending on the amplitude of the ultrasound, these microbubbles can oscillate or implode. The collapse of microbubbles generates shock waves and liquid jets that can damage cell membranes.

Figure 5-3 The oxygen radical theory's mechanism of SDT. Adopted from ref. 2 with permission

Researchers have also explored a therapeutic approach called sonodynamic therapy (SDT). Similar to photodynamic therapy, SDT uses a sensitizing agent and ultrasound to produce reactive species that lead to cell death. SDT has shown promise in reducing solid tumors, and the advantage of ultrasound is its ability to penetrate deeper into tissues compared to light-based therapies. (Figure 5-3)

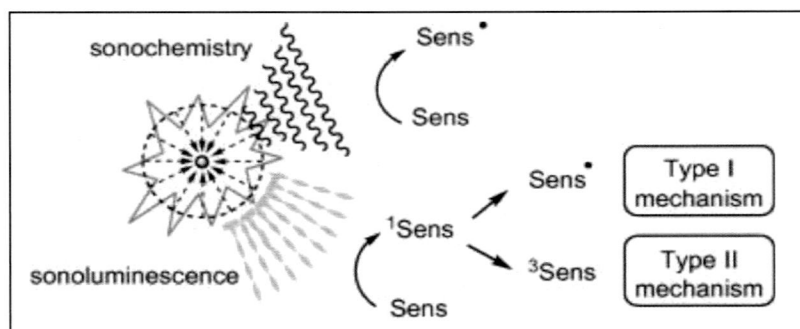

Fig. 5-4. Schematisation of the sonochemistry- and sonoluminescence-mediated generation of cell damage effectors during sonodynamic process. Adopted from ref. 1 with permission

The exact mechanism of SDT is not fully understood, but it is believed that the production of reactive oxygen species (ROS) and free radicals during acoustic cavitation plays a crucial role in damaging cells.

Although the precise mechanism of SDT remains somewhat unclear, it is widely accepted that the main factors causing damage to sonosensitized cells are short-lived species, namely Reactive Oxygen Species (ROS) and free radicals. These species are produced as a result of inertial acoustic cavitation (as shown in Figure 5-4). When the acoustic pressure amplitude reaches a sufficient level, the cavitation microbubbles violently collapse, leading to a dramatic increase in temperature and pressure. Studies have estimated that within nanoseconds, the collapse of microbubbles can generate temperature spikes up to 5000 K and pressures of 250 MPa.

In the localized regions near the collapsing microbubbles, the high liquid shear-forces, shock waves, and localized heating foster sonochemical reactions (sonolysis) and light emission (sonoluminescence). Two hypotheses have been put forward to explain the generation of ROS from acoustic cavitation. One of them suggests that the energy released by the collapsing microbubble promotes the formation of radicals, which then react with oxygen, leading to the production of reactive oxygen species. The second hypothesis suggests that radicals are generated through sonoluminescence, which involves radiation emitted by excited molecules formed during the recombination of radicals from the collapsing microbubble.

In the vicinity of the collapsing microbubble, the emitted light can be absorbed by the sensitizers, triggering a purely photodynamic process. This process can lead to two different outcomes: a Type I process, resulting in the formation of radicals, or a Type II process, where singlet oxygen becomes the primary effector.

Although the exact workings of SDT are not fully understood, researchers widely agree that the damage to sonosensitized cells is caused by short-lived species like ROS and free radicals, which are produced due to inertial acoustic cavitation. The phenomenon involves the violent collapse of cavitation microbubbles, leading to temperature and pressure spikes. In the regions near the collapsing microbubbles, various forces promote sonochemical reactions and light emission. Two hypotheses exist to explain ROS generation from acoustic cavitation, involving either the energy released by collapsing microbubbles or sonoluminescence. The emitted light can be absorbed by sensitizers, initiating a photodynamic process that can lead to the formation of radicals or the activation of singlet oxygen.

The potential of ultrasound in medical science is significant, offering new ways to diagnose and treat various conditions, including cancer. Ultrasound's ability to activate sensitizers and induce cell death through SDT provides a promising avenue for developing novel and efficient cancer treatments with fewer side effects.

Ultrasound is a powerful tool in medicine, used for both diagnosis and treatment. Its unique properties, such as high tissue-penetration, make it a valuable resource in the fight against cancer and other medical conditions. Researchers continue to explore and refine the applications of ultrasound to improve healthcare outcomes for patients.

5.2 Copper Cysteamine Mediated SDT

Copper-Cysteamine Complex (Cu-Cy), due in part to properties, including being insoluble in aqueous solutions, safely, not costly, and easily synthesized for nanoparticulate form, has attracted attention as a new type of nano-drugs. Our research involving of the new types of nanoparticle of Cu-Cy is pale brown crystals, and can be activated by X-Ray or UV. The ideal sensitizer of Cu-Cy has been applied for phototherapy for cancer cells, while free radical species (ROS) generation is much higher using Cu-Cy particles by X-ray activation than produced using PPIX in previous articles. Although X-ray penetration ability is strong, the human body leads to decreased immunity. Other noninvasive and safe approach such as ultrasound irradiation was employed to activation various sensitizers. The present study aims to explore the sonoactivation ability of Cu-Cy in breast cancers both in vitro and in vivo. The sonochemically produced ROS and thereby resulting in apoptosis and necrosis were specially examined. This study provided an alternative approach for activating Cu-Cy using ultrasound, and the future possible application was also discussed in depth.

2. Materials and methods

2.1 Chemicals

Cu-Cy was concentration of 1.2 mM and stored in the dark at 4 °C. Its molecular formula is $Cu_3Cl(SR)_2$ (r =$CH_2CH_2NH_2$) with molecular weight 378.38 g/mol.

Terephthalic acid (TA), 3-(4, 5-dimethylthiazol-2-yl)-2, 5-diphenyltetrazolium bromide tetrazolium (MTT), 2′, 7′-dichlorodihydrofluorescein diacetate (DCFH-DA), and Fluorescein isothiocyanate-dextran 500 KD (FD500) were purchased from Sigma Chemical Company (St Louis, MO, USA). Annexin V-FITC Apoptosis Detection Kit was obtained from Keygen Technology co., LTD (Nanjing, Jiangsu, China).

MDA-MB-231 cells and 4T1 cells were obtained from Resource Center of the Chinese Academy of Science, Beijing, China. All other reagents were commercial products of analytical grade.

2.2 Cell culture and animal model

Human breast cancer MDA-MB-231 cells and 4T1 were cultured in Dulbecco's Modified Eagle's Medium (Gibco, Life Technologies, Carlsbad, CA, USA) supplemented with 10 % fetal bovine serum, 100 U/ml penicillin, 100 U/ml streptomycin and 1 mM L-glutamine. Cultures were maintained at 37°C in humidified atmosphere with a 5 % CO_2 concentration. For all experiments, cells in the exponential phase of growth were used.

The BALB/c mice (female, 18-20 g body weight) were purchased from Fourth Military Medical University (FMMU, Xi'an, China) and were fed in a specific pathogen-free device. After 1 week's acclimation, 0.1 ml of 4T1 cells suspension (1×10^7 cells/ml) was injected near subcutaneously at the right flanks of the mice to induce solid tumors. When the tumor reached a size of 40 mm^3, the tumor-bearing mice were randomly assigned to different groups and ready for experiment. All animal experiments were carried out in accordance with the university's Institutional Animal Care and Use Committee of Shaanxi Normal University (Xi'an, China).

2.3 In vitro experimental protocol

MDA-MB-231 cells re-suspended in a complete culture medium at cell densities of 2×10^5 cells/ml in 35 mm cell culture dish (Corning Inc. Tewksbury MA, USA) for 12 h. Cells were randomly assigned to different groups (Control, Us, Cu-Cy, SDT) and ready for experiment. For Cu-Cy and SDT groups, cells were incubated with Cu-Cy containing medium at 37 °C for 24 h to allow sufficient time for cells uptaking the sensitizer. For Control and Us group, cells were incubated by equal complete culture medium at 37°C for 24 h. Us and SDT groups cells were then exposed ultrasound treatment. For the in vitro ultrasound set-up, a planar transducer was used as previously described, and 0.5W/cm^2 with duty cycle of 20%, duration of 60 s was used for ultrasound treatment.

2.4 Evaluation of ultrasound cavitation

Terephthalic acid (TA) fluorescence method was used to measure cavitational effect. In light of the ultrasonic cavitation of liquid can produce free radicals, TA solution in response to free radicals to result in a fluorescent 2-hydroxyterephthalic acid (HTA). HTA fluorescent intensity indirectly reflected the generation of free radicals during cavitational process. The TA solution (1 mM) reacts with hydroxyl radicals formed during ultrasound (0.5 W/cm^2, 1 min) irradiation with different Cu-Cy concentration (0.06-, 0.1-, 0.3-, 0.6-, 1.2- and 3 μM) for 1min, and the generate HTA was recorded using fluorescence photometer (LS-55, PE, USA) at 426 nm.

2.5 Cell viability measurements

Cytotoxicity of MDA-MB-231 cells treated with Cu-Cy mediated SDT was evaluated by the standard MTT assay. Cells were assigned to different groups: control group (control), 2 μM Cu-Cy alone (Cu-Cy), ultrasound (Us, 0.5 W/cm^2), 0.5 μM Cu-Cy mediate SDT (SDT-0.5 μM), 1 μM Cu-Cy mediate SDT (SDT-1 μM), and 2 μM Cu-Cy mediate SDT (SDT-2 μM). After treatment, cells were cultured in 96-well plates (100 μl/well, Corning Inc., Corning, NY, USA) for 4 h and 24 h, respectively. MTT solution (5 mg/ml, BIO-TEK ELX800, USA) was added to each well and incubated for 4 h, then the MTT mixture was removed and 150 μl DMSO was added to each well. Samples were agitated on a shaker for 20 min, the absorbance was measured using a microplate reader (ELX800, Bio-Tek, USA) at the wavelength of 570 nm. The results were determined as percentage of control [24]. Cell viability was calculated as follows equation:

Cell survival (%) = OD treatment group /OD control group ×100 %.

2.6 Cell apoptosis analysis

The therapeutic efficacy of Cu-Cy mediate SDT on MDA-MB-231 cells was also evaluated by cell apoptosis analysis. The simples were randomly assigned to control, Cu-Cy, Us (0.5W/cm^2), and 1 μM Cu-Cy mediate SDT (SDT-1 μM). After different treatments, the cells were stained with an Annexin V-FITC/PI apoptosis kit following the manufacturer's instructions. 1 μl of recombinant human anti-Annexin V-FITC and 1 μl of propidium iodide (PI) were added to 100 μl of cell suspension. After incubation for 15 min at room temperature in the dark, the cells were analyzed by flow cytometer (NovoCyte^{TM}, ACEA Biosciences Inc., CA, USA).

2.7 Determination of intracellular ROS generation

Intracellular reactive oxygen species (ROS) production with different treatments was assessed using the conversion of non-fluorescent dichlorodihydrofluorescein (DCFH) to fluorescent dichlorofluorescein (DCF) after reaction with cellular ROS as described by previous paper. Following incubation with different concentration of Cu-Cy for 24 h, cells were then exposed to 0.5W/cm^2 ultrasound treatment with pre-incubated DCFH-DA for 20 min. At 1 h post treatment, cells were washed thrice slightly using cold PBS and immediately detected by a flow cytometer.

2.8 Detection of cell membrane permeability

Uptake of FD500 by cells exposed to external stimuli is a common method for revealing cell membrane permeabilization by ultrasound. Once membrane permeability is enhanced by ultrasound, FD500 is the conjugate of fluorescein FITC and dextran with a molecular weight of 500,000 that can freely penetrate the cell membrane. Different groups as described above, MDA-MB-231 cells were sonicated in the presence of 1 mg/ml of FD500. Immediately after ultrasound irradiation exposure, cells were washed thrice with PBS, then the FD500-positive cells were quantified by flow cytometry.

2.9 In vivo ROS imaging

To determine ROS generation in vivo, mice were prepared as described earlier. It should be noted that a focused ultrasound transducer with a frequency of 1.0 MHz and the load power of 2 W was adopted in vivo in this study. The tumor-bearing mice were divided into three groups: Cu-Cy (0.5 mg/kg), Us (2 W, 3 min), SDT-0.5 mg/kg (0.5 mg/kg Cu-Cy, 2 W Us for 3 min). Drug was administered intra-tumorly. 20 min later, 10 μl of the fluorescent probe DCFH-DA (10 mM) was injected directly into the tumor mass. After 30 minutes post-injection, the tumor-bearing mice was exposed directly to the focused ultrasound point for sonication with load power of 2 W and frequency of 1.0 MHz for 3 min. After various treatments, a portion of tumor tissue was collected and cryosectioned at 10 μm thickness, stained with DAPI, fluorescence images of tumor sections were obtained by fluorescence microscopy.

2.10 In vivo antitumor effect

The antitumor efficacy of Cu-Cy mediated SDT was determined by measuring tumor volume as a function of time. For the in vivo antitumor experiments, the tumors were exposed to the focused ultrasound spot for 3 min at 2 W load power with 1.0 MHz frequency. When the tumor volume reached 40-80 mm^3, the tumor-bearing mice were divided into six groups (eight mice per group): control, Cu-Cy (0.75 mg/kg), Us (2 W, 3 min), SDT-0.25 mg/kg (0.25 mg/kg Cu-Cy, 2 W Us for 3 min), 0.5 mg/kg (0.5 mg/kg Cu-Cy, 2 W Us for 3 min) and SDT-0.75 mg/kg (0.75 mg/kg Cu-Cy, 2 W Us for 3 min). Cu-Cy was administrated via the intra-tumor injection to mice every 2 days. The Us irradiating groups were exposed to focused Us at 30 min post injection. The overview protocol is shown in Fig.6 (A). The tumor volume (V = (ab^2)/2, where a and b refer to the largest length and width of tumor, respectively) was recorded and photographed every days until 13 days post treatment. The tumor volume inhibition was analyzed by the expression of $(1 - V/V_0) \times 100\%$ (where V_0 is the tumor volume of the control group, and V represents the tumor volume of the experimental groups). The survival rate of different treatment group was also recorded in a similar experiment.

2.11 Histological examination by H&E staining

Tumor tissues of different groups were fixed with 10% buffered formalin for 24 h. Samples were then paraffin-embedded, sectioned, and stained with hematoxylin and eosin (H&E). Histopathological changes were observed under a Fluorescence Microscope (Nikon Corporation, Tokyo, Japan).

2.12 TUNEL assay of apoptotic cells in vivo

A terminal deoxynucleotidyl transferasemediated dUTP nick-end labeling (TUNEL) assay kit (Beyotime Biotechnology, Shanghai, China) was used to assess the cell apoptosis in the tumor tissues according to the manufacturer's instructions. The tumor tissue was collected and paraffin section at 7 μm thickness. The TUNEL-positive cells (green) were captured by a fluorescent microscopy.

2.13 Statistical analysis

SPSS 19.0 software (SPSS Inc., Chicago) was used for statistical analysis. All data are expressed as the mean ± standard deviation (SD), and the statistical significance was determined using one-way analysis of variance (ANOVA), p-values <0.05, <0.01 and <0.001 were considered statistically significant.

3. Results

3.1 Evaluation of ultrasound cavitation

Firstly, the degree of cavitation was detected by TA (terephthalic acid) method. Fig.5-5(A, B) shows that HTA fluorescence intensity increased significantly after Cu-Cy concentration of 0.5-3 μM and focused ultrasound treatment (0.5 W/cm^2, 1 min), which suggest that medication of Cu-Cy can enhance the effect of ultrasonic cavitation and display dose-dependent effects.

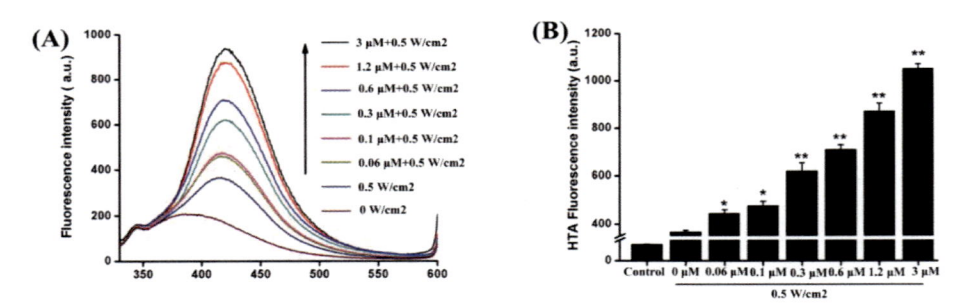

Fig. 5-5 **Evaluation of ultrasound cavitation by TA method**. (A) and (B) Quantification of fluorescence intensity of HTA by fluorescence photometer at 426 nm. In the histogram, *p<0.01, **p<0.01, compared with control. Adopted from ref. 3 with permission

3.2 In vitro efficacy studies

In this study, we explored the sono-activity of Cu-Cy in a dose-dependent manner in vitro. As shown in Fig. 5-6(A), compared with control, Cu-Cy group (2 μM) didn't show obvious cytotoxicity on MDA-MB-231 cells at 4 h and 24 h post treatment. Us alone caused about 30% cell viability loss, while the ultrasound induced cell viability loss was further enhanced with the presence of Cu-Cy. After 24 h post treatment, the survival rate reach to 64.48 %, 34.80 % (p<0.01) and 16.33 % (p<0.001) with the Cu-Cy concentration was 0.5, 1 and 2 μM, respectively, suggesting a synergistic action of cytotoxicity was caused when Cu-Cy was above 0.5 μM when compared to either Cu-Cy alone or US alone. This result also reveals Cu-Cy could be used as a therapeutic agent that applied in sonodynamic killing for tumor cells.

We further adopted flow cytometry to evaluate the induction of apoptosis by SDT treatment. The MDA-MB-231 cells were stained with Annexin V-PE/7-AAD double fluorescent staining to identify necrotic and apoptotic cells. The apoptosis of MDA-MB-231 cells with introduced SDT has an obvious promotion. As shown in Fig. 5-6(B), cells quadrant represented viable cells in the lower-left, both the upper-right and lower-right quadrant indicated the apoptotic cells, and the necrotic cells appeared in the upper-left quadrant. Viable cells in control group was 97.1 %, while it came to Cu-Cy alone and Us alone groups, the percentage dropped to 80.31 % and 79.78 %, respectively. After combined with SDT, the number of viable cells reduce significantly at the same time accompanied by apoptotic cells increasing. The proportion of apoptotic and necrotic cells increased to 32.44 % and 16.84 %, respectively. These results verified that Cu-Cy-SDT was more effective to induce apoptosis and it caused higher cytotoxicity to MDA-MB-231 cells.

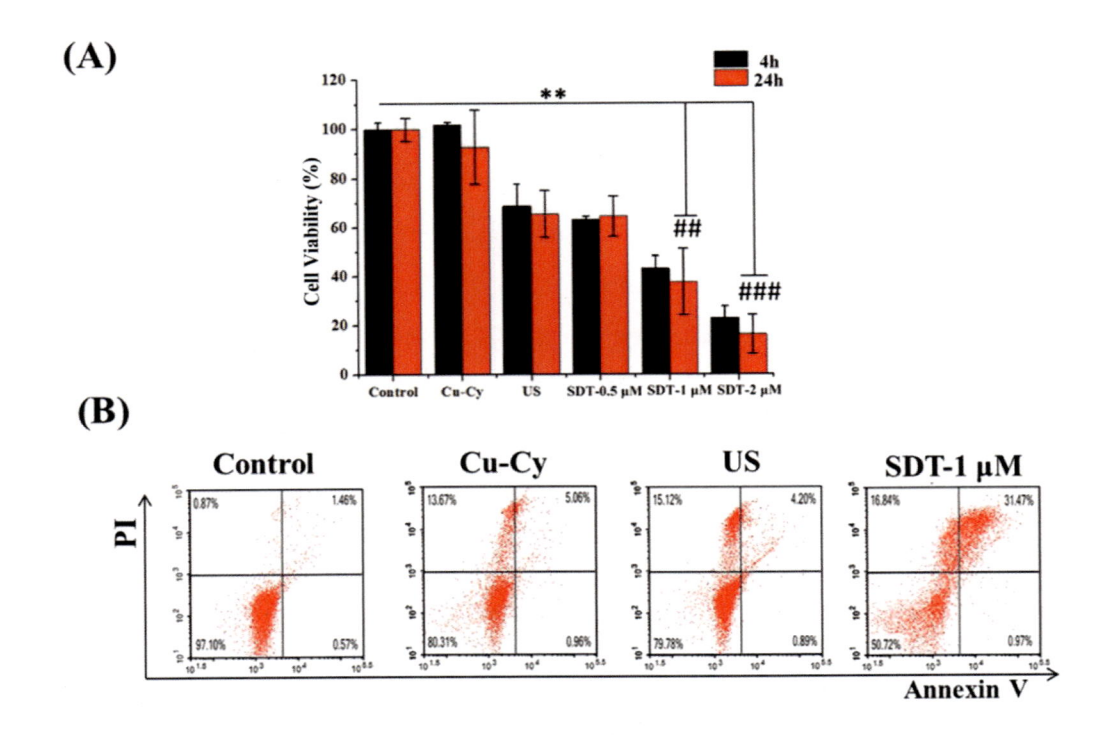

Fig. 5-6 Sonocytotoxicity of Cu-Cy mediate SDT treatment. (A) Cell viability was determined by MTT assay at 4 h, 24 h post-treatment. (B) Apoptosis assessment of MDA-MB-231 cells after different treatment. All data are expressed as percentage of untreated cells, error bars represent S.D. (**p < 0.01 versus control at 4 h, ##p < 0.01, ###p < 0.001 versus control at 24 h). Adopted from ref. 3 with permission

The level of intracellular ROS play an important role in SDT induced cell killing [26]. The more ROS was produced, the more serious damage of tumor cells. It has been reported that Cu-Cy nanostructures could generate a large amount of ROS when irradiated by X-ray for PDT. Therefore, we examined whether Cu-Cy combination SDT treatment can enhance the ROS production in MDA-MB-231 cells. In this study, the leave of intracellular ROS productions with SDT treatments were measure in tumor cells by using DCFH-DA fluorescent probe staining. Result in Fig.5-7 indicates that Cu-Cy alone (2 μM) and Us alone increased cellular ROS level to some extent, while SDT treatment could cause more significant ROS generation which increased with Cu-Cy concentration ranged from 0.5 μM to 2 μM. The result suggests ROS would be a key factor for Cu-Cy-SDT induced cell damage.

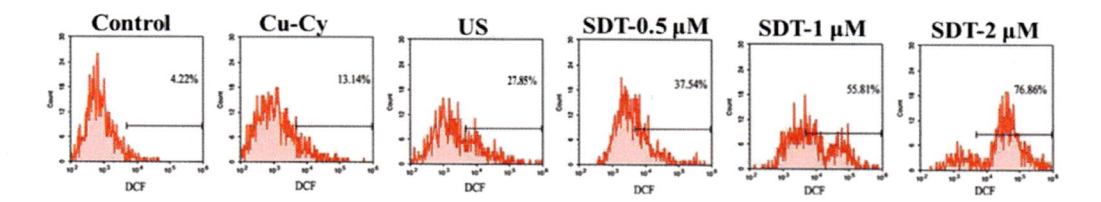

Fig. 5-7 Detection of ROS level using DCFH-DA staining and flow cytometry after different treatment of MDA-MB-231 cells. Adopted from ref. 3 with permission

In this study, the tumor cells membrane permeability was evaluated by FD500-uptake assay under ultrasound. As shown in Fig. 5-8, the proportions of fluorescence intensities of FD500 in MDA-MB-231 cells increased to 15.70 %, 23.57 % and 38.68 % after 0.5, 1, and 2 uM Cu-Cy incubation and ultrasound treatment, respectively. However, the fluorescence intensities of Cu-Cy alone and Us alone have a slight change compared with control. The data indicate that Cu-Cy in this study could cause damage to cell membrane and have concentration dependent effects under Us irradiating.

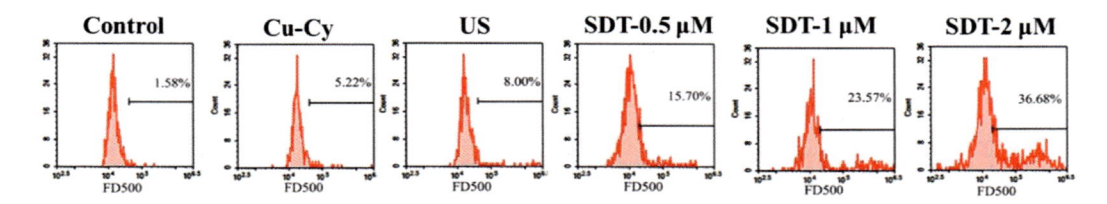

Fig. 5-8 The FD500 was tested with flow cytometry to analysis membrane permeability of MDA-MB-231 cells. Adopted from ref. 3 with permission

3.3 In vivo efficacy studies

The proposed mechanisms of SDT induced cell death mainly focus on the generation of ROS. To investigate the in vivo ROS generation potential in 4T1 tumor-bearing mice, ROS probe of DCFH-DA was injected into tumors before the Us irradiation. The in vivo images (Fig.5-9) reveal that in the tumor amount of ROS (green) was generated by Cu-Cy when US was applied. In contrast, under the same conditions, the tumor tissues were made into paraffin sections and the image by a fluorescence microscope recorded that little ROS was observed in the tumors treated with the no US group of Cu-Cy. This result indicate that Us irradiation can activate Cu-Cy and stimulate ROS generation in vivo.

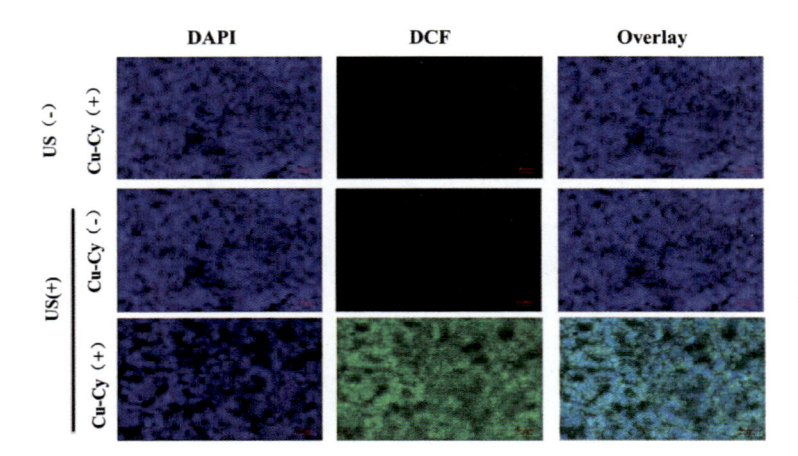

Fig. 5-9 The in vivo ROS generation detected through fluorescence microscopy after different treatment. Adopted from ref. 3 with permission

To assess SDT efficiency against cancer, we further investigate the efficacy of SDT in tumor growth in vivo, which was monitored on 4T1 tumor xenograft in BALB/c mice according to the tumor volume changes. The treatment protocol is shown in Fig. 5-10(A), the tumors was irradiated by US irradiation at 30 min post Cu-Cy in-site injection. The same treatment was repeated four times. At the 13th post treatment, both Cu-Cy and US inhibited tumor growth to a certain extent, in which the tumor-inhibition rate reaches 26.13 % and 36.87 %, respectively. While, the tumor growth in SDT was further inhibited in a Cu-Cy dose dependent manner. The tumor growth was almost restrained in the SDT-0.75 mg/kg group, in which the inhibition ratio was up to 74.43 % compared with control and was more significant than those of SDT-0.25 mg/kg and SDT-0.5 mg/kg group (Fig.5-10D). As show in Fig. 5-10(C), in contrast to the control group, the survival of tumor-bearing mice in SDT-0.25 mg/kg, SDT-0.5 mg/kg and SDT-0.75 mg/kg groups was greatly prolonged with increased dosage, suggesting a potential Cu-Cy mediated SDT property. The body weight of each treatment group was shown in Fig. 5-10(B) with no alterations..

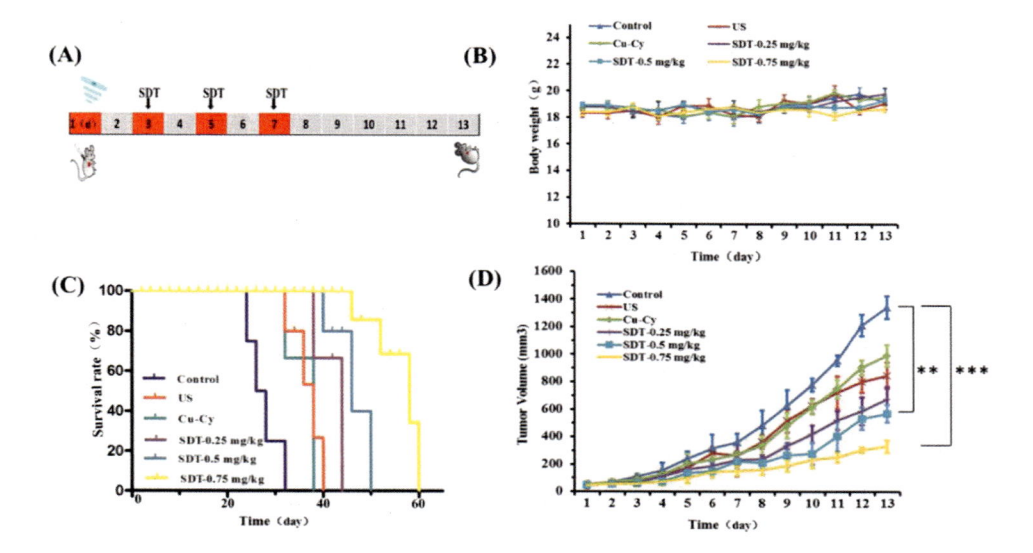

Fig. 5-10 (A) In vivo therapeutic protocol of SDT on mice tumor xenograft. (B) Mice-weight changes as a function of time after different treatments of control, Cu-Cy (0.75 mg/kg), US (2 W, 3 min), SDT-0.25 mg/kg (0.25 mg/kg Cu-Cy plus 2 W US for 3 min), SDT-0.5 mg/kg (0.5 mg/kg Cu-Cy plus 2 W US for 3 min) and SDT-0.75 mg/kg (0.75 mg/kg Cu-Cy plus 2 W US for 3 min). (C) Survival rate for each treatment group. (D) The tumor-volume growth curve as a function of time post different treatments. (**$p < 0.05$, ***$p < 0.01$ versus control). Adopted from ref. 3 with permission

The tumor images at the end of treatments is shown in Fig. 5-11(A), which shows the most decreased tumor size in SDT-0.75 mg/kg groups compared with the other groups. Further histopathological analysis was performed by H&E staining and TUNE assay. The tumor tissues were made into paraffin sections and imaged by a fluorescence microscope. As shown in the H&E-stained of tumor section, Fig. 5-11(B), the portion of purple blue (nuclei stained by hematoxylin) area is less and less with the increase of Cu-Cy dosage, indicating that cancer cells apoptosis and necrosis is increasing. From the TUNEL assay result, Fig. 5-11(C), green fluorescence was observed, which shows the apoptosis of tumor cells of breast tumor tissue sections with the therapeutics at the different dose of Cu-Cy on day 13 after, the number of apoptotic cells stained green in SDT-0.75 mg/kg group is much more than the other groups.

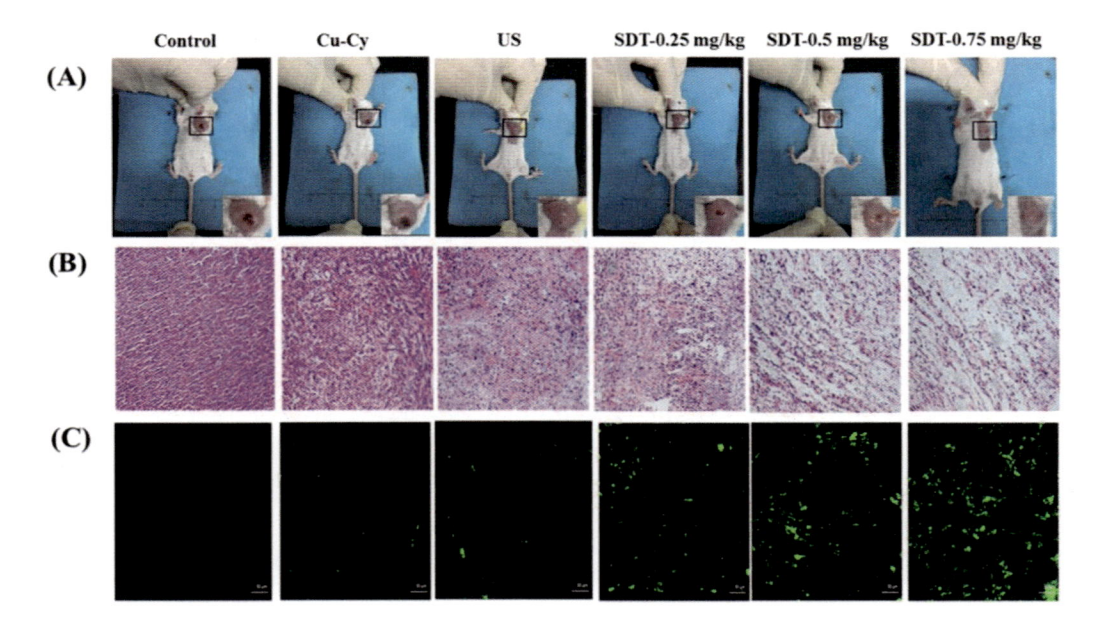

Fig. 5-11 (A) Photographic images of tumor at the end of the treatments. (B) Optical microscopic images of tumor sections stained by hematoxylin and eosin (H&E), (C) TUNEL assay post different treatments. Scale bar represents 50 μm. Adopted from ref. 3 with permission

4. Discussion

With the gradual study on the fundamental mechanisms of different sensitizers in SDT, more and more researchers committed to the development and identification novel sonosensitizer. Most sonosensitizers derive from photosensitizers. For example, the photosensitizers of porphyrin derivatives and phthalocyanines have been used as sonosensitizers in SDT. Previous studies suggest the good potential of Cu-Cy in phototherapy. Here, we attempted to explore the sonoactivity of Cu-Cy and the possible actions in vivo and in vitro.

Firstly, TA method confirmed that Cu-Cy may serve as cavitation nuclei and greatly increased ultrasound induced cavitational effect. This would be a good sign for Cu-Cy combination with ultrasound irradiation. Subsequent in vitro and in vivo studies evidenced the synergy of Cu-Cy and ultrasound treatment. MTT assay showed Cu-Cy-SDT exhibited excellent cytotoxicity on breast cancer cells. Absolutely, similar as other porphyrin sonosensitizers, a proper drug dose and US energy are key to realize this synergetic tumor-cell killing. The results of Annexin V-PI assay in our study demonstrated Cu-Cy mediated SDT mainly led to cell necrosis and apoptosis (Fig. 2(B)). ROS is one of the important factors of the anti-tumor effect in SDT. Excessive ROS triggered by

SDT can damage cell. Our data showed the generation of ROS was increased after MDA-MB-231 cancer cells treated with Cu-Cy mediate SDT. This result was consistent with many reports. Previous studies revealed that most of sensitizers such as porphyrin in both PDT and SDT can generate ROS in tumor cells. Thus, a possible mechanism of Cu-Cy for SDT may be speculated as follows. By receiving US irradiation, Cu-Cy would be activated and changed into the excited state from the ground state in the tumor cells. When the nanoparticals would trend to return to the ground state, the US energy is released and turn into various ROS. On the other hand, the main reason for the Cu-Cy mediate SDT experimental results showing that ultrasound make cell membrane permeability enhance and more nanodrug was transport into the cancer cells to have a higher concentration of Cu-Cy in the sonicated cancer cells and boost the cytotoxicity and the inhibition of tumor growth. ROS was produced, and a series of oxidation reactions happen such as led to destruction of biomembrane structure and function, DNA strand breaks, mitochondrial membrane permeability, effect of intracellular signal transduction and gene expression, causing irreversible damage in tumor cells . According to the above analysis, cells damage enhancement is probably mediated via ROS by ultrasonically activated Cu-Cy, and with the increase of ROS concentration, oxidative stress-induced cell death pathways make the breast tumor cells progressively damaged.

In this case, we further investigated the efficacy of SDT with Cu-Cy in vivo xenografts of 4T1 cancer cells and demonstrated the great tumor growth inhibition. There is obvious phenomenon that necrosis and more apoptotic tumor could be observed by H-E or TUNEL-stained microscopic section of tumors received SDT with Cu-Cy. The same time we also proved that the process of Cu-Cy-mediate SDT generate ROS to increased apoptosis which should not only achieve maximum therapeutic efficacy but also without adverse effects on mice weight. We confirmed for the first time that Cu-Cy-mediate SDT can significantly increase apoptosis and necrosis of tumor cells by generation ROS to inhibit the tumor growth (Fig.5-12), while further mechanisms need deep investigation.

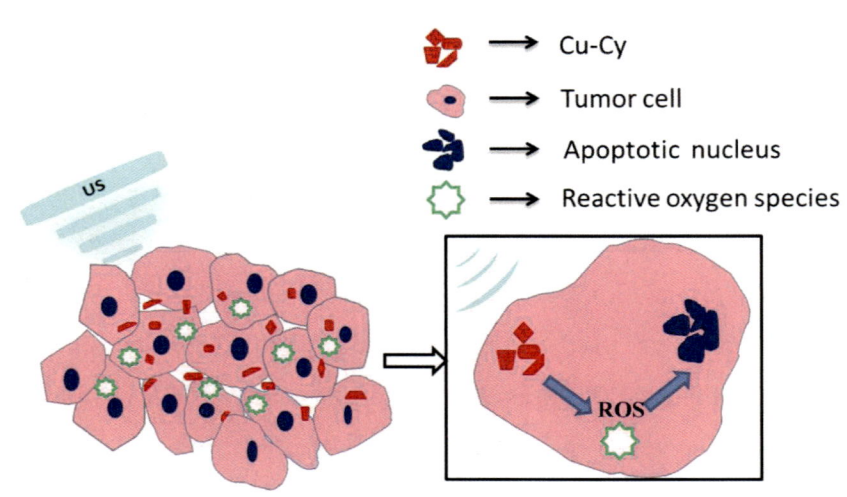

Fig. 5-12 Schematic illustration of the possible mechanisms of Cu-Cy combined with ultrasound. Upon receiving US, Cu-Cy in the tumor cells would receive the US energy and trigger excessive ROS generation to stimulate apoptotic and necrotic responses. Adopted from ref. 3 with permission

Bottom Line

In this study, we have demonstrated that Cu-Cy could be activated by ultrasound irradiation, and which further enhanced ultrasound induced cavitation and ROS generation. Although previous studies have reported its application for phototherapy, this study revealed its potential for SDT, which added the approaches to excite this nano-sensitizer. Thereby, the combination of Cu-Cy and ultrasound irradiation would provide a promising strategy for future cancer treatment.

References for this chapter

1. Loredana Serpe a, Francesca Giuntini, Sonodynamic antimicrobial chemotherapy: First steps towards a sound approach for microbe inactivation, Journal of Photochemistry and Photobiology B: Biology 150 (2015) 44–49

2. Liu Rengenga, Zhang Qianyua, Lang Yuehonga, Peng Zhongzhong, Li Libo, Sonodynamic therapy, a treatment developing from photodynamic therapy, *Photodiagnosis and Photodynamic Therapy 19 (2017) 159–166*

3. Pan Wang, Xiao Wang, Lun Ma, Sunil Sahi, Li Li, Xiaobing Wang, Qingqing Wang, Yujiao Chen, **Wei Chen**, and Quanhong Liu, Nanosonosensitization by using Copper-Cysteamine Nanoparticles Augmented Sonodynamic Cancer Treatment, *Part. Part. Syst. Charact.* 2018, 1700378

Chapter 6

Chemo dynamic Therapy

6-1 Chemodynamic Therapy: Tumour Microenvironment Mediated Fenton and Fenton-like Reactions

Introduction

The treatment for cancer is the most required in the field of medicines as many have side effects and requires a lot of attention as we do not have many alternatives. In order to stop the growth of cancer cells Fenton reaction, which is simply defined as the generation of highly oxidative hydroxyl radicals (•OH) from hydrogen peroxide (H_2O_2), is catalysed by ferrous ion (Fe^{2+}) and has been widely used to remove refractory organics. After extensive research, advanced nanotechnology has created a broad stage for the further development and extension of the Fenton reaction, such as iron-based nanomaterials for the Fenton and Fenton-like reactions, other metal-based nanomaterials, and graphene oxide for the Fenton-like reaction. (Figure 6-1) However, a major issue encountered by scientists is how to broaden the applications of the Fenton and Fenton-like reactions, which would also provide possibilities and has prompted many studies in other fields in addition to the ecological environmental field.

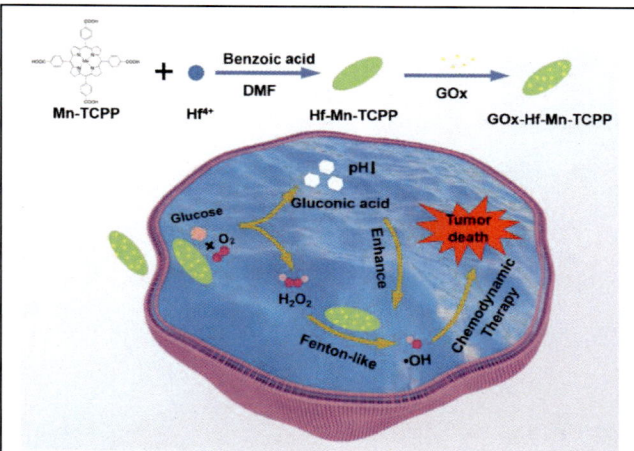

Figure 6-1 Schematic Illustration of the Construction of GOx-Hf-Mn-TCPP and Starving-Enhanced CDT. Adopted from ref. 2 with permission

Characterized by mild acidity, H_2O_2 overproduction, low catalase activity, and hypoxia, the tumour microenvironment (TME) not only provides a suitable environment and nutrition for tumour development and metastasis but also furnishes the "gate" for selective and efficient tumour treatments. In this case, numerous TME-responsive nanomaterials have been developed in recent decades, the majority of which are TME-responsive drug delivery nano carriers that have deficiencies, such as insufficient drug loading and easy leakage to damage normal tissues. Moreover, studies focusing on current clinical treatments would provide researchers with effective guidance to explore more suitable new therapies. For example, radiotherapy generates reactive oxygen species (ROS) in the tumour area through X-rays to destroy the tumour. Certain chemotherapeutic drugs, such as tirapazamine (TPZ) and doxorubicin (DOX), also generate ROS to fight tumours. In addition, the drug artemisinin is a highly effective treatment for malaria. One of the principles underlying the effects of this drug is that the iron in the residual haeme observed in patients with malaria induces the decomposition of artemisinin by catalysing the formation of a peroxide bridge to produce hydroxyl radicals, which are highly active and lethal, subsequently eliminating the malaria parasite. Chemists quickly linked this mechanism to the classical Fenton reaction. After considering these different fields, chemodynamic therapy (CDT), an emerging therapeutic strategy, was recently proposed by our group and defined as in situ treatments using the Fenton reaction or Fenton-like reaction to generate •OH in tumour sites. Briefly, iron-based nanomaterials dissolve ferrous ions under the mildly acidic conditions of the TME and initiate the Fenton reaction to overproduced H_2O_2, generating •OH to trigger apoptosis and inhibit the tumour. Most importantly, this approach ensures normal tissue safety to some degree because the Fenton reaction is substantially suppressed under the slightly alkaline conditions and in the presence of insufficient H_2O_2 in a normal microenvironment. Even so, the potential toxicities of nanomaterials should be taken into consideration for further applications. This strategy not only broadens the applications of the Fenton reaction but also simplifies its potential for clinical translation. Compared with chemotherapy, radiotherapy, photothermal therapy, and photodynamic therapy, CDT has the following advantages: 1) It is highly logical and selective, and 2) is activated by endogenous stimulus. Meanwhile, we also get enlightenment from some drugs as their treatment principles are based on Fenton or Fenton-like reactions. The antitumour principle of bleomycin is that the bleomycin is firstly intercalated in DNA, and then the complex of bleomycin with iron would generate superoxide and hydroxyl radicals to break the DNA strand. At the same time, the cardiotoxicity of anthracycline drugs is mainly from the reactive oxygen species, especially hydroxyl radicals, generated by the binding iron ions with H_2O_2, which also has the potential for CDT. Therefore, studies aimed at the further development of CDT have flourished, which supports the potential utility of CDT for clinical translation.

Development of CDT, the selection of suitable nanomaterials, the modulation of the reaction environment (reduced pH levels, increased amounts of reactants and decreased amounts of glutathione), and the assistance of an exogenous energy source have been used to optimize the effect of CDT, which relies on the guidance of the Fenton or Fenton like reactions and basic chemical principles. Although the majority of the existing CDT agents are iron-based inorganic nanomaterials, other inorganic nanomaterials and organic nanomaterials have also been used to enrich the library. Moreover, nanomaterials used for CDT without low-pH dependence are also satisfactory choices. Nanomaterials that have the ability to exclusively produce protons or H_2O_2 in tumours should also be taken into consideration. Above all, the selection of nanomaterials should consider the issues of more functionality and easy synthesis procedures, which are crucial for applications in the real world. In addition, the efficiency of CDT could also be improved by the consumption of reducing substances in the TME, such as glutathione (GSH), or the modulation of H^+ and H_2O_2 levels by regulating gene expression. Fortunately, several other external energy fields, such as light, heat, ultrasound, electric, or magnetic fields, are desirable to promote the Fenton-like reaction.

6.2 PPIX-Lipo-MnO$_2$ to Enhance Photodynamic Therapy by Improving Tumour Hypoxia

Treating tumours is challenging as the environmental factors support the multiplication of the cancer cells. Photodynamic therapy (PDT) is a promising cancer that consists of three essential components: a photosensitizer, light, and oxygen. Light has extremely poor penetration, and therefore photodynamic therapy is unsuitable for deeply seated cancers. In this direction, considerable progress has been made in recent years. Lack of dissolved oxygen in tumour cells may be responsible for poor radiotherapy efficacy. Most tumours suffer from a lack of oxygen (hypoxia). To enhance the PDT efficacy, it is necessary to develop effective strategies to supply adequate oxygen to reduce hypoxia.

MnO_2 stands as an excellent candidate to improve the tumour hypoxia conditions for PDT. Two important characteristics MnO_2 possesses to enhance the PDT effect of photosensitizers: 1) high specificity and reactivity toward H_2O_2, producing O_2 and H_2O while simultaneously consuming protons, and 2) effectively reducing glutathione levels in the cancerous cells. (Figure 6-2)

Protoporphyrin IX (PPIX) is an FDA-approved photosensitizer with the ability to accumulate in tumours. Because of its amphiphilic nature, PPIX aggregates in the aqueous environment either via π-π stacking or intermolecular interactions between hydrophilic -COOH groups and the hydrophobic porphyrin core. It has been shown that the aqueous solubility of the PPIX could be improved by conjugating it to APTES and poly(styrene-co-4 vinyl pyridine). However, naked PPIX might lead to unwanted toxicity. On the other hand, liposomes offer improved biocompatibility and are an accepted vehicle for drug delivery. As-synthesized PPIX-Lipo and PPlX-Lipo-M were not only highly soluble in aqueous media, but also improved PDT by increasing the oxygen level in cancer cells.

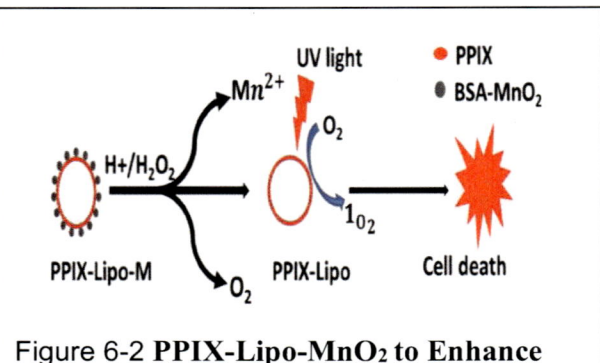

Figure 6-2 **PPIX-Lipo-MnO2 to Enhance Photodynamic Therapy** Adopted from ref. 4 with permission

Synthesis of PPIX-Lipo, BSA-MnO2, and PPIX-Lipo-M

PPIX was encapsulated inside DPPC/Chol liposomes by using a lipid film hydration method. 50 mg/mL of DPPC in chloroform, 7 mg/mL of Chol in chloroform, and 1 mg/mL of PPIX solution in tetrahydrofuran (THF) were separately prepared. Then, 200 μL of the DPPC solution, 100 μL of the Chol solution, and 250 μL of the PPIX solution were mixed. The mixture was vortexed for about 1 min to mix it homogeneously. The mixture was dried to a thin lipid film under a high vacuum using a rotatory evaporator for 2 h. The as-formed thin film was hydrated with DI water at 55°C, rotating at 150 rpm for 1 h. In each 10 min interval of rotation, the mixture was vortexed for 1 min to facilitate the liposome formation. The as-synthesized PPIX-Lipo was then stored in a fridge at 4°C overnight to allow the completion of liposome formation. Unencapsulated PPIX was removed by allowing it to precipitate overnight. Unreacted chemicals were then removed by washing with DI water 3 times. The PPIX-Lipo was then sonicated for 15 min to obtain nano-sized liposomes. The as-synthesized PPIX-Lipo was stored in a fridge protected from light with aluminum foil until further use.

BSA-coated MnO$_2$ (hereafter MnO$_2$) was prepared using a previously reported method with minor modifications. Briefly, 9 mg of KMnO$_4$ was dispersed in 3 mL of 1× PBS and stirred for 5 min. 50 mg of BSA was dispersed in 3 mL of PBS and stirred for 20 min. Then, the KMnO$_4$ solution was added dropwise to the BSA solution and stirred for 2 h at 37 °C. The obtained MnO$_2$ was purified by dialysis using a dialysis bag of 12 kDa cutoff molecular weight against DI water for 24 h. Purified MnO$_2$ was stored at 4 °C for further use. As-synthesized MnO$_2$, was highly soluble and stable in aqueous media for several weeks.

MnO$_2$ was coated onto the liposome surface via physical interactions. PPIX-Lipo and MnO$_2$ were mixed at a respective molar ratio 1:50, and moderately stirred for 3 h at room temperature. During the mixing process, the mixing flask was covered with aluminum foil to protect the mixture protected from incoming light.

Absorption and photoluminescence measurement

The absorption and photoluminescence (PL) spectra were measured using a Shimadzu UV-2450 UV–Vis spectrophotometer and a Shimadzu RF-5301PC luminescence spectrophotometer, respectively. To measure absorption and the PL spectrum of MnO$_2$, PPIX-Lipo and PPIX-Lipo-M, samples were prepared in DI water such that both PPIX-Lipo and PPIX-Lipo-M had an equal concentration of PPIX, and both PPIX-Lipo-M and MnO$_2$ had an equal concentration of MnO$_2$. Typically, PPIX-Lipo and PPIX-Lipo-M had 3 μM of PPIX. In PPIX-Lipo-M, the ratio of PPIX and MnO$_2$ was 1:50 for all further experiments. To demonstrate that MnO$_2$ adsorbed onto the liposome surface, luminescence quenching of PPIX in PPIX-Lipo-M with respect to PPIX-Lipo and the regain in luminescence following the addition of 3 mM of glutathione (GSH) was measured. Photobleaching of PPIX-Lipo and PPIX-Lipo-M was measured after 5 min of UV-light exposure three times. The relative change in luminescence was plotted with UV-light treatment time.

Drug loading efficiency

The luminescence of PPIX dissolved in DMSO was measured at various concentrations, and a calibration curve was established by plotting the integrated PL intensity against its concentration. 2.8 mL of DMSO was added to 200 μL of PPIX-Lipo to disrupt the liposomes, and the integrated PL intensity was measured and plotted against corresponding concentration. The loading efficiency was calculated in percentage by comparing the slope of PPIX and PPIX-Lipo dissolved in DMSO.

In-vitro pH measurement

To demonstrate that our nano-system can react with H_2O_2 under acidic conditions, we measured the change in pH of acidic solutions. First, 100 μM of H_2O_2 was dispersed in pH = 5.6 (HCl solution). Then, MnO_2 was added to the solution. The pH change was monitored in each 1 min intervals by using a digital pH meter.

Singlet oxygen generation measurement

Singlet oxygen produced by PPIX-Lipo and PPIX-Lipo-M with and without 100 μM of H_2O_2 were measured in PBS (pH = 7.4) buffers. The singlet oxygen green sensor (SOSG) was used as a luminescence-based singlet oxygen probe. UV light was excited for 5 min intervals for 5 times, and luminescence intensity was monitored after each excitation. Integrated PL intensity was calculated at each concentration and plotted against the concentration.

Cellular uptake experiment

200,000 cells were cultured in a 35 mm petri-dish and incubated for 24 h to allow cell attachment. Naked PPIX, PPIX-Lipo, and PPIX-Lipo-M were added and incubated for 24 h. Old media were replenished with new media having 1 μM of HOECHST dye to stain the nucleus. The Olympus IX71 fluorescence microscope was used to image the cells. Default DAPI filter (Emi/Exi at 457 nm/350 nm) was used to image the HOECHST dye, while PPIX was imaged using a Emi/Exi 617 nm/ 403 nm filter. Cellular uptake of PPIX-Lipo and PPIX-Lipo-M was confirmed by merging the HOECHST and PPIX channels.

Cell viability study

MTT assay was performed on MCF-7 cell lines. MnO_2 was used in the concentration range of 45 μM to 570 μM, while the concentrations of the PPIX in both PPIX-Lipo and PPIX-Lipo-M varied from 0 μM to 60 μM. The plates were protected from light with aluminum foil to prevent the unwanted excitation of PPIX by light and incubated for 24 h to allow the uptake of the particles by cells. Following the incubation, 5 mg/mL of MTT solution in PBS was diluted to 0.5 mg/mL in the corresponding cell and then applied to each well and incubated for 3 h at 37 °C. DMSO (100 μL) was added to each well to dissolve the formazan crystals. The optical density (OD) was recorded at 540 nm in a microplate reader (Multiskan). Cell viability was determined by comparing OD of the treatment group with OD of the control group as depicted below:

$$\text{Cell viability} = \frac{\text{The OD of the treatment group}}{\text{The OD of the control group}} * 100\% \qquad (1)$$

Each experiment was performed at least three times. Cell viabilities were expressed as mean ± standard deviation.

Hypoxia induction and detection

10,000 cells were seeded into 96-well plates and incubated for 24 h for cell attachment. After the incubation, old media was replaced with new media having 100 µM of cobalt chloride hexahydrate and incubated for 16 h. Hypoxia induction was confirmed using a ROSID® Hypoxia/Oxidative stress detection kit (Enzo Life Sciences) and fluorescence microscopy detection according to the manufacturer's instructions.

PDT effect study

10,000 cells/well were seeded in each experiment. Five equal concentrations of PPIX-Lipo and PPIX-Lipo-M were added to the 96-well plates and incubated for another 24 h. Then, the OD of solubilized formazan crystal was recorded at 540 nm in the microplate reader. PDT effect was determined by using Eq. (1). At least three independent experiments were performed, and cell viabilities were expressed as mean ± standard deviation. One-way ANOVA was performed to determine the significant difference with $p < 0.05$.

Results

Synthesis of PPIX-Lipo, BSA-MnO$_2$, and PPIX-Lipo-M

Using thin-film hydration method as illustrated in Fig. 6-3, PPIX was encapsulated between the lipid bilayer of the liposomes. PPIX-Lipo had a reddish color and is soluble in water (Fig. 6-4a(ii)), while naked PPIX was black and precipitated in DI water as displayed in Fig. 6-4a(i). Luminescence of naked PPIX and PPIX-Lipo under UV light are depicted in Fig. 6-4b(i and ii), respectively. PPIX-Lipo showed a bright red luminescence, but bare PPIX did not have luminescence under UV light. As-synthesized MnO$_2$ nanoparticles were highly soluble and stable in an aqueous solution for several weeks. MnO$_2$ nanoparticles were then coated to the liposomal surface via physical interactions. MnO₂ is adsorbed onto the liposome surface via hydrophobic effect as BSA has a strong tendency to interact with cholesterol and DPPC of the liposome. As shown in Fig. 2a(iii) and b(iii), the luminescence of PPIX-Lipo-M was quenched compared to that of PPIX-Lipo. MnO₂ has a wide range of absorption from 200 nm to 700 nm, which coincides with PPIX emission spectra. Consequently, MnO₂ adsorbed onto the liposomal surface could effectively quench the luminescence of PPIX via FRET energy transfer and/or an inner filter effect.

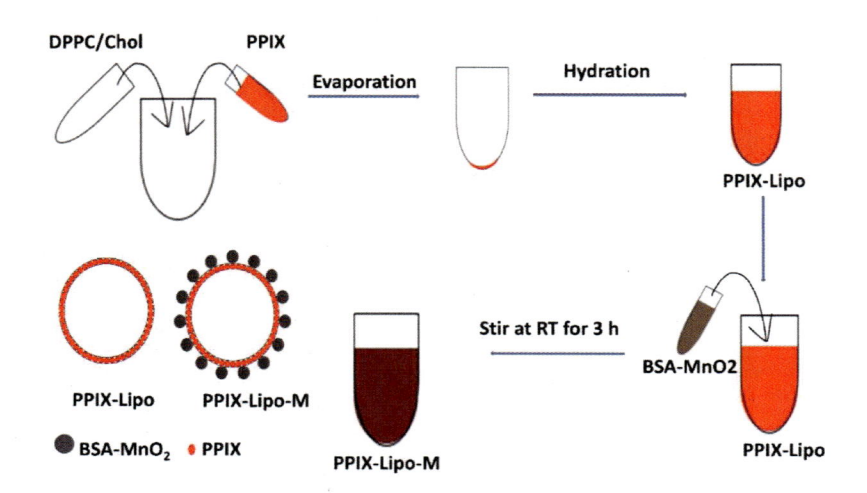

Figure 6-3: Schematic of synthesis of PPIX-Lipo and PPIX-Lipo. Adopted from ref. 4 with permission

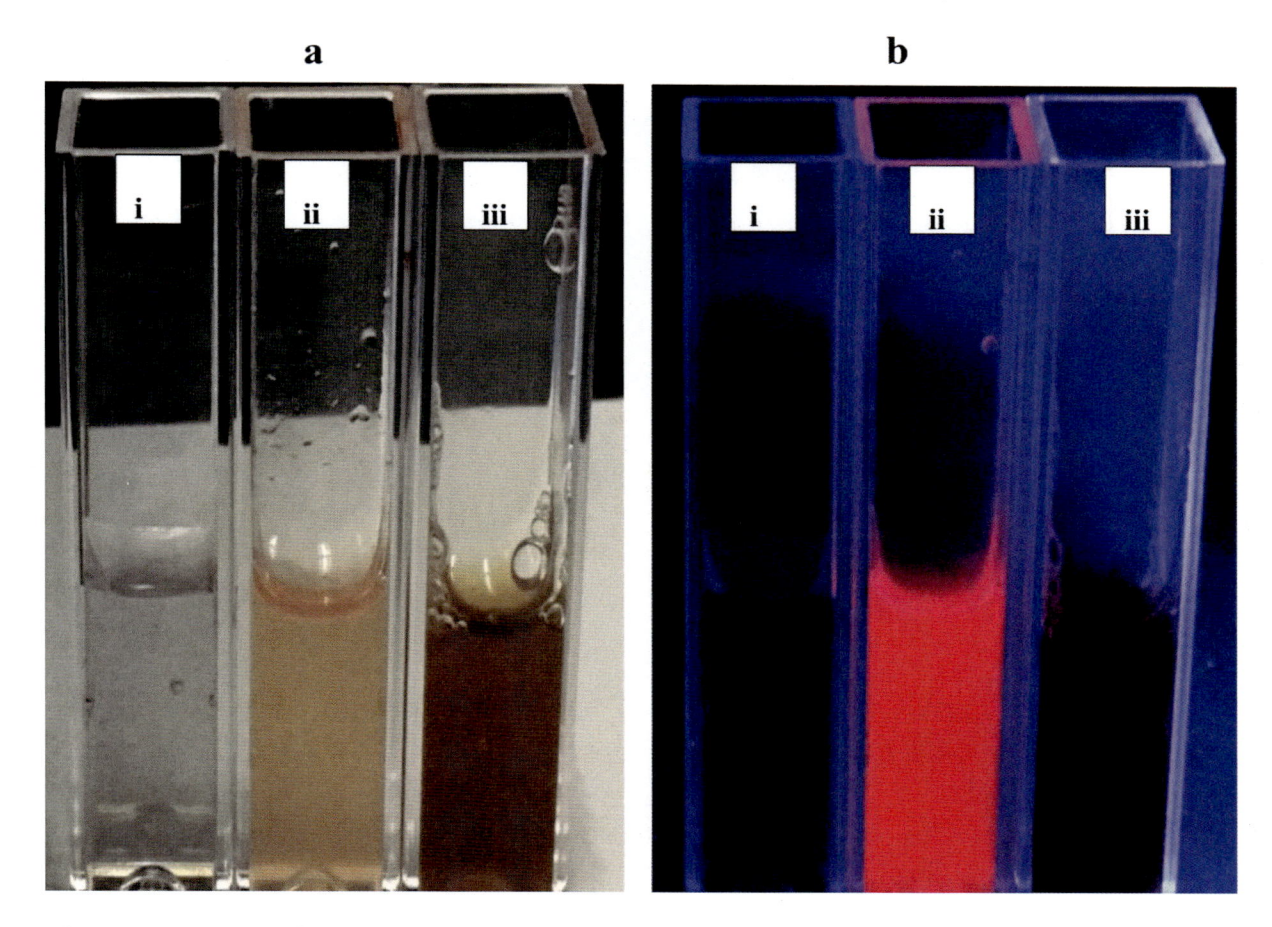

Figure 6-4 Images of bare PPIX(i), PPIX-Lipo(ii), and PPIX-Lipo-M(iii) under (a) room-light and (b) UV-light respectively. Adopted from ref. 4 with permission

UV–vis absorption and photoluminescence spectra measurement

UV–Vis absorption spectra of PPIX-Lipo, PPIX-Lipo-M, and MnO_2 are shown in Fig. 6-5a. PPIX-Lipo-M has increased absorptions in the 200–400 nm region in UV region, which indicates the conjugation of PPIX and MnO_2. Adsorption of MnO_2 on PPIX-Lipo surface was further confirmed by measuring the quenching of the luminescence of PPIX by MnO_2 (Fig. 6-5b). MnO_2 adsorbed onto the liposome surface is expected to improve its resistance against photobleaching. We measured the change in luminescence after 5 min of UV light exposure to both PPIX-Lipo and PPIX Lipo-M (Fig. 6-5c). As anticipated, it was observed that PPIX-Lipo lost its luminescence by 25% within 15 min of cumulative UV light application, while PPIX-Lipo-M lost only 9% of its luminescence. The improved resistance against photobleaching could be attributed to the MnO$_2$ adsorbed onto the liposome surface.

The encapsulation efficiency of PPIX into the liposome was determined by comparing the PL intensity of PPIX-Lipo and bare PPIX. Both PPIX-Lipo and PPIX were dissolved in DMSO. As shown in Fig. 6-5d, the slope (integrated PL intensity per unit micromolar concentration) of PPIX-Lipo was found to be 2151.9 ± 58.9 arb. unit/μM, whereas that of PPIX was 2770 ± 180.3 arb. unit/μM. Comparing these two slopes, it was calculated that 78 % ± 7% of PPIX was encapsulated in the liposome.

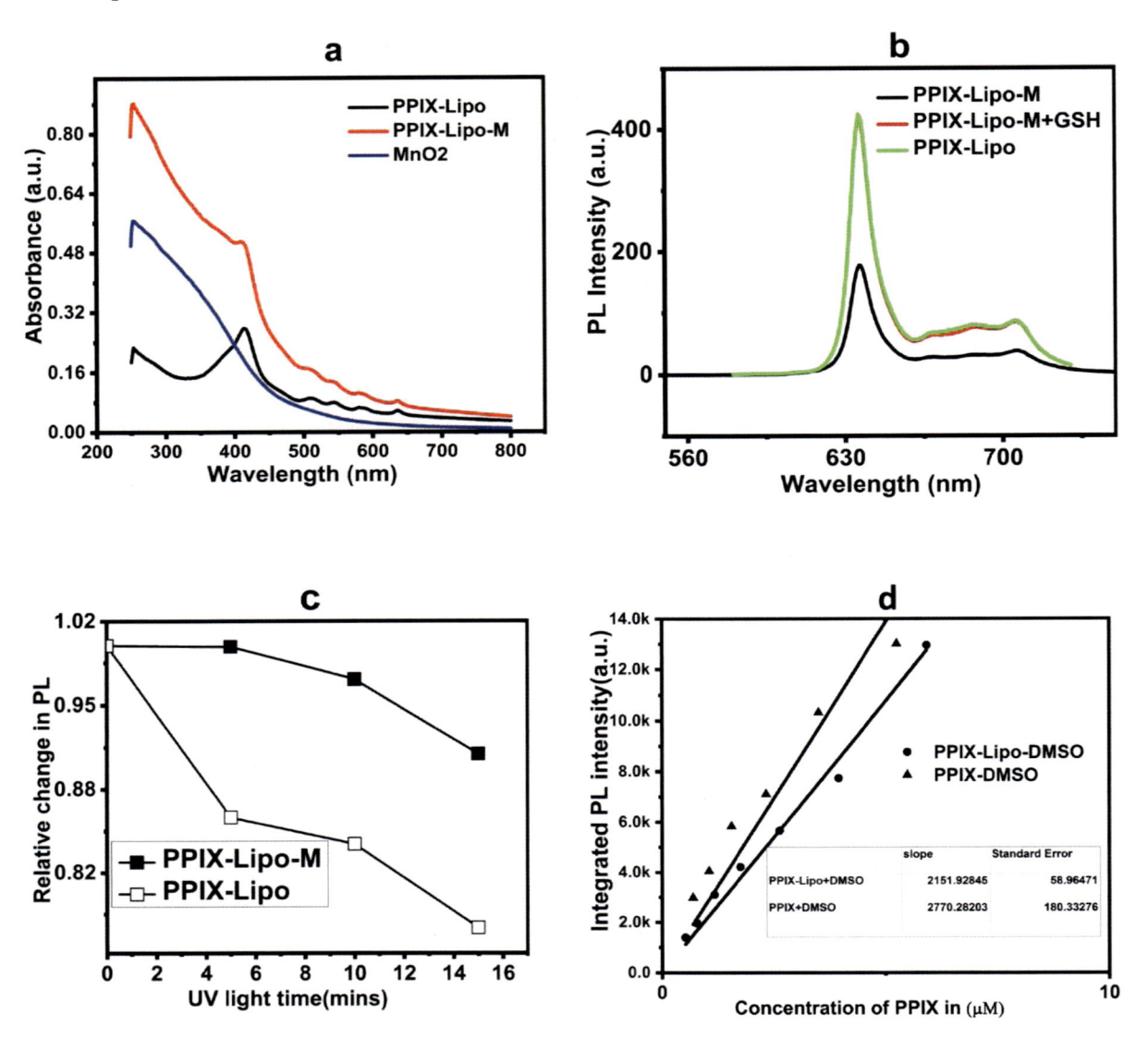

Figure 6-5: (a) UV-Vis absorption spectra of PPIX-Lipo, PPIX-Lipo-M and MnO$_2$. PPIX-Lipo is more symmetric about 420 nm, whereas PPIX-Lipo-M has raised absorption in the range of 200 nm-350 nm. (b) PL spectra of PPIX-Lipo with or without 3 mM GSH. PPIX-Lipo-M regained its luminescence in the presence of GSH. (c) PL quenching of PPIX-Lipo and PPIX-Lipo-M under UV light excitation. (d) determination of encapsulation efficiency. Adopted from ref. 4 with permission

Singlet oxygen measurement

Most cancer cells have an enhanced level of H$_2$O$_2$. MnO$_2$ reacts with H$_2$O$_2$ under acidic conditions and produces oxygen. SOSG is used to determine singlet oxygen generation by PPIX-Lipo and PPIX-Lipo-M with and without H$_2$O$_2$ under UV light excitation. In the absence of H$_2$O$_2$, PPIX-Lipo produced more singlet oxygen than PPIX-Lipo-M. In the presence of H$_2$O$_2$, PPIX-Lipo-M produced more singlet oxygen than PPIX-Lipo because of extra oxygen produced by MnO$_2$ reacting with H$_2$O$_2$.

pH change induced by MnO$_2$

MnO$_2$ reacts with H$_2$O$_2$ under acidic conditions efficiently, and it may help to increase pH of the tumour microenvironment. The data shows that with the addition of 150 µM of MnO$_2$ to an acidic solution containing 100 µM of H$_2$O$_2$, pH increased from 5.6 to 7.2 within 20 min.

Cellular uptake

Cellular uptake study of PPIX-Lipo and PPIX-Lipo-M to MCF-7 cell lines are presented in Fig. 6-6. The blue channel represents the HOECHST-stained nucleus. The red channel represents the luminescence from PPIX. HOECHST and PPIX channels were merged to confirm the cellular uptake. Confocal images (Fig. 6-6) reveal that PPIX-Lipo gets into the cell; bright red luminescent PPIX-Lipo can be seen localized in the same plane as the nucleus.

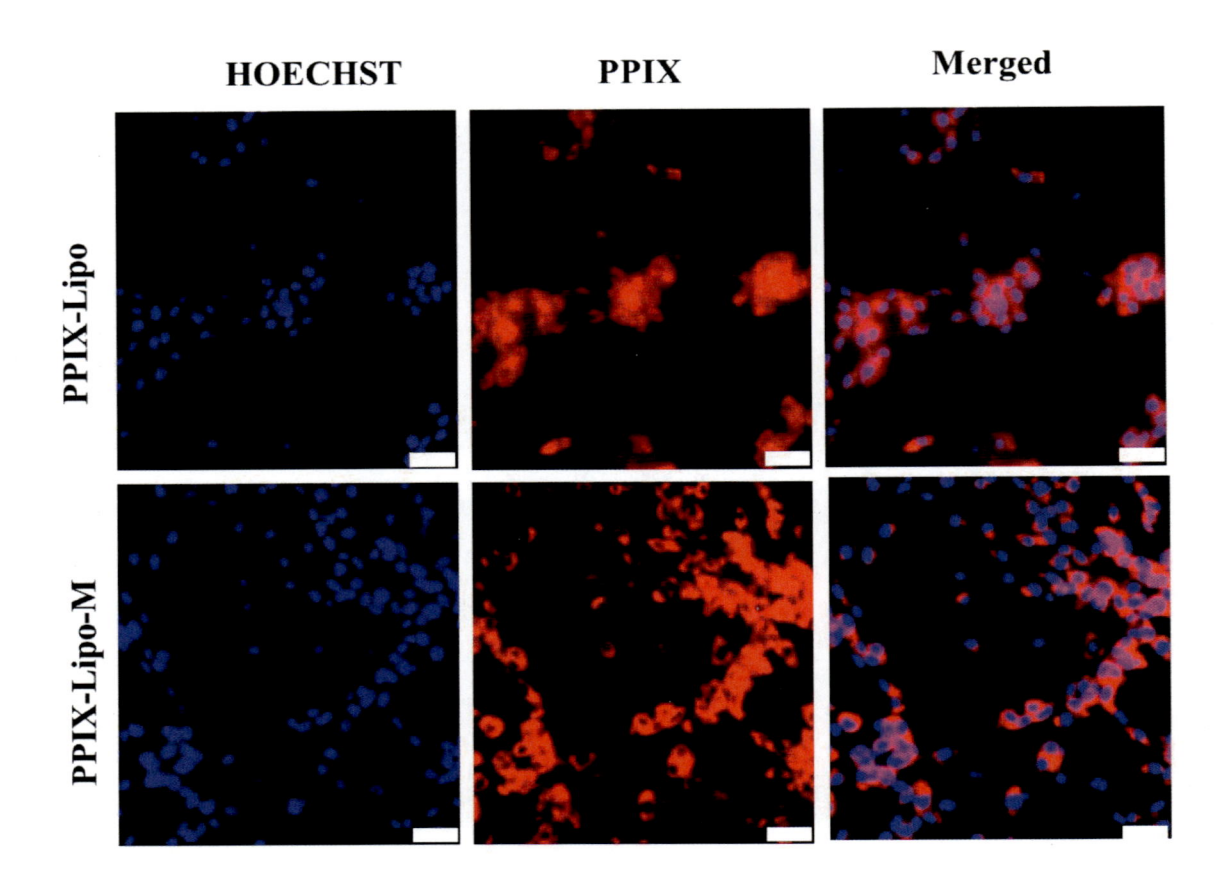

Figure 6-6: Cellular uptake study of PPIX-Lipo and PPIX-Lipo-M into MCF-7 cancer cells by using fluorescence microscopy. PPIX-Lipo and PPIX-Lipo-M were applied to MCF-7 following 24 hours incubation. HOECHST dye was applied 5 minutes before imaging to stain nuclei. (Scale bar: 50 µm). Adopted from ref. 4 with permission

Cellular viability study

Using MTT assay, cell viability of PPIX-Lipo, PPIX-Lipo-M, and MnO_2 was determined (Fig. 6-7). The concentrations of the PPIX were varied from 0 to 60 µM for both PPIX-Lipo and PPIX-Lipo-M. All the plates were protected from light by covering them with aluminum foil. The concentrations below 3 µM had minimal dark toxicity (Fig. 6-7b).

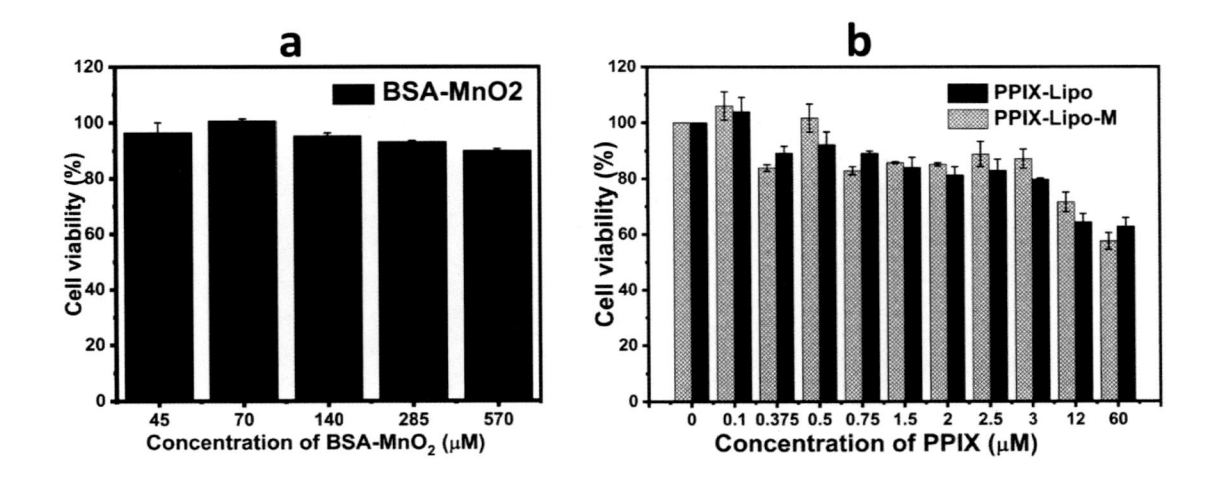

Figure 6-7: Cell viability study of MnO2, PPIX-Lipo, and PPIX-Lipo-M treated MCF-7 cell lines. Cells were incubated with the particles for 24 hours and were protected from light with aluminum foil. MnO2 does not show substantial toxicity to MCF-7 cell lines up to 570 μM concentration. PPIX-Lipo and PPIX-Lipo-M both have more than 80 % cell viability at and below 3 μM. No significance difference was observed between the toxicity of PPIX-Lipo and PPIX-Lipo-M. Adopted from ref. 4 with permission

Hypoxia induction and detection

Cobalt chloride is known as a hypoxia inducing agent *in vitro* and *in vivo*. A 50 to 100 μM concentration has been reported as non-toxic and efficient at inducing hypoxia. The use of cobalt chloride allows us to open the plate and to apply UV light outside the incubator without interrupting hypoxia. It induces hypoxia by occupying of the HIF-α binding domain of a von Hippel-Lindau protein, thereby preventing the degradation of HIF-α.

The hypoxia induction was confirmed by using an ROS-ID® Hypoxia/Oxidative stress detection kit (Enzo Life Sciences) and fluorescence microscopy detection according to the manufacturer's instructions. The control group was incubated with regular media, while the hypoxia group was incubated with media containing 100 μM of cobalt chloride for 16 h. The non-luminescent probe becomes red fluorescent under hypoxic conditions. It takes advantage of the nitroreductase activity present in hypoxic cells, which converts nitro-group to hydroxylamine and amino group and releases the red-luminescent probe. A can be seen in Fig. 6-8, the cobalt chloride treated cells shows the bright red luminescence from hypoxia red, whereas the cells incubated without cobalt chloride do not show red luminescence from hypoxia red. The result implies the successful induction of hypoxic conditions in the MCF-7 cell lines.

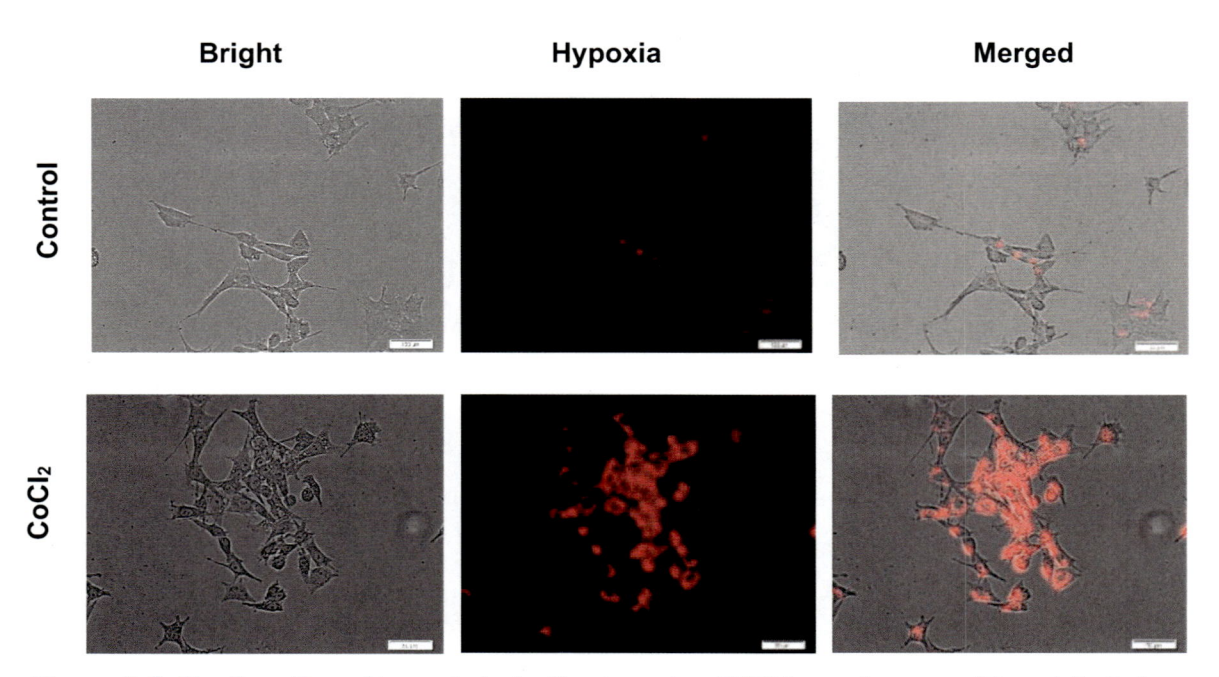

Figure 6-8: Confirmation of hypoxia induction by using ROS-hypoxia assay (Enzo Life Sciences) on MCF-7 cell lines. The red luminescence confirms cellular hypoxia. The increase in red luminescence of the assay in cobalt chloride treated cell indicates successful induction of hypoxia. (Scale bar: 50 μm). Adopted from ref. 4 with permission

PDT effect study

Normoxic conditions

Fig. 6-9a depicts the PDT effect of PPIX-Lipo and PPIX-Lipo-M to the MCF-7 cell lines under normoxic conditions. Under normoxia, it was observed that the PPIX-Lipo killed more cells than the PPIX-Lipo-M (Fig. 6-9a). Normoxia is regarded as a condition where the cellular oxygen level is at its normal value of 38 mmHg to 160 mm Hg. Cell culture media, which are incubated in an incubator with 95% O_2 and 5% CO_2, is expected to have normoxic conditions. Under normoxic conditions, the PPIX-Lipo may produce larger amounts of singlet oxygen than PPIX-Lipo-M, which is consistent with what was observed during the singlet oxygen measurement. Higher singlet oxygen production by PPIX-Lipo can be attributed to the fact that PPIX-Lipo-M does not have direct access to the light due to MnO_2 being adsorbed onto the liposome surface. PPIX-Lipo has smaller size than PPIX-Lipo-M, which might result in higher cellular uptake of PPIX-Lipo and hence better efficacy of PPIX-Lipo.

Hypoxic conditions

In Fig. 6-9b, for 1.5 and 2 µM concentration groups, PPIX-Lipo-M killed more cells than PPIX-Lipo. The IC-50 value of PPIX-Lipo-M (1.625 µM ± 0.27 µM) was significantly lower than that of PPIX-Lipo (2.21 µM ± 0.09 µM) (Fig. 6-9c), which indicates that during hypoxic conditions, PPIX-Lipo-M performs better than PPIX Lipo. The addition of MnO_2 to PPIX-Lipo can aid in overcoming the hypoxic conditions of the cancer cells by generating oxygen by reacting with endogenous H_2O_2. Higher production of singlet oxygen species by PPIX-Lipo-M kills more cells.

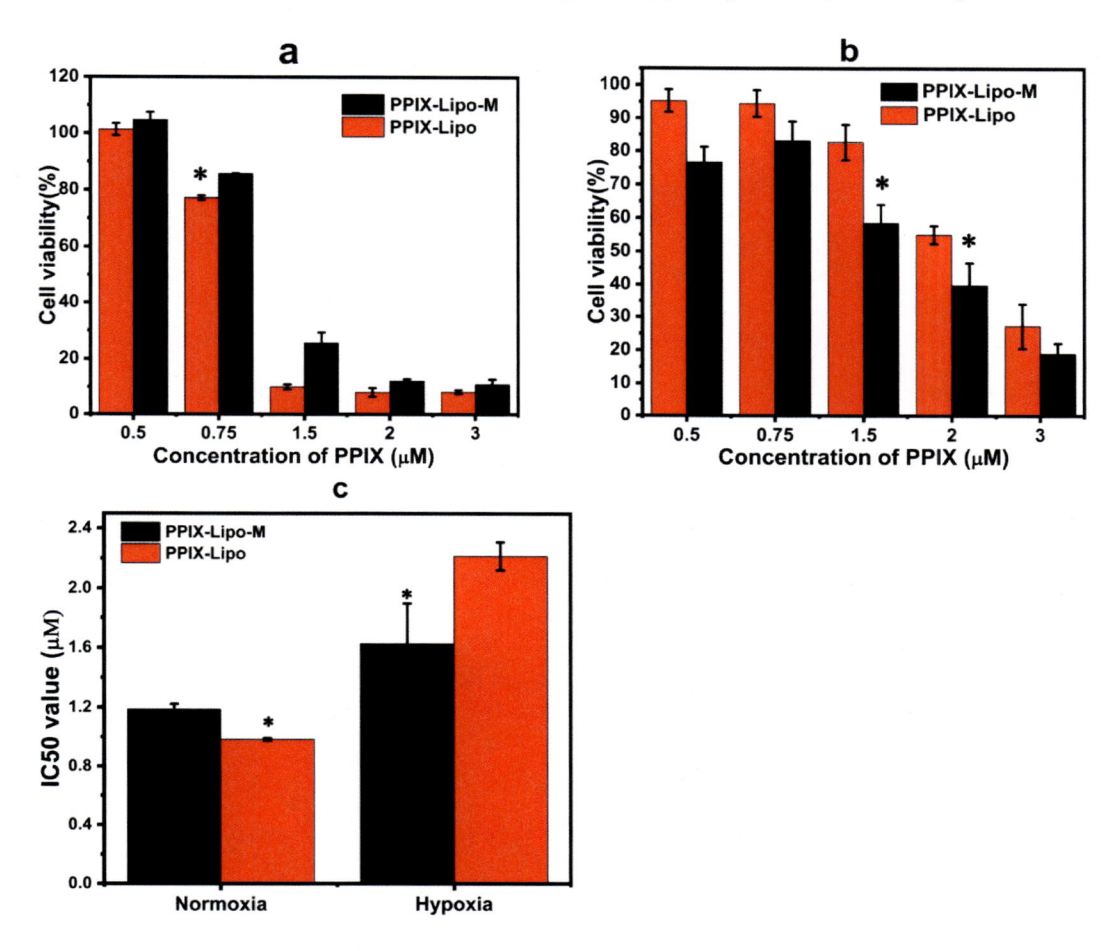

Figure 6-9: Study of PDT effect of PPIX-Lipo and PPIX-Lipo-M under (a) normoxia, (b) hypoxia, and (c)IC-50 values of PPIX-Lipo and PPIX-Lipo-M to MCF-7 cell lines and incubated for 24

hours. Commercial UV-light was used for 5 minutes as an excitation source. * indicates $p < 0.05$ significant difference from the corresponding group. Adopted from ref. 4 with permission

Discussions

Tumours have a unique environment called the tumour microenvironment (TME) which helps for the sustained growth, invasion, and metastasis of cancer cells. Characteristics of TME are hypoxia, lower pH, and elevated levels of both glutathione and H_2O_2.

MnO_2 possesses several characteristics to enhance the PDT effect of photosensitizers; it has high specificity and reactivity toward H_2O_2, producing O_2 and H_2O while consuming protons in the reaction.

As shown in Fig. 5b, MnO_2 can react with GSH and H_2O_2 under acidic conditions producing oxygen as well as increasing pH value. The reaction scheme of MnO_2 with H_2O_2 is presented below:

$$MnO_2 + 2H_2O_2 \rightarrow Mn^{2+} + O_2 + 2H_2O$$

$$MnO_2 + 2H_2O_2 \xrightarrow{H^+} Mn^{2+} + O_2 + 2H_2O$$

Following the reaction, the MnO_2 nanoparticles disintegrate into Mn^{2+} ions which can easily be cleared via renal clearance.

PPIX is an FDA-approved photosensitizer. Liposomes were utilized for drug delivery because of their known capacity to encapsulate both hydrophilic and hydrophobic drugs. The amphiphilic nature of PPIX causes it to aggregate in the aqueous environment either via π-π stacking or intermolecular interactions between the hydrophilic -COOH group and the hydrophobic porphyrin core.

It is generally accepted that liposome encapsulation reduces drug toxicity. PPIX is encapsulated into liposomes (PPIX-Lipo) and then conjugated with BSA coated MnO_2 to fabricate the PPIX-Lipo-M nano-system. Liposomal encapsulation drastically improved the solubility of PPIX. As compared to naked PPIX, PPIX-Lipo had much better cellular uptake that enhanced its photodynamic effect. PPIX-Lipo-M can improve the efficacy of photodynamic therapy by supplying oxygen to the cancer cells.

Cobalt chloride is used to induce cellular hypoxia, a reliable and economical alternative to the hypoxia chamber. The use of cobalt chloride allowed us to handle the cell plates easily and apply UV-light outside the incubator without disturbing hypoxia. PPIX-Lipo-M is less effective than PPIX-Lipo under normoxia conditions. However, when hypoxia was created, PPIX-Lipo was not effective due to the lack of oxygen. In contrast, PPIX-Lipo-M could produce oxygen due to the reactions between MnO_2 and H_2O_2. Accordingly, PPIX-Lipo- M produces significantly more singlet oxygen than PPIX-Lipo.

The Bottom Line

In conclusion, PPIX-Lipo was coated with MnO_2 nanoparticles. The coating of MnO_2 on the PPIX-Lipo surface was confirmed by measuring the PL quenching effect of MnO_2 on PPIX- Lipo. Hypoxia was successfully induced to MCF-7 cell lines by incubating them with cobalt chloride for 16 h. PPIX-Lipo-M could solve hypoxia issues in the tumour microenvironments by converting the H_2O_2 into oxygen, thereby improving the efficacy of photodynamic therapy.

6.3 Copper-Cysteamine Nanoparticles as a Heterogeneous Fenton-Like Catalyst for Highly Selective Cancer Treatment

One of the most effective ways to enhance the selectivity of cancer drugs is to fabricate drugs that can be activated by cancer-specific stimuli as most of the conventional cancer drugs lack selectivity leading to the manifestation of toxic effects on healthy cells, resulting in numerous side effects. The tumour microenvironment (TME) is characterized by mild acidity, elevated H_2O_2 levels, hypoxia, low catalase activity, and elevated levels of GSH.

Fenton reactions refer to the process in which Fe and its salts catalyze the conversion of H_2O_2 to •OH. If other cations, such as Cu, Ag, Mn, and Au, participate in the catalytic conversion, then such reactions are referred to as Fenton-like reactions. Considering elevated levels of H_2O_2 and slightly acidic pH in TME, Fenton and Fenton-like reactions can be exploited to achieve highly selective cancer treatment. The nanocatalysts used without external additives needed to be administered at high doses in order to achieve desired therapeutic outcomes. Cu-based materials are an efficient Fenton catalyst and are used in developing new cancer treatments.

Highest reaction rate of Cu^{1+} with H_2O_2 (10^4 M^{-1} s^{-1}) is considerably higher than that of Fe^{2+} (63 M^{-1} s^{-1}). Cu^{2+} based heterogeneous nanocatalyst that can be activated by GSH and H_2O_2 following a logic "AND" gate; however, this catalyst requires a high dose of 200 µg/mL for optimum efficacy. Higher levels of copper could cause damage to vital organs, including the brain and liver. Therefore, if Cu-based catalysts are to be used for cancer therapy, then we must find a way to lower their effective dose such that they may be physiologically tolerable. One way to improve the efficiency of a heterogeneous Cu-based catalyst is developing the catalyst that has copper in its reduced state (Cu^{1+}) rather than in its oxidized state (Cu^{2+}) as the reaction rate of Cu^{1+} is approximately 22 times faster than that of Cu^{2+} (eqs 1 and 2).

$$Cu^{1+} + H_2O_2 \rightarrow Cu^{2+} + \bullet OH + OH^- \;(k = 1 \times 10^4 M^{-1}S^{-1}) \quad (1)$$

$$Cu^{2+} + H_2O_2 \rightarrow Cu^{1+} + \bullet HO_2^- + H^+ \;(k = 460 M^{-1}S^{-1}) \quad (2)$$

Copper-cysteamine (Cu-Cy) nanoparticles (NPs) are assessed for their heterogenous Fenton-like activity and their potential use in highly selective cancer therapy. The Cu-Cy NP being activatable by multiple excitation sources, is already a promising candidate for a new nanomedicine to combat cancer. Cu-Cy NP is a novel sensitizer having Cu^{1+} instead of Cu^{2+}, which can be stimulated by X-rays, UV-light, microwaves, and ultrasound to produce various types of ROS for cancer treatment. Furthermore, Cu-Cy can be used to inactivate bacteria upon UV light activation. The •OH produced by Cu-Cy NPs and H_2O_2 (100 μM) in aqueous solutions were systematically explored at different pHs and doses using coumarin as an •OH detecting probe.

Study of Fenton-Like Reaction in Aqueous Solution

1. Hydroxyl Radical (•OH) Measurement

Cu-Cy NPs were examined for their ability to participate in Fenton-like reactions using coumarin as the •OH detection probe. A typical testing solution contained an appropriate amount of Cu-Cy, H_2O_2, and 0.1 mM coumarin at different pH values (7.4, 6.5, and 5.5). The PL spectrum of coumarin with excitation 332 nm was monitored at various time intervals for up to 6 h. The PL intensity of coumarin at 452 nm was plotted against various time intervals to serve as a semiquantitative •OH detection.

2. Stability Study A standard calibration curve between Cu^{2+} concentration and absorbance by using $CuCl_2 \cdot 2H_2O$ as a source of free Cu^{2+}. One mg/mL of Cu-Cy and 100 μM of H_2O_2 were mixed and incubated for 24 h at room temperature. Then, the mixture was centrifuged at 12 000 rpm for 30 min, and the supernatant was used to detect any free copper leached from Cu-Cy. A 3 mL testing solution was prepared by mixing 1200 μL of the supernatant of the sample, 300 μL of PEI, 300 μL of Bronstate-Robinson buffer, and 1200 μL of DI water. The absorption of the testing solution was collected, and the calibration equation A= 4093.964C ± 0.03327 was used to determine the concentration of Cu^{2+}. $CuCl_2$ (0.2 mM), a source of free Cu^{2+}, was used as a positive control.

The stability of Cu-Cy during the Fenton-like reaction was also assessed by monitoring PL intensity of Cu-Cy incubated with or without H_2O_2 under different pHs at various time points up to 24 h. The XRD patterns and FTIR spectra of Cu-Cy incubated with or without H_2O_2 (pH 7.4 and 5.5) for 24 h were also collected in order to determine the stability of Cu-Cy NPs during the Fenton-like reaction.

In Vitro ROS Measurement

2′,7′-Dichlorofluorescein diacetate (DCFH-DA) was employed to detect intracellular ROS levels after Cu-Cy treatment. 2×10^5 cells per imaging plate were cultured and incubated for 24 h. Then, the old media was replaced with new media with or without Cu-Cy (30 μg/mL) and incubated overnight. On the next day, the cells were treated with serum-free media containing 20 μM of DCFH-DA and incubated for 1 h. Afterward, the cells were replaced with regular media and imaged using an Olympus IX-71 fluorescence microscope (495/515 nm filter), keeping the same exposure time and sensitivity throughout the experiment.

The DCF intensities were quantified using ImageJ software as follows: first, the background luminescence of each image was subtracted. Next, the "Threshold" function was applied to select only DCF luminescence in the cellular body. Finally, "Measure" function was used to obtain the average gray value of the DCF luminescence.

In Vitro Selective Toxicity Study

1. Oxygen Consumption Rate Assay

The effect of Cu-Cy on the mitochondrial function of the cancer cell lines (KYSE-30 and DM6) and normal (HET1A) cells were evaluated by measuring the oxygen consumption rates (OCR) via the Seahorse XFp analyzer. The cells were seeded in XFp culture microplates (Seahorse Bioscience, North Billerica, MA). Each plate was seeded with 3×10^4 cells/well in 80 μL of culture medium. Following 2 h of incubation, various concentrations of 120 μL of Cu-Cy was added so that a final concentration of 45, 30, 22.5, and 11.25 mg/L in a 200 μL culture medium were achieved. The plates were then incubated overnight in a humidified incubator (37 °C, 5% CO_2). The control group was supplemented with 120 μL of the respective medium. On the next day, the culture media was replaced with freshly prepared Seahorse Assay Media (Seahorse Bioscience, Billerica, MA) and incubated in a non-CO_2, 37 °C incubator for 1 h.

After measuring the basal OCR, a number of mitochondrial modulators were sequentially injected. First, 2 μM of oligomycin (an ATP synthase inhibiter) was added to determine the respiration contributed by proton leakage. After that, a mitochondrial uncoupler (FCCP(0.5 μM)) was used to force the cells to operate at their maximal respiration rates. Finally, Rotenone/antimycin (0.5 μM), a mitochondrial oxidative phosphorylation inhibitor, was used. Various respiration parameters were obtained by using the manufacturer's-built software (Wave). To compare the effect of Cu-Cy on OCR values of different cell lines, they were expressed as the percentage of the respective control group (without Cu-Cy).

2. Live/Dead Cell Assay

Live/dead assay was employed to evaluate cell viability. Two ×10^5 cells were seeded in a 35 mm Petridish and then incubated at 37 °C in a humidified atmosphere of 5% v/v CO_2 for 24 h. Then, 1 mL of new media containing desired concentrations of Cu-Cy NPs were added to the Petri-dishes. The cell samples were stained with 0.25 μmol/L of calcein-AM and 5 μmol/L of ethidium homodimer-1 (Invitrogen, Waltham, MA) for 45 min. Fluorescent images were taken by using an Olympus IX-71 fluorescence microscope. The results of the live/dead assay were quantified using the "Particle analyzer" feature of the ImageJ software.

Bright-Field Imaging

Olympus IX-71 fluorescence microscope was used to observe the changes in the morphology of the cell lines following the Cu-Cy treatment.

MTT Assay

The cytotoxicity of Cu-Cy to cancer and normal cell lines was further evaluated using MTT assay. 1×10^4 cells/well were seeded in 96 well plates and incubated for 24 h. A stock solution of a desired concentration of Cu-Cy was prepared in DI water. 100 μL of various doses of Cu-Cy NPs were applied and incubated for 24 h. Afterward, the old media was replaced with 100 μL of MTT solution and incubated for 3 h. Then, 150 μL DMSO was used to solubilize formazan crystals, and the absorption of the purple-colored formazan crystals was measured using a microplate reader (Multiskan). Cell viability was then calculated as presented in the following equation:

$$\text{cell viability} = \frac{\text{the absorbance of the treatment group}}{\text{the absorbance of the control group}} \times 100\%$$

Selectivity was quantified by determining selectivity index as follows:

$$\text{selectivity index} = \frac{IC-50 \text{ of normal cells}}{IC-50 \text{ of cancer cells}}$$

RESULTS AND DISCUSSION

Characterization of As-Synthesized Cu-Cy

An excess amount of cysteamine can reduce Cu^{2+} of $CuCl_2$ to Cu^{1+}, resulting in highly crystalline copper(I)-cysteamine nanoparticles (Cu-Cy NPs). Figure 6-10A illustrates UV-visible absorption spectrum Cu-Cy NPs in DI water. As displayed in Figure 6-10B, the PL spectrum of Cu-Cy has two emission peaks at 607 and 633 nm, with an excitation peak at 365 nm. Figure 6-10C presents images of Cu-Cy dispersed in DI water under ambient light (left) and UV light (right). Figure 6-10D depicts the power XRD pattern of Cu-Cy. The HRTEM (Figure 6-10E) depicts the high crystallinity of as-synthesized Cu-Cy NPs. A representative TEM image of Cu-Cy NPs used in this work is presented in Figure 6-10F.

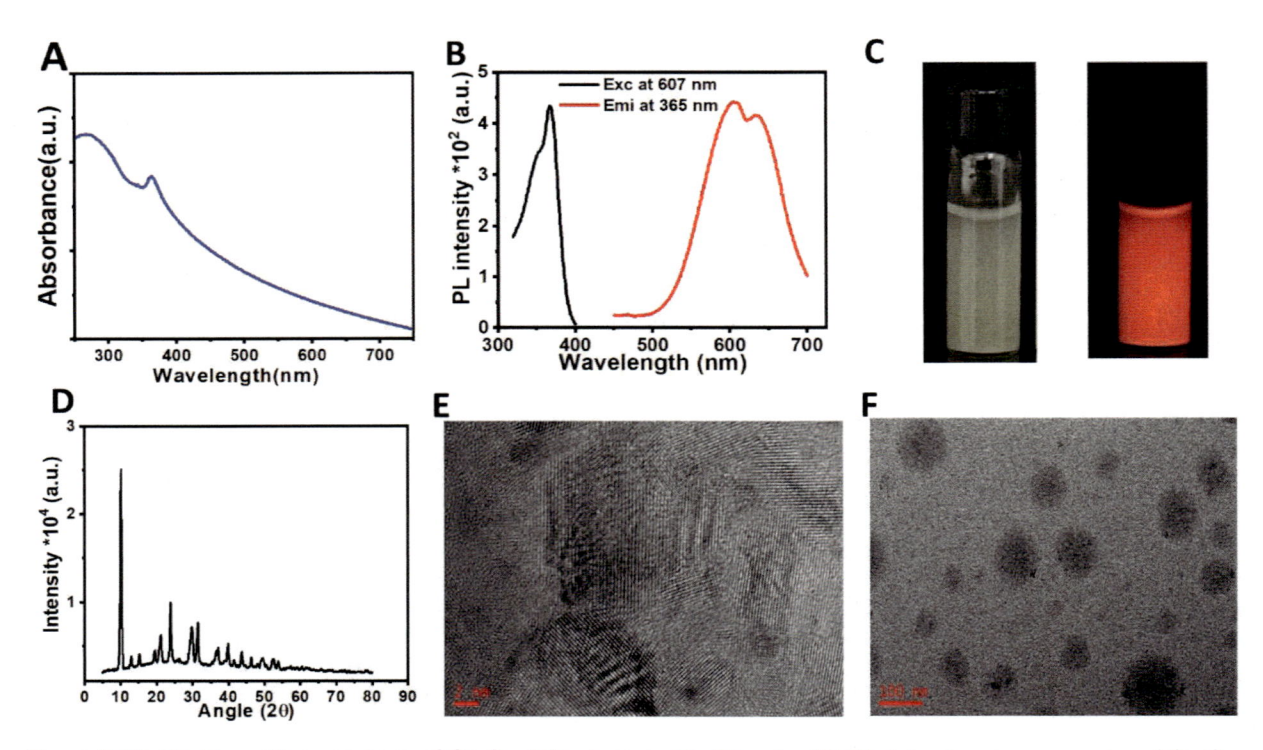

Figure 6-10 (A) Absorption spectrum of Cu-Cy NPs dispersed in DI water (B) Photoluminescence spectra of Cu-Cy with excitation and emission peaks taken at 365 nm and 607 nm, respectively (C) Image of Cu-Cy dispersed in DI water under ambient light (Left) and UV light(Right). (D) XRD pattern of Cu-Cy powders (E) HRTEM image of Cu-Cy. (F) A representative TEM image of Cu-Cy used in this study. Adopted from ref. 3 with permission

Study of Fenton-Like Reaction Mediated by Cu-Cy

It is no secret that Cu^{1+}/Cu^{2+} can actively catalyze H_2O_2 to produce •OH via a Fenton-like reaction. Consequently, Cu-Cy NPs are expected to act as a heterogeneous Fenton-like catalyst for the conversion of H_2O_2 to •OH. The •OH generated by various concentrations of Cu-Cy (0–300 µg/mL) and H_2O_2 (100 µM) is presented in Figure 6-11A. The PL intensity of 7-hydroxycoumarin increased with the increase in the Cu-Cy dosages, suggesting a higher level of •OH formation with increases in the Cu-Cy dose. Likewise, the •OH generated by various concentrations of H_2O_2 (0−1 mM) and Cu-Cy (100 µg/mL) demonstrated a clear correlation between •OH generation and H_2O_2 concentration. The results suggest that •OH generation depends upon the dose of the catalyst (Cu-Cy) and H_2O_2. Furthermore, when compared to pH 7.4, the •OH generation enhanced by 4 and 8 folds at pH 6.5 and pH 5.5, respectively. A detailed statistical analysis of •OH production at different pH after 6h of reaction is displayed in Figure 6-11D. The analysis showed that Cu-Cy + H_2O_2 produced significantly more ($p < 0.001$) •OH at pH 6.5 and 5.5 as compared to pH 7.4. These results collectively indicated that Cu-Cy NPs can exploit low pH and higher levels of H_2O_2 in cancer cells to yield substantial amounts of •OH, leading to the subsequent destruction of cancer cells.

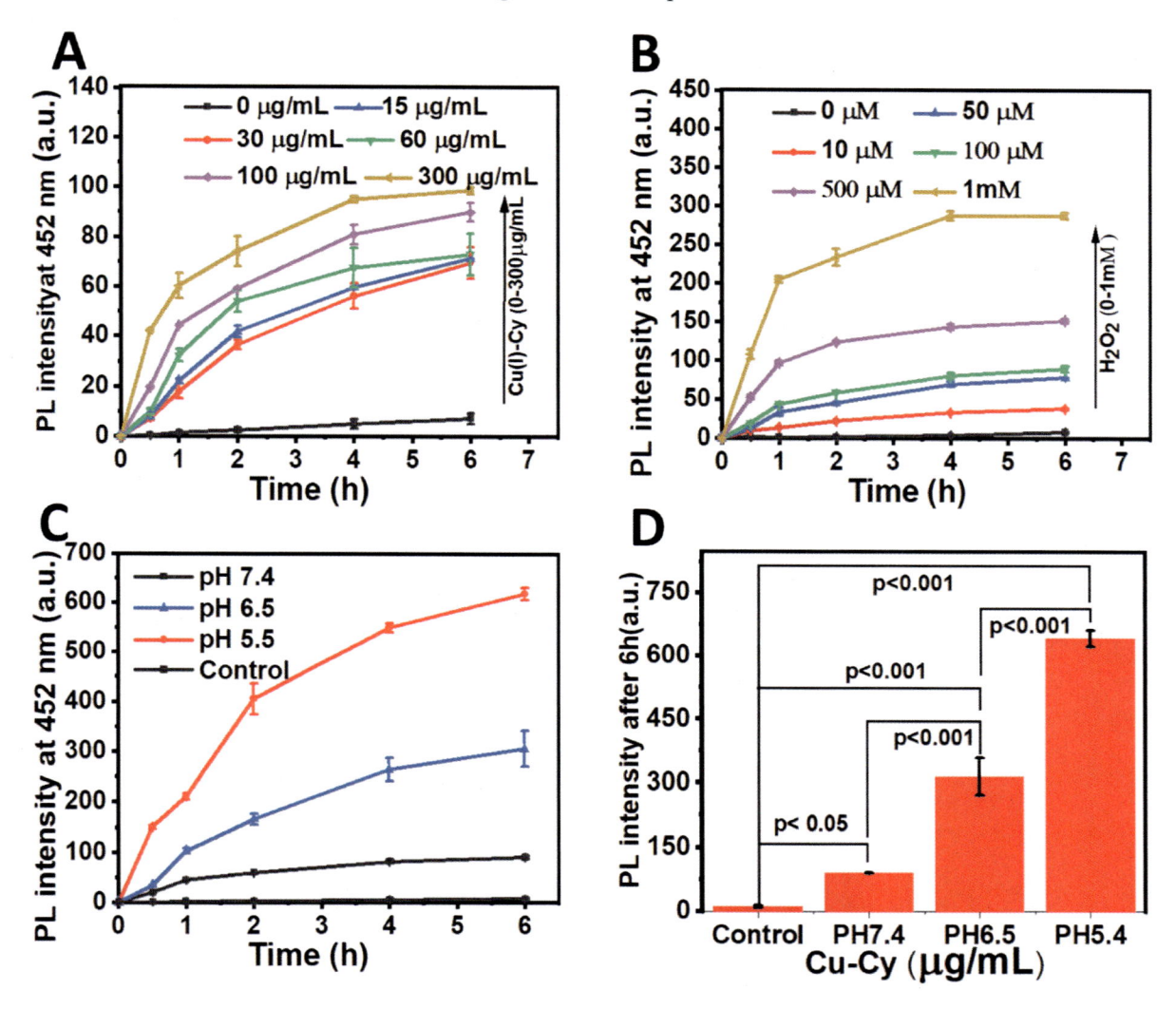

Figure 6-11. Measurement hydroxyl radical generated by Cu-Cy/ H_2O_2 using coumarin as a probe. The •OH produced by (A) Cu-Cy (0-300 µg/mL) and H_2O_2 (100 µM) and (B) Cu-Cy (100 µg/mL) and (0-1mM H_2O_2) at various time intervals. (C) The •OH generated by Cu-Cy (100 µg/mL)+ H_2O_2 (100 µM) at different pH conditions and (D) stastical analysis of •OH production after 6h of (C). The data are presented as Mean±SEM of three independent experiments. Adopted from ref. 3 with permission

Stability Study during Fenton-Like Reaction

A spectrophotometric method was employed to measure the free Cu^{2+} leached from Cu-Cy dispersion (1 mg/mL). This method is capable of measuring only free Cu^{2+} by making a PEI-Cu^{2+} complex that has a strong absorption at 275 and 630 nm. The stability of Cu-Cy during the Fenton-like reaction was further assessed by monitoring the PL intensity of Cu-Cy incubated with or without H_2O_2 up to 24 h. As depicted in Figure 6-12A, there was no apparent difference in PL intensity between the control group, Cu-Cy + H_2O_2 and Cu-Cy + H_2O_2 + pH 5.5 after 24 h incubation. From this result, we can infer the high stability of Cu-Cy during the reaction with endogenous levels of H_2O_2 (100 μM). The excellent stability of Cu-Cy also suggests that it can continuously convert endogenous H_2O_2 to •OH for many cycles, acting as a replenishable source of •OH in cancer cells.

The stability of Cu-Cy during the Fenton-like reaction was further assessed by monitoring the PL intensity of Cu-Cy incubated with or without H_2O_2 up to 24 h. As depicted in **Figure 6-12B**, there was no apparent difference in PL intensity between the control group, Cu-Cy + H_2O_2, and Cu-Cy + H_2O_2 + pH = 5.5 after 24 h incubation. From this result, we can infer the high stability of Cu-Cy during the reaction with endogenous levels of H_2O_2 (100 μM). The excellent stability of Cu-Cy also suggests that it can continuously convert endogenous H_2O_2 to ˙OH for many cycles, acting as a replenishable source of ˙OH in cancer cells.

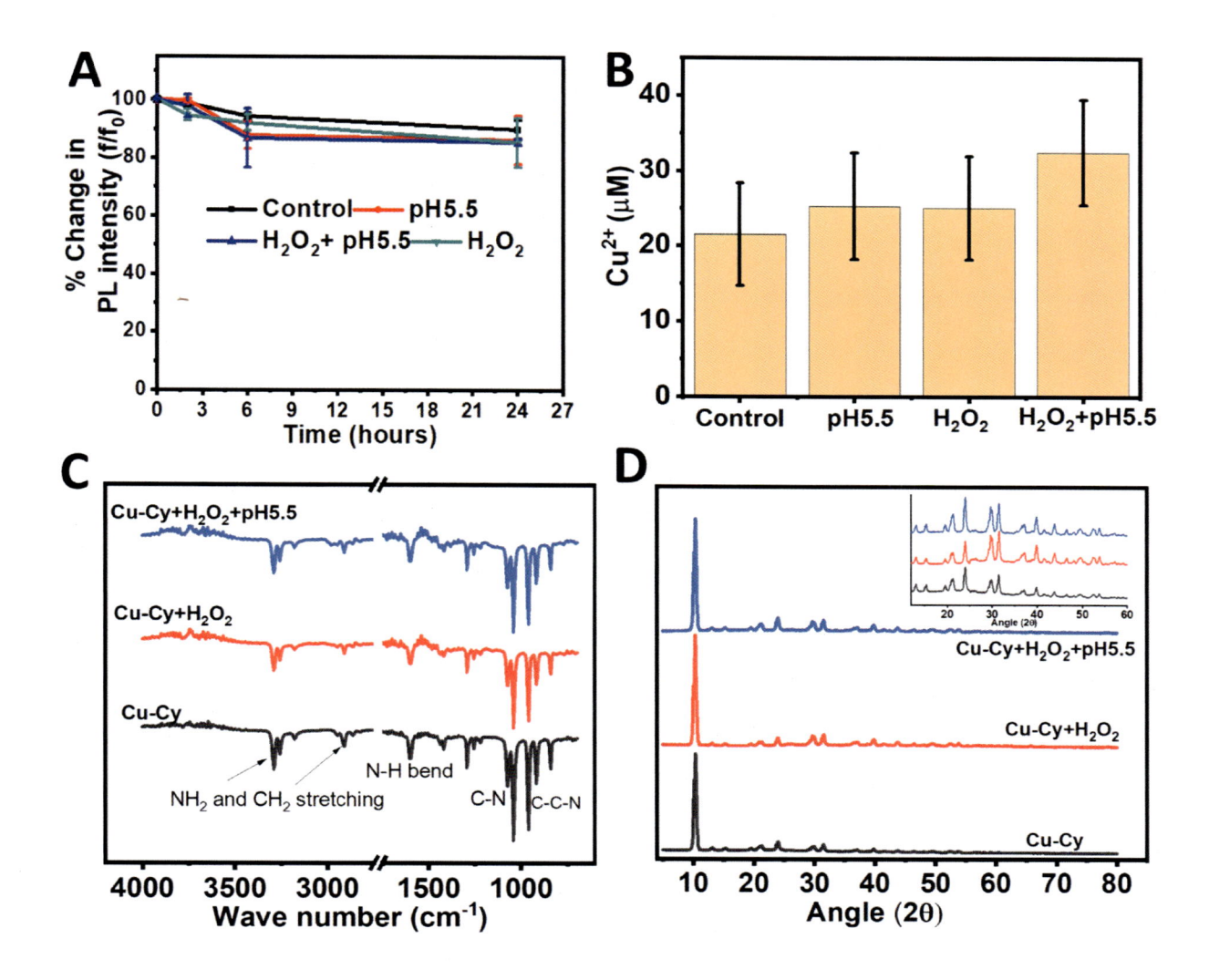

Figure 6-12. Stability test of Cu-Cy following the Fenton-like reaction. (A) Free Cu^{2+} detected in the supernatant of the Cu-Cy (1 mg/ mL) following the incubation with H_2O_2 (100 μM) upto 24 h. (B) The PL intensity change of Cu-Cy following the incubation with H_2O_2 upto 24 h. (C) FTIR spectra and (D) XRD pattern of Cu-Cy before and after Fenton-like reaction for 24 h. Adopted from ref. 3 with permission

As shown in Figure 6-12C, the FTIR spectra of Cu-Cy matched with previously reported results. The peaks at 3300 cm^{-1}, 2800 cm^{-1}, and 1600 cm^{-1} correspond to NH_2 stretching, CH_2 stretching, and N−H bending, respectively. Additionally, the peaks that are in the range of 700−1300 cm^{-1} correspond to C−N and C−C−N vibrations. As can be seen in Figure 6-12C, the FTIR spectra of Cu-Cy after the incubation with H_2O_2 at pH 7.4 and H_2O_2 (100 μM) at pH 5.5 for 24 h did not noticeably change, indicating its high stability during Fenton-like reactions. Likewise, no change was noticed in the XRD pattern of Cu-Cy following the incubation with H_2O_2 (100 μM) at pH 7.4 and H_2O_2 (100 μM) at pH 5.5 during 24 h, further confirming the high stability of Cu-Cy (Figure 3D). Overall, Cu-Cy exhibits high stability during the Fenton-like reaction, making it a potential candidate for Fenton-reaction mediated cancer therapy.

Intracellular ROS Measurement

As shown in Figure 6-13A, the luminescence of DCF in HDF was not noticeably different for cells with or without Cu-Cy treatment, suggesting that Cu-Cy did not induce noticeable ROS generation in HDF (normal cells). In contrast, Cu-Cy treated DM6 (cancer cells) showed noticeably higher luminescence than DM6 cells without Cu-Cy (control). Figure 6-13B represents the quantification of the DCF luminescence. The fluorescence (FL) intensity of DCF in Cu-Cy treated DM6 cells is significantly higher ($p < 0.01$) than that of the control. On the other hand, no such difference was noticed for HDF cells treated with or without Cu-Cy. A similar outcome was observed for a breast cancer cell line (MCF-7); the FL intensity of DCF was substantially higher in Cu-Cy treated cells than in the control group, implying higher levels of ROS in Cu-Cy treated cell lines. These results suggest that Cu-Cy can selectively produce higher amounts of ROS in cancer cells than in normal cells, most likely due to elevated levels of H_2O_2 and low pH in cancerous cells.

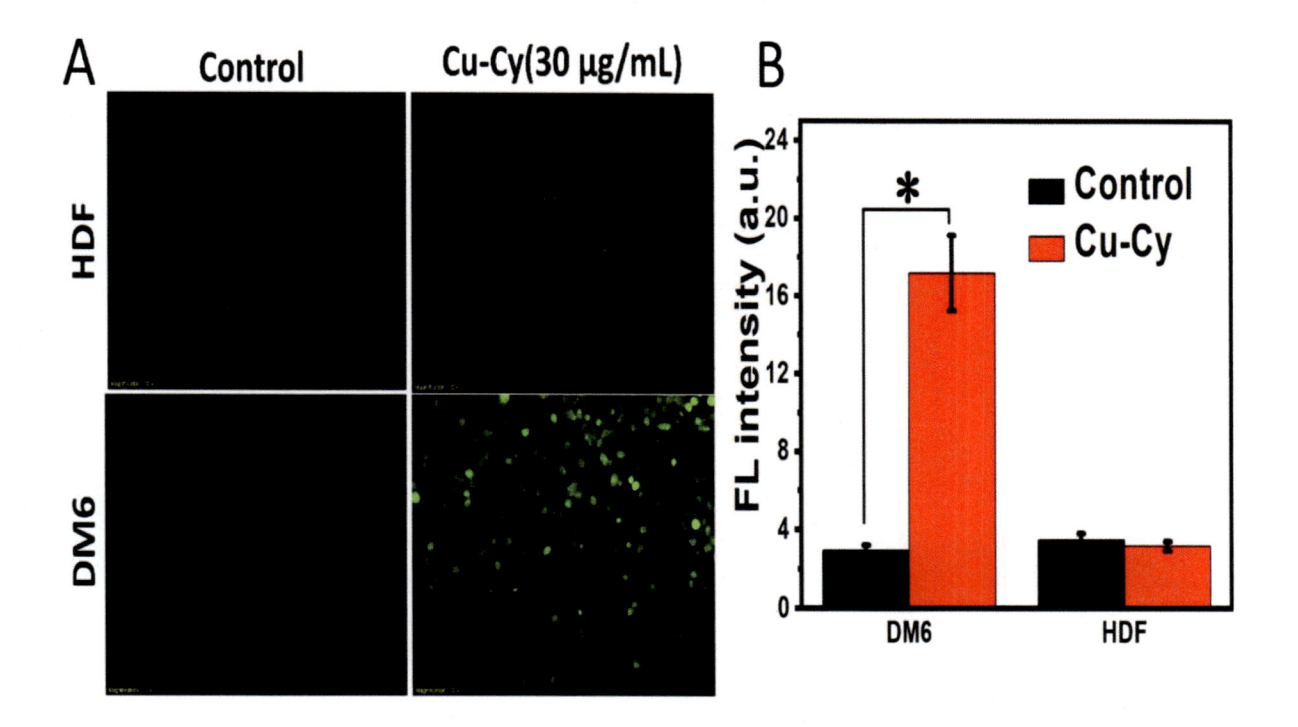

Figure 6-13. Intracellular ·OH detection using DCFH-DA. (A) Representative images (B) Quantification of ROS level. The cells pre-incubated with or without Cu-Cy for 12h were treated with 20 μM DCFH-DA for 1 h. The green luminescence of DCF was imaged using 495/515 nm filter of Olympus IX-71 and quantified using imageJ. (p< 0.01) Adopted from ref. 3 with permission*

Live/dead cell assay

A live-dead cell assay was performed to further evaluate the cytotoxicity of Cu-Cy NPs in cancer and normal cells. The live/dead assay consists of calcein-AM and ethidium homodimer-1 to stain live and dead cells, respectively. The calcein-AM stains nucleus and cytoplasm in the ratio of 3:1, indicating that it is a suitable dye for staining the whole cell body. Calcein-AM can also be used as a reliable probe for staining early apoptotic cells. Apoptotic cells undergo slow and systemic changes in cell morphology; in its early stage, the nucleus and cytoplasm condense to become round in shape while keeping the plasma membrane intact. Therefore, the apoptotic cells retain the calcein with stronger luminescence than that in viable cells.

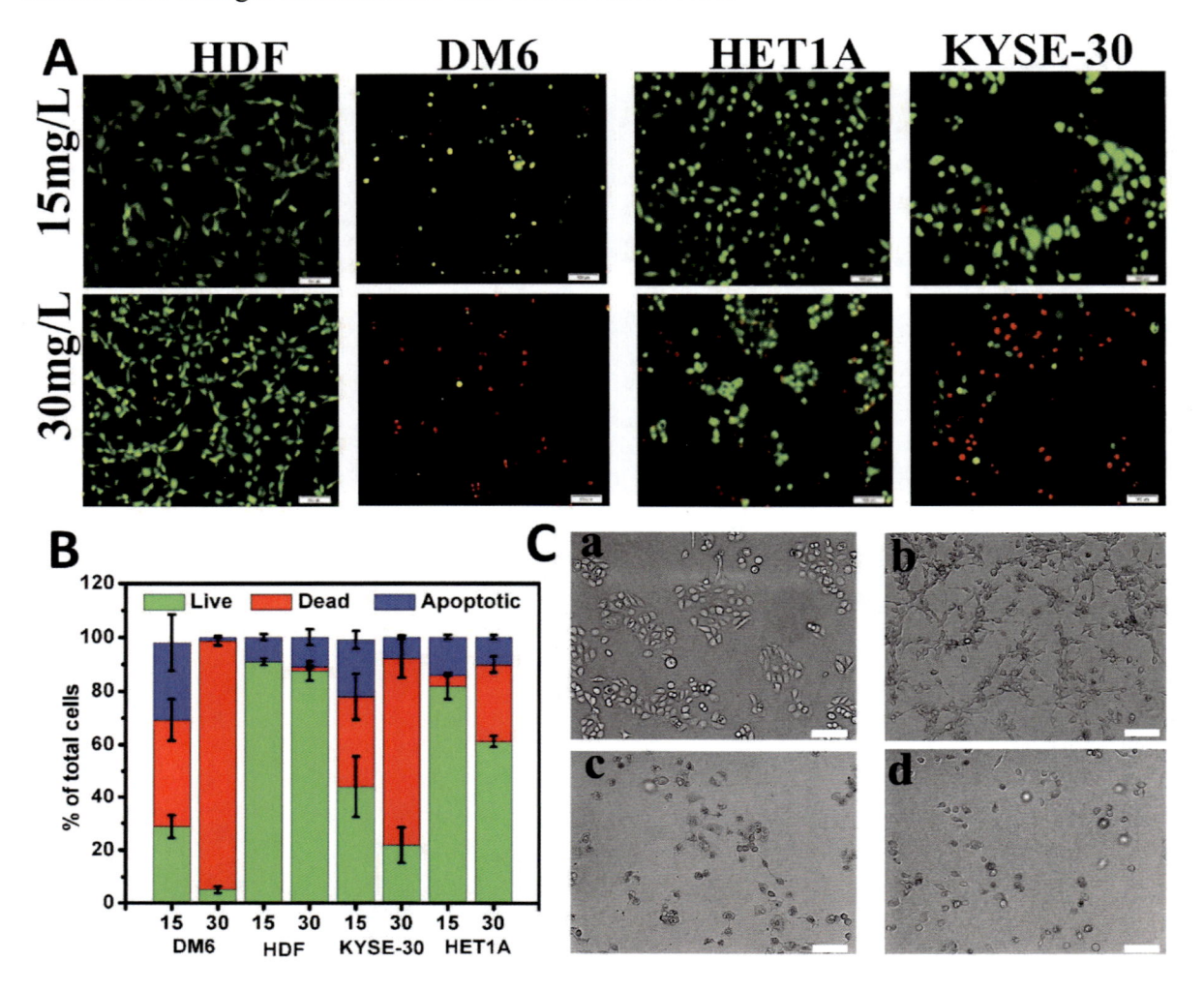

Figure 6-14. (A) Live/dead assay to assess toxicity of Cu-Cy to cancer (DM6 and KYSE-30) and normal (HDF and HET1A) cell lines: Green and red channels are from calcein-AM (Live) and Ethidum homodimer (Dead), respectively. (B) Quantification for the cell viability and early apoptosis using imageJ. (C) Bright-field imaging to observe morphological changes of the Cu-Cy (15 µg/mL) treated normal cancer cancer cell lines: **(a)** HET1A, **(b)** HDF, **(c)** KYSE-30, and **(d)** DM6. Scale bar : 100 µm.

Adopted from ref. 3 with permission

As depicted in **Figure 6-14A,** most of the Cu-Cy treated cancer cell lines (DM6 and KYSE-30) were EthD-1 positive (dead). In addition, among the calcein positive cells, a large number of cells turned into a round-shaped structure, a characteristic feature of early apoptotic cells. On the other hand, the Cu-Cy treated HET1A and HDF cells were mostly calcein positive and retained their structure, suggesting low toxicity of Cu-Cy towards normal cells.

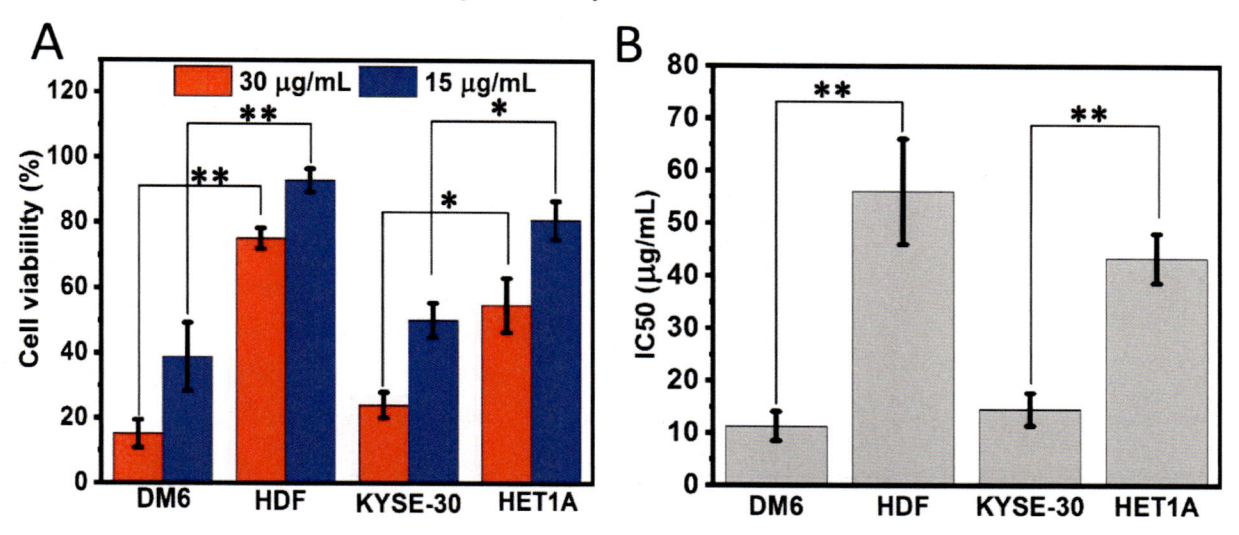

Figure 6-15: Evaluation of cytotoxicity of Cu-Cy to different cell lines using MTT assay. (A) Cell viability of different cell lines with Cu-Cy treatment . (B) IC-50 value calculation. (* p< 0.05, ** p< 0.01) Dopted from ref. 3 with permission

We also attempted to quantify live, dead, and apoptotic cells by using the particle analyzer feature of imageJ. For each image, the green (live) and red channels (dead) were merged, and representative images are presented in **Figure 6-14B**. As evident from **Figure 6-14B**, Cu-Cy NPs induced significant cytotoxicity to cancerous cells (DM6 and KYSE-30); most of the cells are either dead or apoptotic after 24h of incubation. On the other hand, under similar experimental conditions, most of the normal cells were viable with intact cell bodies.

3.6.4. Bright-field imaging of Cu-Cy treated cells

We further carried out bright field imaging to monitor morphological differences among both normal and cancer cells, following the Cu-Cy (15 mg/L) treatment **(Figure 6-14C)**. It can be seen that normal cell lines (HET1A and HDF) retained their structure after incubation with Cu-Cy for 24 h. The intact structure indicates low cytotoxicity of Cu-Cy towards normal cell lines. On the contrary, Cu-Cy treated cancer cell lines (DM6 and KYSE-30) showed a significant loss in their structure and were generally more roundly shaped. This indicates that Cu-Cy is highly toxic to cancer cell lines, but it has minimal toxicity to normal cell lines.

3.6.5. MTT assay

The selective toxicity of Cu-Cy was also explored by conducting MTT assays on two cancer cell lines (DM6 and KYSE-30) and corresponding normal cell lines (HDF and HET1A). As depicted in **Figure 6-**

15A, normal cells treated with Cu-Cy had higher cell viabilities than those of cancer cell lines. DM6 cell lines have 15 % and 39 % viability at 30 and 15 μg /mL of Cu-Cy, respectively, which is significantly lower (p < 0.01) than that of HDF (77 % and 90 % at 30 and 15 μg/mL, respectively). Similarly, cell viabilities of KYSE-30 (22 and 50% at 30 and 15 μg/mL, respectively) are significantly lower (p<0.05) than that of HET1A (58 and 80 % at 30 and 15 μg /mL, respectively). Likewise, low cell viabilities were observed for Cu-Cy (8 % and 27 % for 30 and 15 μg /mL Cu-Cy, respectively) treated breast cancer cells (MCF-7).

The IC-50 value of Cu-Cy against DM6 and KYSE-30 (11 and 14 μg/mL, respectively) are significantly lower (p< 0.01) than HDF and HET-1A (56 and 44 μg/mL, respectively) (**Figure 6-15B**). The IC-50 value of Cu-Cy against the MCF-7 cell was found to be 8 μg/mL . To the best of the authors' knowledge, an IC-50 value of 11 μg/mL to cancerous cells is the lowest reported among heterogeneous Fenton and Fenton-like nanocatalyst for cancer therapy thus far. In addition, the average selectivity index was calculated to be 4.5, which is comparable to most Fenton based chemo-dynamic cancer drugs.

   a. **Cytotoxicity after 24 h treatment b. is a molecular complex.**

Overall, Cu-Cy NPs' performance is markedly better than most heterogeneous Fenton-like nano-catalysts reported so far, which require high doses and exogenous additives to achieve desired cytotoxicity The excellent performance of Cu-Cy can be attributed to the existence of copper in its reduced state (Cu^{1+}) rather than in the oxidized state Cu^{2+}. The Cu^{1+} in Cu-Cy can directly participate in Fenton-like reaction and generates •OH rapidly as illustrated in **Eqn.1-2**. In cancer cells, the redox reactions between Cu-Cy and over present H_2O_2 can continue for many cycles, resulting in a ROS level that is beyond what the cell can withstand and thereby inducing cell death. However, due to the lower production of H_2O_2 in normal cells, the Cu-Cy NPs can not generate a high level of ROS to reach the cell-death threshold (**Figure 6-16**).

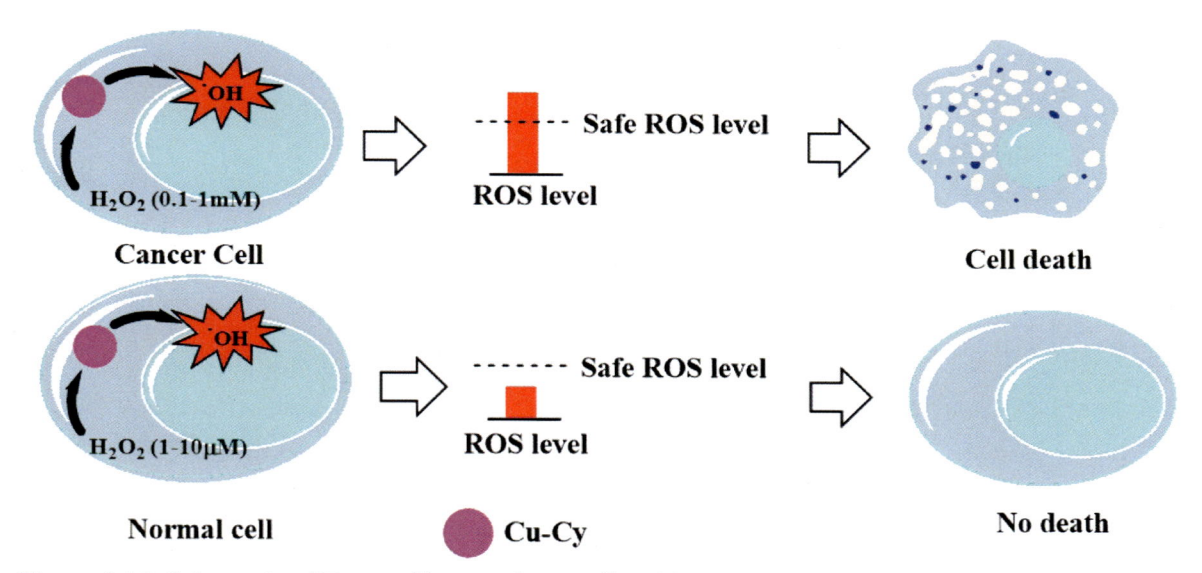

Figure 6-16. Schematic of Fenton-like reaction mediated by Cu-Cy. Cu-Cy NPs can undergo Fenton-like reaction with overproduced H_2O_2 in cancer cells resulting in ROS levels that is above the safe ROS level, causing cell death. On the other hand, owing to lower level of H_2O_2, Cu-Cy is harmless to normal cells. Adopted from ref. 3 with permission

Bottom Line

We investigated the Cu-Cy NPs for heterogeneous Fenton-like reactions facilitated cancer therapy with high selective toxicity. Our results suggest that Cu-Cy NPs, which have Cu^{1+} instead of Cu^{2+}, can catalyze over-produced H_2O_2 in cancerous cells to produce significantly higher levels of ROS, thereby inducing significantly more cancer cell destruction than healthy cells. The catalytic effect of Cu-Cy dramatically increased in slightly acidic conditions, which further contributes towards high selectivity owing to the acidic nature of tumor cells. The excellent stability of Cu-Cy, its low average IC-50 value (11 µg/mL), and high selectivity (4.5) towards cancer cells direct us to believe that Cu-Cy NPs could be a promising candidate of the translational nano-medicines in the context of cancer treatment with low systemic toxicity.

6.4 Chemodynamic Therapy Via Generation of Singlet Oxygen through the Russell Mechanism in Hypoxic Tumors and glutathione Depletion

Due to its low invasiveness and great selectivity, photodynamic therapy (PDT), which is based on $^1O_2$ created by the reaction between tissue oxygen and the photosensitizer (PS) during illumination, has gained widespread interest in cancer treatment. However, some existing flaws are difficult to overcome, including oxygen reliance, limited penetration depth of external light, and decreased therapeutic efficacy due to $^1O_2$ scavenging by increased glutathione (GSH). To overcome the inhibitory effects, different nanoscale O_2-evolving or GSH-depleting photodynamic agents have been developed to alleviate tumour hypoxia or decrease GSH levels. Additionally, several ways have been devised to generate $^1O_2$ or free radicals through thermal breakdown of substances exposed to near-infrared light. Nonetheless, the techniques remain constrained by their reliance on an external light source, even when local light activation improves selectivity.

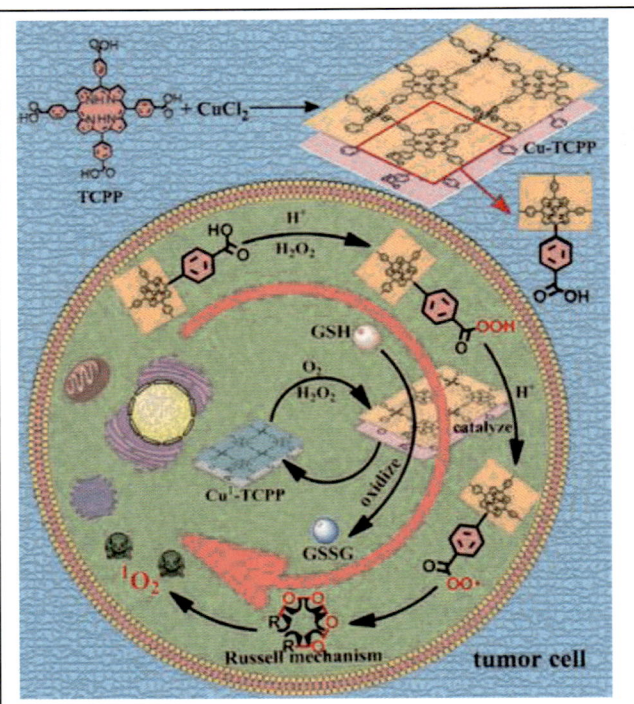

Figure 6-17 Cu-TCPP (tetrakis(4-carboxyphenyl)porphyrin) meditated CDT. Adopted from ref. 5 with permission

To accomplish specific tumour therapy, hypoxia, acidity, and high H_2O_2 and GSH levels in the tumour microenvironment (TME) have been widely explored. For example, Fenton or Fenton-like reactions utilising TME to generate free radicals or $^1O_2$ could be used to delicately surpass the penetration constraint and achieve selectivity. However, the fact that existing techniques have minimal therapeutic efficacy or require sophisticated catalyst syntheses would greatly impede their clinical translation. According to the Russell mechanism, $^1O_2$ can be created by reactions of biological hydroperoxides in the presence of a trace quantity of metal ion or enzyme. Significantly, the majority of biological hydroperoxides can be synthesised via the peroxidation of reactive oxygen species (ROS). This indicates a possible alternative to photodynamic agents that are light- and oxygen-dependent.

Cu-TCPP (tetrakis(4-carboxyphenyl)porphyrin) nanosheets, for example, which are composed of Cu^{2+} and the TCPP ligand, have demonstrated exceptional properties in photo-electrochemical cells, biosensors, and tumour therapy. (Figure 6-17) It was reported that $^1O_2$ may be created spontaneously by Cu-TCPP nanosheets via the Russell process (Figure 6-17), which can be employed for selective tumour treatment without relying on oxygen or external light as is the case with current photodynamic therapy (PDT) approaches. As illustrated in Figure 6-18A, the TCPP ligands of internalised nanosheets may be peroxidized with H_2O_2 at an acidic pH, a condition that closely resembles that of TME, and then reduced to peroxyl radicals (ROOC) in the presence of peroxidase-like Cu-TCPP nanosheets and a trace amount of Cu^{2+} ions. Following that, $^1O_2$ can be created via ROOC's spontaneous recombination reaction. As a result, hyperoxic cancers can be targeted specifically with minimal adverse effects. Additionally, the depletion of GSH by the inserted Cu^{2+} ions boosts therapeutic efficacy. This finding gives information on a novel process for the creation of $^1O_2$.

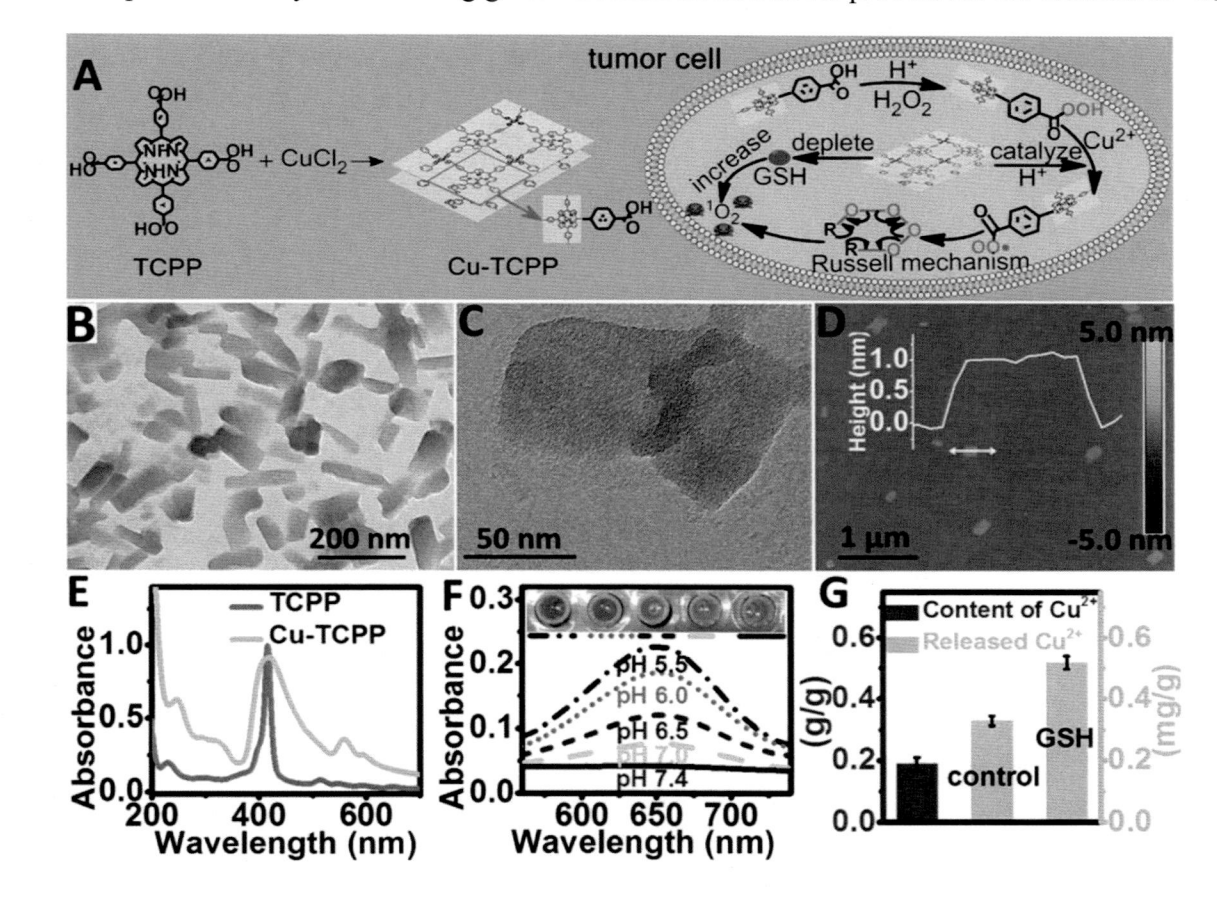

Figure 6-18. A) Synthesis and therapeutic mechanism of the Cu-TCPP nanosheets. B) TEM, C) HRTEM, and D) AFM images of the nanosheets with their height (inset). E) UV/Vis spectra of TCPP and Cu- TCPP nanosheets. F) pH dependent UV/Vis spectra of mixtures of Cu- TCPP nanosheets, TMB, and H_2O_2 with photographs of these mixtures (inset). G) Content and release (spontaneously or with GSH) of Cu^{2+} in the Cu-TCPP nanosheets determined by ICP. Adopted from ref. 5 with permission

Cu-TCPP nanosheets as generated exhibited rectangle-like structures with an average length of 106 nm, an average width of 37 nm, and a thickness of 1 nm (Figure 6-18B-D) They were distributed in water with a hydrodynamic diameter of around 148 nm and a zet potential of @39.2 mV, which is an acceptable size for nanosheet distribution into cancer cells. The four absorption peaks of TCPP in the UV/Vis spectra for the Q b and Cu-TCPP nanosheets were reduced to two (Figure 6-17E), indicating that the copper ions were coordinated in the porphyrin centres of TCPP, as confirmed by IR spectroscopy.

In this study, researchers wanted to see how well a new treatment using tiny particles called Cu-TCPP nanosheets could work on tumors inside the bodies of mice. They injected these nanosheets into mice with tumors through their veins, along with another group of mice that didn't receive the treatment (control group see Figure 6-19). They found that the tumor growth in the mice treated with the nanosheets was significantly slowed down in the first 5 days. After that, the tumors started to shrink gradually, and the mice didn't seem to lose weight or show any side effects.

When the researchers looked at the tumor tissue under the microscope, they saw that the nanosheets caused the tumor cells to die, while normal tissues remained unharmed. This indicated that the Cu-TCPP nanosheets were effective in treating tumors without harming healthy tissues. The nanosheets achieved this by producing a substance called $^1O_2$ specifically in the tumor environment and depleting another substance called GSH.

The researchers also examined the blood of the treated mice and found that there were no significant changes in their health compared to the healthy mice that didn't have tumors. This suggested that the treatment didn't negatively affect the overall health of the mice.

Additionally, when the researchers looked at the organs of the treated mice, they noticed that the nanosheets accumulated in the liver and spleen. This accumulation, along with the nanosheets' relatively short time in the bloodstream, indicated that the mice's bodies were likely clearing out most of the nanosheets through natural processes.

Overall, these findings showed that the Cu-TCPP nanosheets were effective in slowing down tumor growth and were safe for the mice, making them a promising potential treatment for tumors.

Additionally, the 2D Cu-TCPP MOF effectively converted all of the depleted GSH in the solution to oxidised glutathione (GSSG), as the GSH content in the supernatant of the Cu-TCPP with GSH mixture decreased from approximately 76 percent to 5% within 5 hours, while the GSSG content increased from approximately 24 percent to 75 percent due to the oxidation of Cu^{2+} in Cu-TCPP. Additionally, the Cu-TCPP nanosheets converted GSH to GSSG successfully in HeLa cells (Figure 6-18B), even when the intracellular GSH level was pre-enhanced by the GSH promoter, N-acetyl-l-cysteine (NAC). Further addition of H_2O_2 to the solution of Cu-TCPP and GSH resulted in the appearance of a weak 1:1:1:1 quartet signal in the electron spin resonance (ESR) spectrum in the presence of the COH scavenger DMSO following the addition of the trapping agent 5,5-dimethyl-1-pyrroline N-oxide (DMPO) at the initial time point (0 h), which disappeared after 6 h. (Figure 6-18C). However, with addition of DMPO, weak 1:2:2:1 quartet signals were obtained at 0 and 6 hours for a combination of superoxide dismutase (SOD, scavenger of O_2^-), Cu-TCPP, H_2O_2, and GSH. These findings indicated that O_2^- was created first and then vanished, whereas COH was produced throughout the process, despite the fact that COH had no interaction with free Cu^{2+}. In light of our and earlier findings, the following mechanism of GSH depletion was proposed:

$$2\,Cu^{II}-TCPP + 2\,GSH \rightarrow 2\,Cu^{I}-TCPP + GSSG \qquad (1)$$

$$Cu^{I}-TCPP + O_2 \rightleftharpoons Cu^{II}-TCPP + O_2^{\cdot -} \qquad (2)$$

$$Cu^{I}-TCPP + H_2O_2 \rightarrow Cu^{II}-TCPP + {\cdot}OH + OH^- \qquad (3)$$

$$O_2^{\cdot -} + H_2O \rightarrow {}^1O_2 + H_2O_2 + 2\,OH^- \qquad (4)$$

This process suggested that GSH may be depleted as a result of the Cu^{2+} and Cu^{1+} cyclic conversion in the Cu-TCPP and that the Cu-TCPP nanosheets may deplete GSH, preventing it from successfully scavenging $^1O_2$. These findings reveal unequivocally that the Cu-TCPP nanosheets were extremely effective at preventing tumour growth while remaining biocompatible.

The Bottom Line

To summarize, Cu-TCPP nanosheets that form $^1O_2$ when reacting with H_2O_2, which is abundant in TME, and cycle-depleting GSH. As a result of their selective generation of $^1O_2$ and resistance to $^1O_2$ scavenging by GSH, the tailored Cu-TCPP nanosheets are capable of inducing tumour death in vitro and in vivo without causing adverse effects. This strategy removes the need on oxygen and external light stimulus required for PDT, providing some inspiration for the creation of cancer therapy techniques in hypoxic tumors.

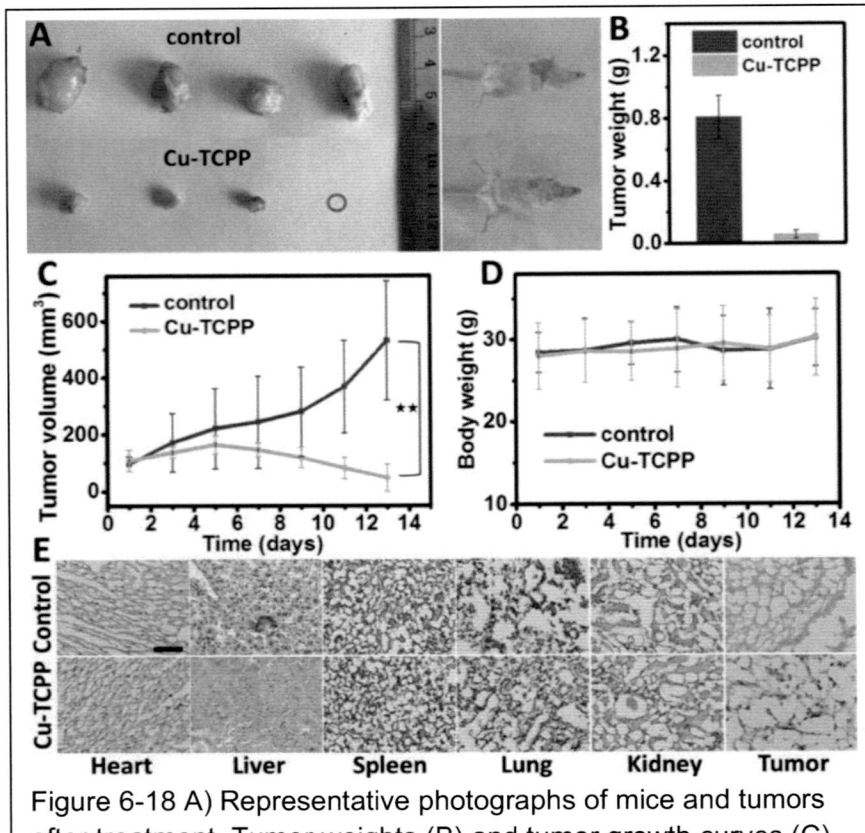

Figure 6-18 A) Representative photographs of mice and tumors after treatment. Tumor weights (B) and tumor growth curves (C) of each group (n=5/group, **P<0.01). D) Mice weight growth curves of each group. E) H&E stained images of normal tissues and tumor tissues of each group. Scale bar: 40 μm. The mice treated with PBS were used as the control group. Adopted from ref. 5 with permission

References for this chapter

1. Zhongmin Tang, Yanyan Liu, Mingyuan He, and Wenbo Bu, Chemodynamic Therapy: Tumour Microenvironment-Mediated Fenton and Fenton-like Reactions, Angew. Chem. Int. Ed. 2019, 58, 946 – 956

2. Yingyan Liu, Kaixiu Chen, Yapu Yang, and Pengfei Shi, Glucose Oxidase-Modified Metal–Organic Framework for Starving-Enhanced Chemodynamic Therapy, *ACS Applied Bio Materials* **2023** *6* (2), 857-864

3. Lalit Chudal, Nil Kanatha Pandey, Jonathan Phan, Omar Johnson, Liangwu Lin, Hongmei Yu, Yang Shu, Zhenzhen Huang, Meiying Xing, J. Ping Liu, Minli Chen, Wenzhi Song, and **Wei Chen**, Copper-Cysteamine Nanoparticles as a Heterogenous Fenton-like Catalyst for Highly Selective Cancer Treatment, *ACS Applied Biomaterials,* 2020, 3: 1804−1814

4. Lalit Chudal, Nil Kanatha Pandey, Jonathan Phan, Omar Johnson, Xiuying Li, **Wei Chen**, Investigation of PPIX-Lipo-MnO$_2$ to enhance photodynamic therapy by improving tumor hypoxia, *Mater. Scie. Eng. C,* 2019, 104: 109979

5. Chao Wang, Fengjuan Cao, Yudi Ruan, Xiaodan Jia, Wenyao Zhen, and Xiue Jiang, Specific Generation of Singlet Oxygen through the Russell Mechanism in Hypoxic Tumors and GSH Depletion by Cu-TCPP Nanosheets for Cancer Therapy, Angew. Chem. Int. Ed. 2019, 58, 9846 −9850

Chapter 7

Photothermal Therapy

7.1 The use of heat for cancer destruction

Nanotechnology has drastically changed the landscape of several industries, including but not limited to the field of medicine and medical research. With the advent of nanomedicine, targeted drug delivery systems have seen a boom leading to the invention of various site-specific, selective, and even receptor-targeted options for imaging and therapy. Particles in the nano-size range possess novel properties which change their physical and chemical properties significantly, for example – semiconductors, have altered optical properties such as luminescence. These changes may lead to brighter luminescence and easier tunability of the emission color of semiconductor nanoparticles. Luminescent nanoparticles have tremendous potential for use in cancer detection and imaging. The key features of luminescent nanoparticles, such as small size, water-solubility, good photostability, narrow emission bandwidth, and enhanced surface functionalities, render it a potential candidate for *in vivo* applications such as targeted delivery to specific disease sites. Moreover, they can be employed in accessing different cellular compartments for selective imaging and/or therapy.

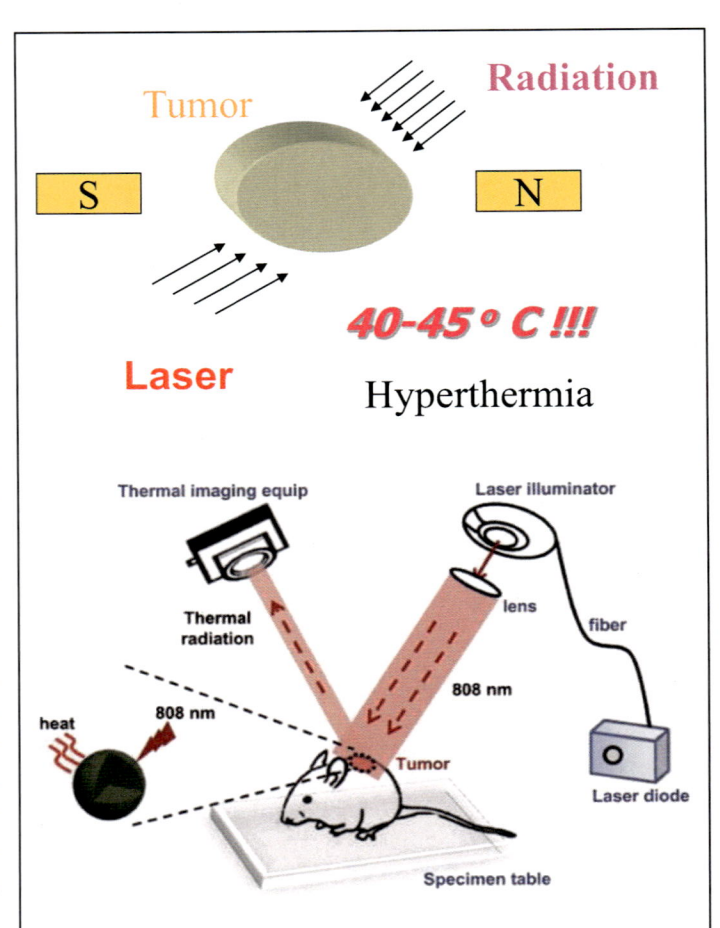

Figure 7-1: A schematic illustration to use heat for cancer treatment. Adopted from refs. 5 and 8 with permissions

Hyperthermic therapy is the use of heat between 40 and 45°C to damage cancer cells while preventing the surrounding cells from being affected, often used to increase the effectiveness of other treatment modalities, such as chemotherapy or radiation therapy. At higher temperatures (>45°C), just thermal energy alone may be used to directly ablate cancer cells **as illustrated in Figure 7-1.** To deliver the heat for hyperthermic therapy and thermal ablation various modes of thermal energy such as microwave, radiofrequency, magnetic field, focused ultrasound or even laser stimulation can be used. Irrespective of the energy source chosen, a sufficient amount of heat must be generated in a specific disease volume over a given period of time to activate and achieve efficient treatment. One major obstacle to achieving successful hyperthermic/thermal ablation therapy is that cancer cells aside, even healthy tissues can absorb electromagnetic and ultrasound energies. Therefore, the healthy tissues between the tumor and the external energy source can also get heated up, resulting in a limited therapeutic window. The application of functional nanoparticles that interact with the external energy sources to mediate the thermal effect may significantly help in overcoming this limitation, thanks to the virtue of nanoparticles by which they can be selectively directed to the cancer cells.

7.2 Au Nanostructures Mediated PTT

A variety of functional nanoparticles have been examined as potential thermal mediators. It has been demonstrated that magnetic nanoparticles can improve hyperthermic cancer treatment. Gold nanoparticles, nanoshells, and hollow nanospheres have all been investigated for thermal ablation therapy induced by a near-infrared (NIR) light, hence the term photothermal ablation therapy (PTA). These gold nanostructures exhibit strong absorption of NIR light between a range of 700 and 1100 nm, in which light can penetrate deeply into the tissues. The intense absorption is attributed to the surface plasmon phenomenon, and the absorption maximum is related to the particle size and shape, and the dielectric constant of the surrounding matrix, such as the solvents and the core material in the core-shell gold nanostructures.

AuNPs-mediated photothermal therapy (PTT) is a treatment gaining popularity for both research in labs and medical use. It's a promising method for treating breast cancer because it can use light to generate heat inside the cancer cells. This is better than traditional heat treatments. However, there are some challenges that need to be addressed before it becomes widely used. One problem is that the treatment is not very specific to cancer cells, so it may affect healthy cells too. Also, the effectiveness of converting light to heat is not very high, and sometimes the light cannot penetrate deep into the tissues.

Despite these challenges, there have been some important breakthroughs in using AuNPs for PTT, especially for breast cancer treatment. Scientists can now create AuNPs of different sizes and shapes with specific properties that can target and treat breast cancer cells. While, how to improve the performance of AuNP-based

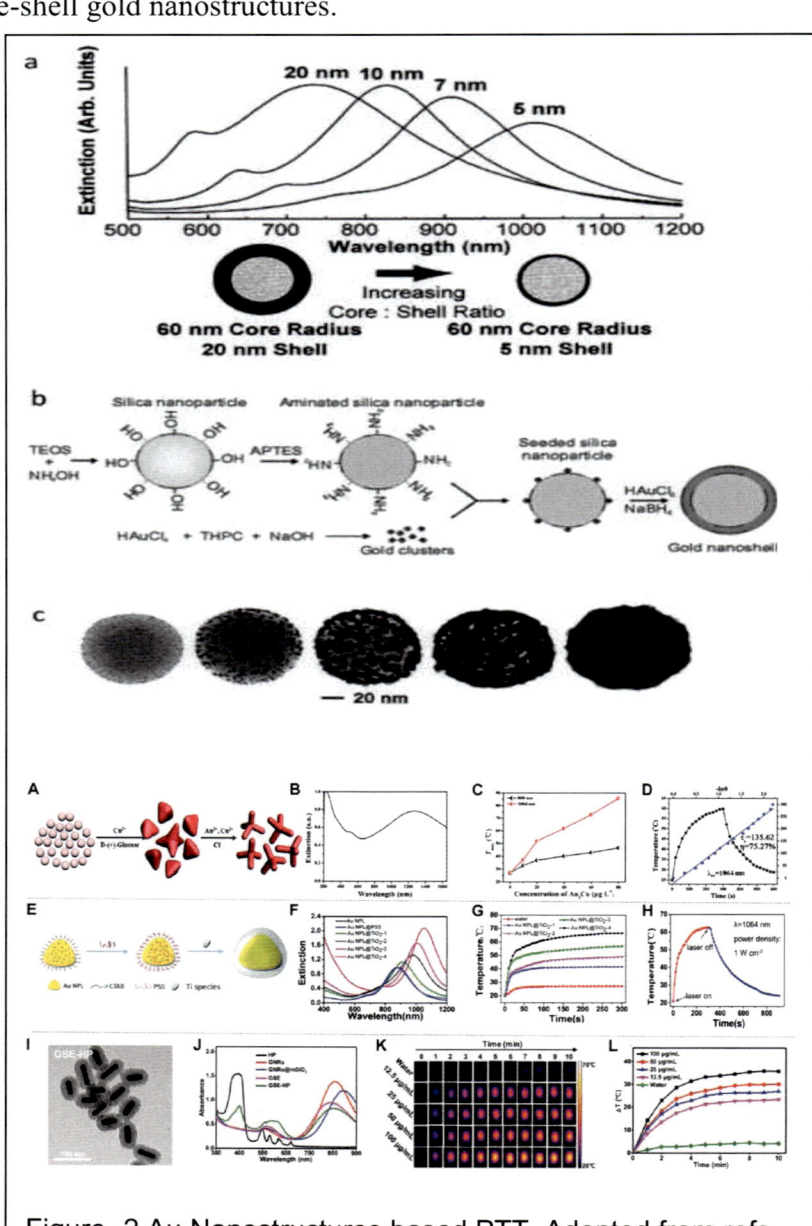

Figure -2 Au Nanostructures based PTT. Adopted from refs. 1 and 2 with permissions

PTT is still a challenging issue. This includes ways to diagnose and target cancer cells more effectively using AuNPs. AuNP-mediated PTT shows great promise for treating cancer, and with further research and improvements, it could become a valuable treatment option in the near future."

7.2 CuS Nanoparticles Based PTT

Semiconductor copper sulfide (CuS) nanostructures display interesting electrical, optical and catalytic properties, with potential applications in photodegradation of pollutants, biological labeling, laser light monitoring, and eye protection, and DNA detection. As a semiconductor, the infrared absorption in CuS nanoparticles is fundamentally different from that displayed by gold nanostructures. The former is derived from energy band–band transitions, while the absorption from gold nanostructures results from surface plasmons. In this study, the hypothesis that the interaction of CuS nanoparticles with NIR light could generate heat, which could be harnessed for PTA of cancer cells is put to test. One of the pioneer studies, this is the first report on the use of semiconductor nanoparticles for PTA therapy to the best of our knowledge.

MATERIALS & METHODS

MATERIALS

Thioglycolic acid (TGA), $CuCl_2 \cdot 2H_2O$, and thioacetamide were purchased from Sigma-Aldrich (MO, USA). Roswell Park Memorial Institute (RPMI)-1640 culture medium, calcein AM and EthD-1 LIVE/DEAD® viability kit were obtained from Invitrogen (Eugene, OR, USA). Gold nanoparticles (20 nm) were prepared by adding 5 ml of sodium citrate (25 mM) into a boiling aqueous solution of $HAuCl_4$ (0.25 mM). The mixture was stirred until the solution turned into a red wine color, indicating the completion of the reaction. Human cervix adenocarcinoma HeLa cells and human embryonic kidney 293 (HEK293) cells were obtained from American Type Culture Collection (VA, USA).

NANOPARTICLE SYNTHESIS & CHARACTERIZATION

Thioglycolic acid-stabilized CuS nanoparticles were synthesized as follows. Cupric chloride was dissolved in distilled water and Thioglycolic acid was added to this solution with constantly stirring the mix, followed by pH adjustment to 9.0 using a 1M solution of sodium hydroxide. The pH-balanced solution was then transferred to a three-necked flask (fitted with a septum and valves) followed by degassing with argon bubbling for a duration of 20 minutes. Then, a mix of thioacetamide solution in distilled water was added to the solution and heated at a constant temperature of 50°C for a duration of two hours for promoting the growth of nanoparticles.

Further examination of the nanoparticles for properties such as the size and shape was conducted by x-ray diffraction (XRD) and high-resolution transmission electron microscopy (HRTEM) techniques. The crystalline structure, size, and shape of the nanoparticles were observed by x-ray diffraction (XRD), using a Siemens Kristalloflex 810 D-500 x-ray diffractometer (Karlsruhe,

Germany). The nanoparticles in the solution were placed onto holey carbon-covered copper grids for HRTEM observation. The HRTEM images of the particles were obtained with a JEOL JEM-2100 electron microscope (Tokyo, Japan). The absorption spectra for the nanoparticles were recorded using a Shimadzu UV-2450 UV-vis spectrophotometer (Kyoto, Japan).

PHOTOTHERMAL EFFECT IN AQUEOUS SOLUTION

To gauge the photothermal effect of the nanoparticles, a continuous laser wave from a fiber-coupled diode laser was used. The laser, with a center wavelength of 808 ± 10 nm. A 5-m, 600-µm core BioTex LCM-001 optical fiber (Houston, TX, USA), was used to transfer laser light from the laser unit to the target. This fiber had a lens mounting at the output that allowed the laser spot size to be changed by changing the distance from the output to the target. The output power was independently calibrated using a hand-held optical power meter (Newport model 840-C, CA, USA) and was found to be 1.5 W for a spot diameter of 1.3 mm (~113 W/cm2) and a 2-Amp supply current. For measuring temperature changes mediated by CuS nanoparticles, 808-nm NIR laser light was delivered through a quartz cuvette containing the nanoparticles. A thermocouple was inserted into the solution perpendicular to the path of the laser light. The temperature was measured over a period of 15 minutes using water as a control.

IN VITRO PHOTOTHERMAL ABLATION OF CANCER CELLS WITH CuS NANOPARTICLES

This study involved HeLa cells derived from cervical cancer cells, for evaluating photothermal ablation with CuS nanoparticles. The HeLa cell line was chosen for this study as a result of the potential use of NIR light with a colposcope to illuminate cervical cancer and pre-cancerous lesions. HeLa cells were seeded onto a 96-well plate, one day prior to the experiment. The cells were washed thrice with Hanks balanced salt solution (HBSS, Sigma-Aldrich), followed by incubation with CuS nanoparticles at 37°C for a period of 2 hours. Post incubation, the culture media with nanoparticles was removed and the cells were resupplied with fresh phenol red-free RPMI-1640. The cells were then irradiated with a NIR laser centered at 808 nm at an output power of 0, 24, or 40 W/cm^2 for 5 minutes or 64 W/cm^2 for 3 minutes. The diode laser was coupled in a way that delivered a circular laser beam of 2 mm in radius, covering the central area of the microplate well, followed by automatic power calibration.

After laser irradiation, the cells were resupplied with RPMI-1640 containing 10% fetal bovine serum and were incubated at 37°C for 24 hours. The cells were then washed with Hanks balanced salt solution, HBSS, and stained with calcein-AM for visualization of live cells and with EthD-1, Ethidium homodimer for visualization of dead cells, according to the manufacturer's suggested protocol (Invitrogen). The cells were then examined under a Zeiss Axio Observer. Z1 fluorescence microscope (Carl Zeiss MicroImaging GmbH, Göttingen, Germany). A Tecan microplate reader with Magellan software (Männedorf, Switzerland) was used to measure the fluorescence intensity of each well. The percentage of viable cells in each well was calculated according to the manufacturer's protocol. Each experiment was performed in triplicate. Differences in viability between each treatment and the control (i.e., no laser, no nanoparticles) were analyzed using Student's t-test, with $p < 0.05$ considered to be statistically significant.

CYTOTOXICITY

To evaluate the cytotoxicity of the CuS nanoparticles, HEK293 cells were used to represent a normal cell line. The cells were continuously exposed to the CuS nanoparticles or 20-nm gold nanoparticles for 48 hours and were evaluated for cell viability using a tetrazolium salt (WST-1) assay kit (Takara Bio, Inc., Shiga, Japan). The working mechanism of WST-1 (4-[3-(4-iodophenyl)-2- (4-nitrophenyl)-2H-5-tetrazolio]-1,3-benzene disulfonate) similar to that of 3-[4,5-dimethylthiazol- 2-yl]-2,5-diphenyltetrazolium bromide (MTT), by reacting with the mitochondrial succinate-tetrazolium reductase forming the formazan dye. The WST-1 reagent produces a water-soluble formazan unlike the water-insoluble product of the MTT assay.

To conduct the evaluation, exponentially growing HEK293 cells were dispensed into a 96-well flat-bottom plate. After allowing 24 hours for cell attachment, each concentration of nanoparticle solution or an aqueous solution of $CuCl_2$ was diluted appropriately in fresh media and added to the microwells, three wells per concentration. Then, cell viability was determined by the addition of the WST-1 solution. The plate was further incubated for an additional period of 2 hours at 37°C and 5% CO_2 concentration, allowing viable cells to convert the WST-1 into a colored, soluble dye, by using mitochondrial dehydrogenase enzymes. The soluble salt was then released into the media. Absorbance at 430 nm was measured against a background control of blank using a microtiter plate reader (Molecular Devices, Sunnyvale, CA, USA). Data were presented as mean absorbance ± standard deviation.

RESULTS & DISCUSSION

Copper sulfide nanoparticles were readily synthesized in an aqueous solution by allowing $CuCl_2$ and thioacetamide to react in the presence of TGA at pH 9. TGA served to stabilize the resulting CuS nanoparticles.

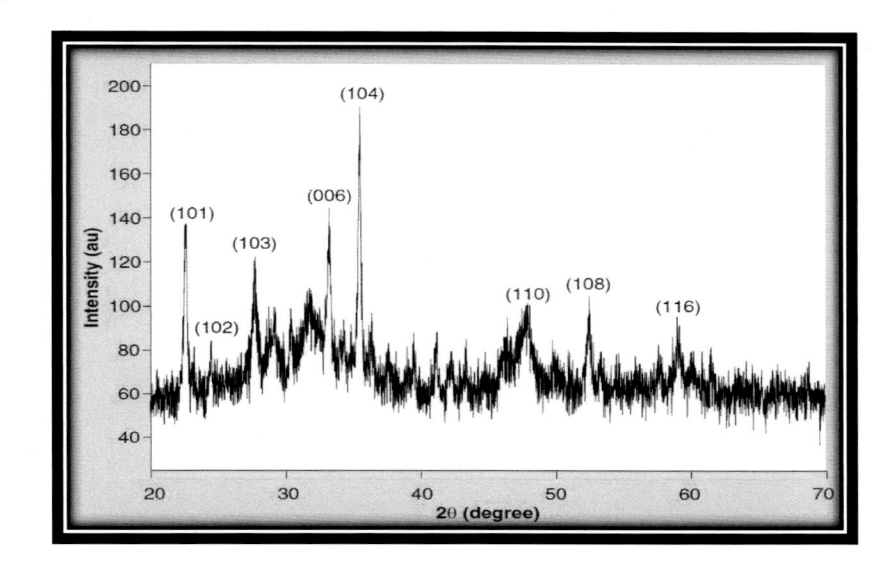

Figure 7-3 – Represents the X-ray diffraction pattern of copper sulfide nanoparticles. Adopted from ref. 3 with permission

Figure 7-3 shows the XRD pattern of CuS nanoparticle powder deposited from the aqueous solution, which is in agreement with that of the standard powder diffraction pattern of CuS with a hexagonal structure. The diffraction lines are indexed as labeled in **Figure 7-3** for the hexagonal phase of CuS. The key indication for the formation of nanoparticles is the broadening of the diffraction peaks, as seen above. The absence of any obvious impurity peaks is an indication of acquiring high-quality covellite CuS particles.

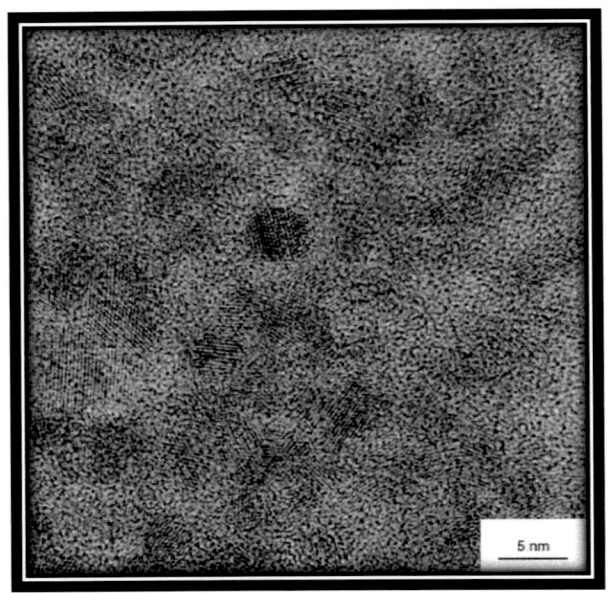

Figure 7-4 – Represents a High-resolution transmission electron microscope image of copper sulfide nanoparticles. Adopted from ref. 3 with permission

Figure 7-4 shows the HRTEM images of CuS nanoparticles. The average size of the formed nanoparticles was approximately 3 nm with a uniform size distribution. Assuming a density of 4.6 g/cm^3, each CuS nanoparticle is estimated to contain approximately 3260 CuS 'molecules'. The nanoparticles were observed to have a hexagonal structure and the crystal lattice fringes from the (102) and (103) lattice planes could be observed. The lattice spacing of the (102) plane measured from the images is approximately 0.30 nm and that of the (103) plane was approximately 0.28 nm. These observed properties are very close to the lattice spacing of the (102) plane (0.305 nm) and of the (103) plane (0.282 nm) of previously reported hexagonal CuS nanostructures.

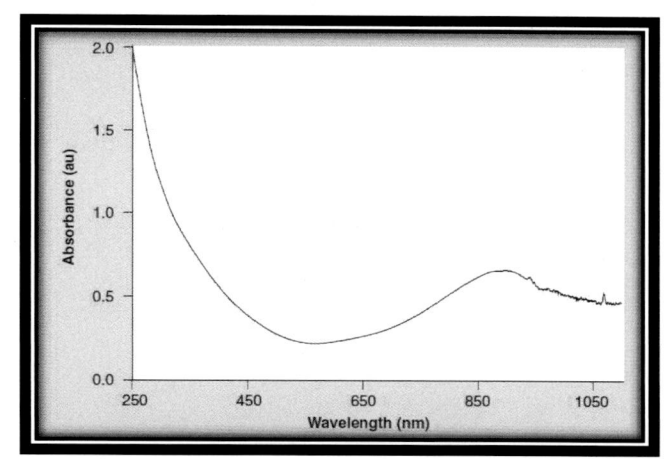

Figure 7-5 – **Represents the optical absorption spectrum of copper sulfide nanoparticles. Adopted from ref. 3 with permission**

Figure 7-5 shows the optical absorption spectrum of CuS nanoparticles. The effect of quantum size confinement, a defining characteristic of nanoparticles was confirmed by the short-wavelength absorption edged at approximately 500 nm, which was a significant blue shift from the energy gap of bulk CuS. The sample shows an increased absorption band in the NIR region, with maximum absorption at 900 nm. Based on the absorbance measurement, the absorption coefficient value (e) was estimated to be approximately 2×10^7 Mcm^{-1} at 900 nm. The peak absorption of the study sample was assigned to the overlapping d–d transition of Cu^{2+} in a trigonal environment, exhibiting approximately a 20-nm blue shift, whereas the blue shift of other CuS nanoparticles reported in the literature was approximately 5 nm, thus the blue shift observed in the synthesized nanoparticles was significantly greater in comparison to that reported in earlier studies. This observed higher blue shift in the absorption spectrum of the sample is speculated to be due to the weakening of the crystal field strength, owing to the smaller size of the synthesized nanoparticles in comparison to the previously studied CuS nanoparticles. Owing to the smaller size of our nanoparticles, fewer ions were coordinated at sites near the surface than in the bulk CuS. In addition, interaction with distant neighboring ions was much weaker or non-existent in smaller CuS nanoparticles compared with that in bulk CuS. Thus, it is expected that the crystal field interaction of these ions is weaker in smaller nanoparticles. As a result, the lowest excited state of the d electrons is upshifted and the d–d transition is shifted to the blue region. No shoulders were observed at 450 nm, which is a typical absorption peak of the Cu2S phase. Put together, these results, the XRD and HRTEM data, indicate that the synthesized CuS nanoparticles are of high purity and quality. The intense absorption by CuS nanoparticles of the NIR should enable their use in PTA therapy.

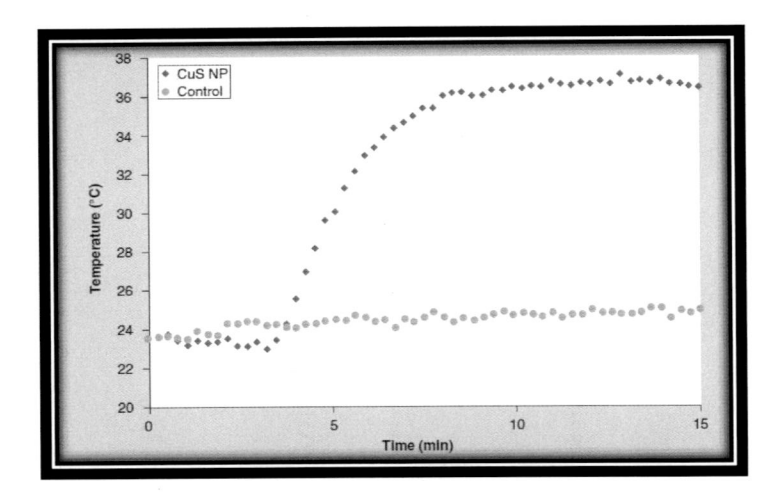

Figure 7-6 – Represents the temperature measured over a period of 15 minutes of exposure to 808-nm near-infrared light at an output power of 24 W/cm^2. The concentration of CuS NPs in water was 770 µM equivalent CuS. CuS: Copper sulfide; NP: Nanoparticle. **Adopted from ref. 3 with permission**

Figure 7-6 displays the temperature of an aqueous solution containing CuS nanoparticles as a function of the time of exposure to a laser beam at 808 nm. To test the photothermal properties of the synthesized CuS nanoparticles, the temperatures of an aqueous solution containing CuS nanoparticles and that of pure water were recorded under exposure to a NIR laser beam at 808nm. It was observed that the temperature increased to 12.7°C over a period of 5 minutes, while no change was observed in the temperature of pure water. Thus, CuS nanoparticles can mediate photothermal effects at 808 nm in the NIR region, albeit to a smaller extent than those induced by gold core-shell nanostructures. Since the absorption of CuS nanoparticles peaks at 900 nm, it is anticipated that the photothermal effect mediated by CuS nanoparticles at the peak absorbance wavelength of 900 nm would be much stronger than that obtained at 808 nm. Since in reality, it is very difficult to obtain gold core-shell nanostructures with a peak absorption of more than 850 nm, CuS nanoparticles that absorb light at wavelengths greater than 850 nm may have quite interesting applications, especially where photothermal response at a higher laser wavelength is needed.

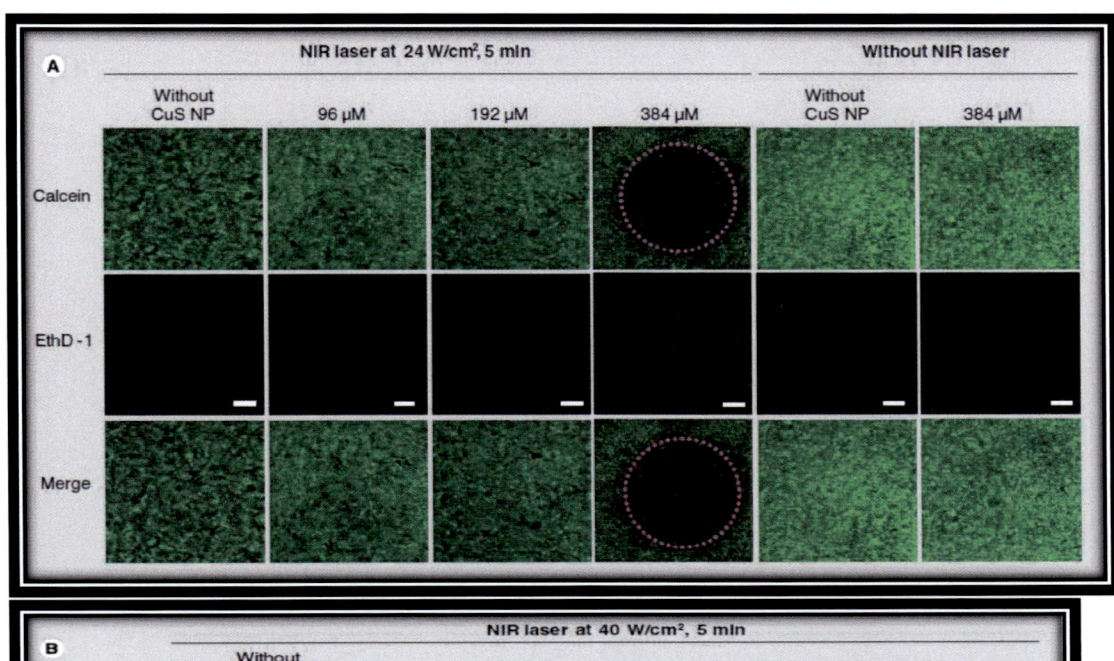

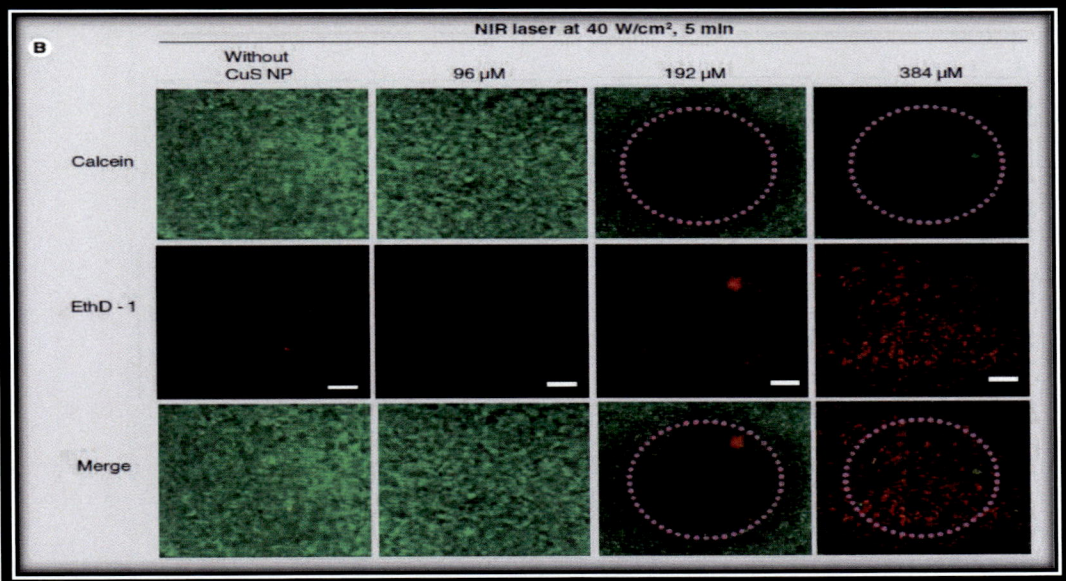

Figure 7-7 – Represents the cell viability after near-infrared irradiation.

(A) HeLa cells were treated with different concentrations of CuS NPs and NIR light (808 nm) at 24 W/cm2 for 5 minutes. B) Following irradiation with the NIR laser beam at higher power (40 W/cm2 for 5 min), cell death was observed at a
After treatment with NPs at a concentration of 384 μM CuS plus NIR laser, most cells were dead in the zone of exposure (circled area). lower concentration of 192 μM CuS, and the cell death calcein, dead cells were stained red with EthD-1. Bar = 200 μm. By contrast, after treatment with NIR laser alone, NPs alone or NPs at concentrations of 192 μM CuS followed by NIR laser, cells retained normal morphology and few dead cells were observed. CuS: Copper sulfide; EthD-1: Ethidium homodimer-1; NIR: Near-infrared; NP: Nanoparticle.
Adopted from ref. 3 with permission

To estimate the cell lysis induced by the photothermal effects of CuS nanoparticles, HeLa cells were employed. HeLa cells were chosen because of the possibility of NIR light being delivered colposcopically to illuminate cervical cancer and precancerous lesions in the cervix. The cell line was derived from cervical cancer cells. The cells were incubated with CuS nanoparticles for 2 hours, followed by irradiation with a NIR laser centered at 808 nm. As shown in **Figure 7-7**, 24 hours post laser treatment, the cells treated with CuS nanoparticles plus a NIR laser experienced substantial cellular death. In fact, at a CuS concentration of 384 µM and output power of 40 W/cm^2, cell death expanded beyond the zone of laser exposure, indicating the spread of heat outside the area of laser irradiation (**Figure 7-7**). While, there was no apparent cell death observed in cells treated with CuS nanoparticles, either alone or with just laser. Quantitative analysis of cell viability showed that at the laser power of 24 W/cm^2 for 5 minutes, the percentage of viable cells was 55.6 ± 5.8% when cells were pre-treated with CuS nanoparticles at a concentration of 384 µM CuS.

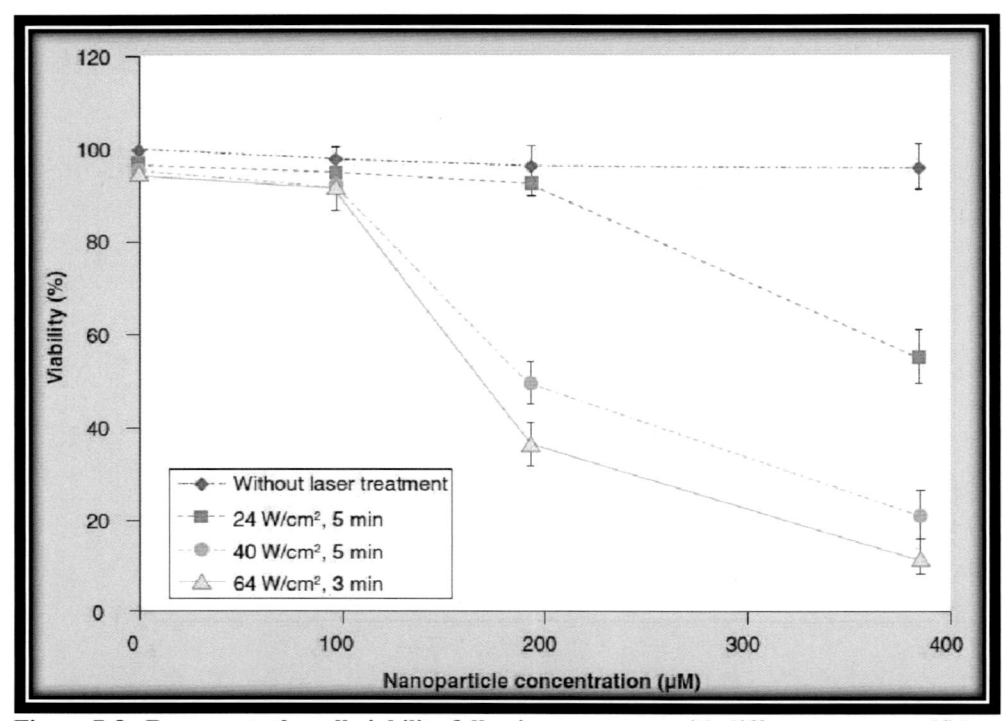

Figure 7-8 - **Represents the cell viability following treatment with different copper sulfide nanoparticle concentrations and different near-infrared laser doses.** The values are presented as mean ± standard deviation from triplicate samples. **Adopted from ref. 3 with permission**

At the same nanoparticle concentration, the cell viability decreased to 21.2 ± 5.6% and 12.2 ± 3.7% when the laser power was increased to 40 W/cm^2 for 5 minutes and 64 W/cm^2 for 3 minutes, respectively. A similar trend was found when the nanoparticle concentration was increased and the laser power was maintained (**Figure 7-8**). These data indicate that the extent of cell death caused by the photothermal effect mediated by CuS nanoparticles is a function of the concentration of the nanoparticles and the output power of the laser used.

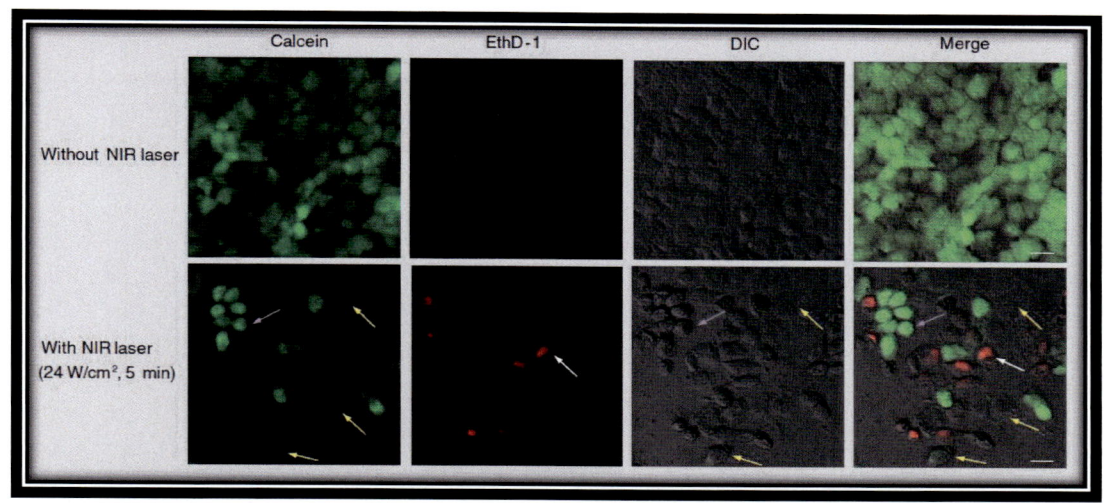

Figure 7-9 - Represents the Microphotographs of cells incubated with copper sulfide nanoparticles (384 μM copper sulfide) followed by near-infrared laser irradiation (24 W/cm², 5 min). Without laser treatment, the cells were viable and polygonal. By contrast, most cells treated with the NIR laser shrank and had spherical morphology (purple arrows). Some cells lost viability, as evidenced by calcein-negative staining (yellow arrows). Others lost membrane integrity, as indicated by positive staining with EthD-1 (white arrows). Bar = 20 μm. DIC: Differential interference contrast; EthD-1: Ethidium homodimer-1; NIR: Near-infrared. **Adopted from ref. 3 with permission**

Morphologically, the untreated HeLa cells were observed to be polygonal in shape, and a few cells were stained red with ethidium homodimer-1 (EthD-1). However, post-treatment with CuS nanoparticles (384 μM CuS) and the NIR laser, many cells that stained positive with calcein (green) became more rounded in shape (purple arrows, **Figure 7-9**), possibly as a result of the condensation of skeletal proteins. On the other hand, some cells lost their viability, as indicated by calcein-negative staining (yellow arrows, **Figure 7-9**). The rest of the cells stained positive with EthD-1, which indicates loss of cellular membrane integrity (white arrows, **Figure 7-9**).

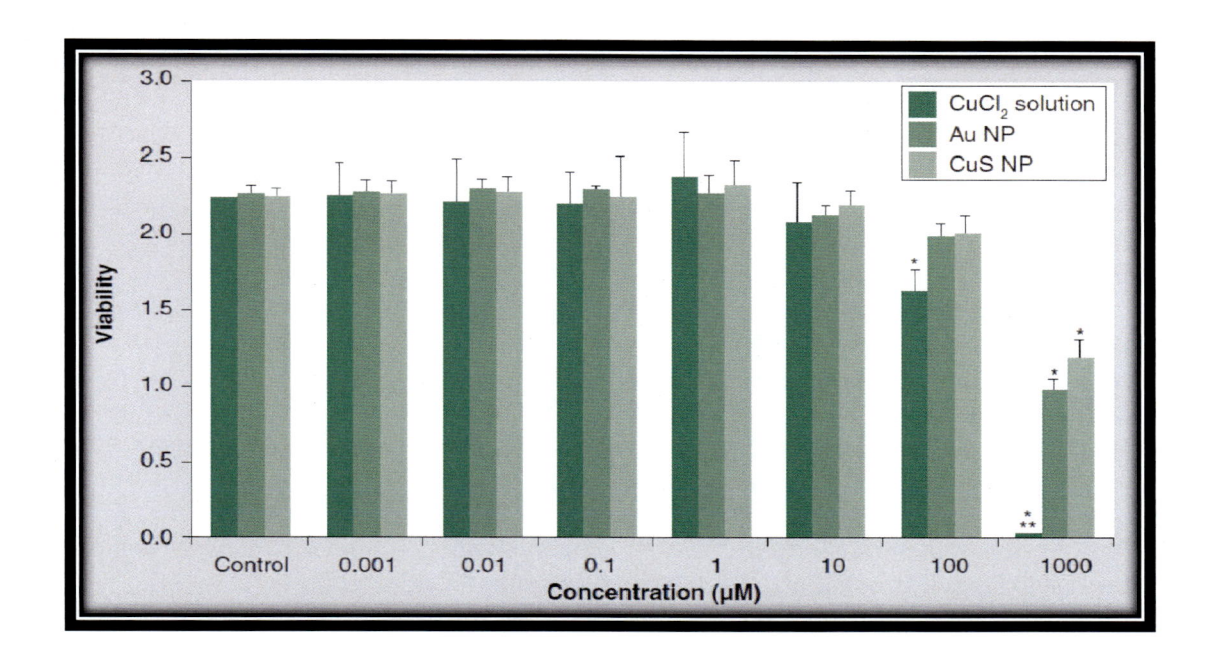

Figure 7-10 – Represents the cytotoxicity of copper sulfide nanoparticles in HEK293 cells.
The cells were incubated in a culture medium containing NPs at concentrations ranging from 1 nM to 1 mM for 48 hours. CuCl2 solution and 20-nm Au NPs were included in the study. Cell viability is expressed as the absorbance at 430 nm. Control: untreated cells. Data represent mean ± standard deviation. *p < 0.05 compared with untreated control, **p < 0.05 compared with CuS Nanoparticles, Au: Gold; CuS: Copper sulfide; NP: Nanoparticle. **Adopted from ref. 3 with permission**

The cytotoxicity of CuS nanoparticles in HEK293 cells was compared with that of 20-nm gold nanoparticles, the widely accepted biocompatible nanomaterials (Figure 7-10). The size of these gold nanoparticles was determined by transmission electron microscopy (TEM) and dynamic light scattering methods. Both CuS and gold nanoparticles (20 nm) were observed to have no cytotoxic effect on the cells at concentrations up to 100 µM post 48 hours of incubation. At the highest concentration tested (1 mM), both nanoparticles caused a significant decrease in cell viability. The aqueous solution of $CuCl_2$, which was used for the preparation of CuS nanoparticles, was observed to be significantly more cytotoxic than its corresponding CuS nanoparticles at equivalent concentrations of CuS, i.e. greater than 100 µM. Almost all cells were found to be dead after treatment with the aqueous solution of $CuCl_2$ at 1 mM. These observations suggest that the cytotoxicity profiles of CuS nanoparticles and gold nanoparticles are fairly comparable. One study found that mesoporous silica nanoparticles could enhance MTT formazan exocytosis in HeLa cells, giving an overestimation of the cytotoxicity of mesoporous silica nanoparticles. However, no such phenomenon was observed with the WST-1 assay, which is similar to the MTT assay since in both assays tetrazolium salt reduction is driven by intracellular NADH contents. However, the formazan dye produced by enzymatic cleavage of the tetrazolium salt WST-1 is water-soluble and does not form crystals, whereas reduced MTT forms water-insoluble dye. Another study reported the interactions between single-walled carbon nanotubes and various dyes, including MTT and WST-1, used to assess the cytotoxicity, to be resulting in false-positive toxicity. However, there were no potential interactions were observed between the dye molecules and CuS nanoparticles by the current study's authors. Consistent with this notion, no morphological changes were observed at a CuS concentration of up to 384 µM (Figure 7-9).

The advantages of CuS nanostructures are numerous in comparison to those of gold nanostructures, such as the cost of manufacture as gold is way more expensive. Other advantages include obtaining d-d transitions at higher wavelengths of 900nm, to attain NIR absorption for *in vivo* applications. To attain NIR absorption, gold nanoparticles are to be altered to special structures such as hollow nanospheres, nanoshells or nanorods, etc., and the plasmon absorption maximum of gold nanoparticles shifts when compared with *in vitro* observations, thus complicating the treatment conditions. This is not the case with CuS nanostructures, making it a better option, as they are not only cost-effective and sans complexities, their pharmacokinetic properties are more favorable for targeted delivery post systemic administration than that of gold nanostructures. Finally, one of the key advantages is of size, as the smallest gold nanostructure exhibiting NIR absorption reported to date is 40 nm, whereas CuS nanostructure is of 3nm, comparatively very small, which increases the odds of being delivered to the targeted site and even renal clearance and eventual elimination from the system.

Limitations of CuS nanoparticles include their relatively low photothermal conversion efficiency. In the present study formulation, both the concentration of CuS nanoparticles and the laser energy required to cause sufficient cell death in the *in vitro* monolayer setting are exorbitantly high for *in vivo* applications. Therefore, further improvement of the physicochemical properties of CuS nanoparticles is needed. The authors believe there is sufficient scope to increase the absorbance of CuS nanoparticles. In addition, another strategy to increase their absorbance is coating the CuS nanoparticles with zinc sulfide shells, for core-shell nanostructures can further confine the excitons in the core nanoparticles. The study authors have future plans for synthesizing CuS/ zinc sulfide core-shell structures, intending to increase the absorbance as well as the heating efficiency. Further, the absorbance at 900 nm is approximately 1.5-times stronger than that at 808 nm, thus the efficiency can be enhanced if laser irradiation of 900 nm is used for the treatment.

Bottom Line

The present study suggests that CuS nanoparticles with strong absorption in the NIR region are promising new nanomaterials for Photothermal Ablation treatment of cancer. It was observed that following irradiation by a NIR laser beam at 808 nm, the temperature in CuS nanoparticle aqueous solution is increased as a function of exposure time and nanoparticle concentration. CuS nanoparticles were seen to induce photothermal destruction of HeLa cells in a laser dose- and nanoparticle concentration-dependent manner and displayed minimal cytotoxic effects with a profile similar to that of gold nanoparticles. The unique optical property of quantum size confinement, small size, low cost of production, and low cytotoxicity make CuS nanoparticles a promising and new type of nanomaterials for cancer Photothermal Ablation. Further studies on the *in vivo* pharmacokinetics, biodistribution, photothermal ablation efficiency, and systemic toxicity are warranted.

FUTURE PERSPECTIVE

As a new type of agent for photothermal treatment of cancer, CuS nanoparticles have many advantages, as reported in this research. The most favourable features are the low costs, simple and easy preparation, and small size for targeting. In addition, the intrinsic *d–d* transition of Cu^{2+} determines its merits for practical application. The only challenging issue is their weak absorbance, as a high-powered laser is required for activation. This is particularly true when the therapy is for *in vivo* applications. Once this problem is solved, their application is vast and may change the direction for photothermal treatment of cancer. The selection of proper lasers at approximately 900 nm to fit the absorption peak and the improvement of the nanoparticle qualities (surface passivation and size distribution), particularly the development of core-shell nanostructures to enhance the oscillator strength, are the possible solutions for enhancement. Numerous studies have shown that *in vivo* delivery of laser light at the NIR region is not a problem. In fact, NIR can penetrate intact skull and skin in mice. Therefore, the treatment based on CuS nanoparticles is promising and will be the focus of our future studies.

7.4 Au/CuS Nanocomposites with Local Field Enhancement for PTT

Cancer nanotechnology is a rapidly growing field that focuses on the development and application of nanomaterials for cancer detection, imaging, diagnosis, treatment, and prevention. Photothermal therapy (PTT) is a method of treating cancer that involves the application of heat between 41 and

45 degrees Celsius to kill cancer cells. The brilliance of PTT is its dual targeting mechanism—it targets both the agents and the light utilised locally to activate them. This method efficiently minimises adverse effects and the possibility of causing injury to adjacent healthy tissue. Nanoparticles, nanoshells, nanocages, hollow nanospheres, nanoplexes, and carbon nanotubes have all been widely explored for PTT therapy in cancer treatment. CuS nanoparticles have a large absorption range between 700 and 1100 nm, and we previously established that when they interact with near infrared light, they generate heat that may be used to PTT cancer cells. CuS nanoparticles have significant benefits over Au nanostructures as a novel type of agent for photothermal cancer treatment. The most advantageous characteristics are the inexpensive cost, ease of preparation, and compact size for targeting. Since our initial publication on CuS nanoparticle-based PTT,20 CuX nanoparticle-based PTT (X = S, Se, and Te) has been a popular topic. However, the PTT efficiency when CuS nanoparticles are used as transducers is lower than when Au nanostructures are used, and this efficiency must be increased for practical applications. The purpose of this study is to determine the effect of Au nanoparticle surface plasmon coupling on the efficacy of CuS nanoparticle-PTT in Au/CuS nanocomposites for cancer treatment. A surface plasmon is an electromagnetic field that is concentrated at the metal-dielectric interface. 25 Surface plasmons can significantly raise the electric field at the surface, hence increasing the rate of any processes that are field-dependent. Due to the fact that the field enhancement caused by surface plasmon resonance is projected to be 1,000 times greater than the incident field, it can be exploited to boost any light excitation or transition processes occurring at interfaces. Metallic nanoparticles' surface plasmon resonances are currently being used for a number of purposes, including molecular sensing, luminescence amplification, Raman effect enhancement, and near-field optical imaging. Due to the resulting localised field amplification, it is reasonable to predict that stimulation of surface plasmons in metal nanoparticles put on a semiconductor would boost optical absorption of light photons within the semiconductor region adjacent to each nanoparticle. In semiconductors and in the optical absorption spectra of molecular adsorbates, surface plasmon enhanced optical absorption has been reported. These enhancement effects have been used to raise the photocurrent in Si-pn junctions, the output of light-emitting diodes,34 and the efficiency of solar cells or photovoltaics. Although Sun et al.36 previously documented the synthesis of Au/CuS core–shell nanoparticles,36 local field augmentation of CuS absorption and the use of local field enhanced

CuS nanoparticles for cancer cell killing have never been reported earlier. For the first time, we report on the augmentation of CuS absorbance in the local field for cancer treatment.

DETAILS OF THE EXPERIMENT

To validate the hypothesis of enhancing the local field of CuS nano-PTT, we created Au/CuS nanocomposites and evaluated them in vitro for cancer treatment. The nanocomposites are prepared in two phases utilizing a modified technique for the synthesis of Au/CuS coreshell nanoparticles. To begin, Au nanoparticles are produced, followed by their coating with CuS shells. The seeded growth method is used to create gold nanoparticles nanopolyhedra. To make the seeds, a freshly prepared, ice-cold 0.01 M NaBH4 solution (0.6 mL, 0.006 mmol) is added to a 0.01 M HAuCl4 (0.25 mL, 0.0025 mmol) and 0.1 M Cetyltrimethylammonium Bromide combination solution (CTAB, 7.5 mL, 0.75 mmol). The resulting solution is rapidly inverted for 2 minutes and then allowed to cool to room temperature for 1 hour before use. The growth solution is made by adding 0.1 M CTAB (6.4 mL, 0.64 mmol), 0.01 M HAuCl4 (0.8 mL, 0.008 mmol), and 0.1 M ascorbic acid (3.8 mL, 0.38 mmol) to water in a sequential fashion (32 mL). The seed solution stabilised with CTAB is diluted tenfold with water. The diluted seed solution (0.02 and 0.06 mL, respectively) is then added to the growth solution to initiate the formation of Au nanoparticles nanocubes and nanopolyhedra. The resulting solution is gently inverted for 10 seconds and then allowed to stand undisturbed overnight. In the second step, 0.002 g (0.0060 mmol) of nickel thiobenzoate, i.e., (PhCOS)2Ni (made using Ni(NO3)2 6H2O, thiobenzoic acid, and AgNO3) is dissolved in 10 mL of previously prepared washed Au nanopolyhedra dispersion. Following that, 0.01 M Cu(NO3)2 solution is added. Cu^{2+} content in the solution is maintained at 300 M. The resulting solution of the mixture is transferred to an autoclave and heated to 140°C for 3 hours. After removing the container from the autoclave, it is allowed at ambient temperature overnight to cool, and then the nanoparticle solution is dialyzed to remove any unreacted compounds.

To investigate the photothermal ablation capacity of Au/CuS nanocomposites in vitro, breast cancer MCF-7 cells (Michigan Cancer Foundation–7) were used. Prior to undertaking photo thermal ablation tests, an MTT assay was used to determine the nanoparticles' toxicity. After three washes with phosphate buffered saline (37°C), the cells were replaced with media. MCF-7 cells were seeded at a density of 2,000 cells per well in a 96-well plate (using 90 L medium) and incubated for 48 hours at 37°C and 5% CO_2. Following incubation, the cells were examined under a microscope (ZEISS IM-35) to see whether they remained attached prior to being treated with nanoparticles. For 24 hours at 37°C and 5% CO_2, the cultured cells were incubated with a control (phosphate buffered saline) and 25% of the concentration of Au/CuS nanoparticle solution (this is the highest concentration of nanoparticle solution utilised in photothermal therapy).

At 37°C and 5% CO_2, the cultivated cells were treated for 24 hours with 25, 10%, and 2.5 percent concentrations of the original 2.4 µM Au/CuS nanoparticle solution. After incubation was complete, the nanoparticle-containing culture media were removed and replaced with fresh media. The cells were subsequently irradiated for 5 minutes with a 980 nm near infrared laser (Opto Engine LLC) operating at 0.125 or 0.2 W/cm^2. After irradiation, the culture media were withdrawn and replaced with new medium, and the cell viability was determined using the MTT assay. Cell viability was determined using the MTT test. Each well received 10 µl of a 5 mg/ml MTT solution and was incubated for 4 hours at 37°C and 5% CO2. After removing the supernatant, the cells were lysed with 100 µl dimethyl sulfoxide. To test cell survival, absorbance at 570 nm was measured using a microplate reader. Additionally, imaging was used to determine the number of surviving and dead cells following photothermal treatment. In this scenario, the cultivated cells were incubated for 24 hours at 37°C and 5% CO_2 with concentrations of 25, 10, and 2.5 percent of the initial Au/CuS nanocomposite solution (2.4 M). After incubation, the nanocomposites-containing culture media were removed and replaced with new media. The cells were then irradiated for 5 minutes with a 980 nm near infrared laser operating at 0, 5, 10, or 20 W/cm^2. The cells were then rinsed with phosphate buffered saline and stained with calcein AM for live cell visibility and with Ethidium Homodimer-1 (EthD-1) for dead cell visualisation, as recommended by the manufacturer (Invitrogen). The cells were photographed using a fluorescent microscope from Olympus, the DP72.

Outcomes & Analysis

It is visible in Figure 7-11 high resolution transmission electron microscope (HRTEM) photos. Clear lattice fringes can be seen in the cores under HRTEM, showing a high degree of crystallinity, and the d-spacing of 0.24 nm matches to the gold (111) lattice planes. In some nanoparticles surrounding the Au nanoparticles, crystal lattice fringes from the (102) and (103) lattice planes of CuS may be detected. The plane measured from Figure has a lattice spacing of around 0.282 nm, while the plane (102) has a lattice spacing of roughly 0.30 nm. These results are quite consistent with the lattice spacing of the (103) plane (0.282 nm) and the (102) plane (0.305 nm) of previously reported hexagonal CuS nanostructures. The TEM observations demonstrate the creation of Au/CuS nanocomposites, and the structure of our nanocomposites is comparable to that of previously described Au/CuS core–shell nanostructures. However, given their observable structure, it is more fair to refer to them as nano composites.

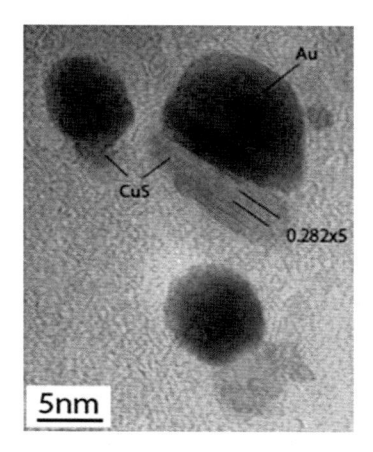

Fig. 7-11. Transmission electron microscopy images of Au/CuS nanocomposites. **Adopted from ref. 4 with permission**

The creation of Au/CuS nanocomposites can be confirmed further by examining the optical absorption spectra of Au, CuS, and Au/CuS nanoparticles, as illustrated in Figure 7-12, where the concentration of Au or CuS is the same in each sample. Au nanoparticles exhibit a 531 nm absorption peak, CuS nanoparticles exhibit a 981 nm absorption peak, and Au/CuS nanocomposites exhibit two absorption peaks at 531 and 981 nm. It's rather fascinating to see how much absorbance is increased in Au/CuS nanocomposites. CuS nanoparticles' absorption peak at 981 nm is raised approximately 2.2 times. To determine the mechanism of the enhancement, we investigated the optical absorption spectra of Au and CuS nanoparticle mixtures and found no enhancement in their mixtures, as illustrated in Figure 7-12. This implies that the enhancement in the absorption of Au/CuS nanocomposite is due to the local field enhancement caused by Au nanoparticle surface plasmon coupling, as previously reported.

As a result of the improved absorption intensity in Au/CuS nanocomposites due to the local field, the PTT efficacy may be increased. To demonstrate the enhancement, photothermal treatment of MCF-7 (Michigan Cancer Foundation–7) breast cancer cells with Au/CuS core–shell nanoparticles at three different laser output powers (5, 10, and 15 W/cm^2) and three different concentrations (2.5, 10, and 25% of the original Au/CuS nanocomposites concentration, 2.4 M) was performed. A 980 nm near infrared laser was utilised in this investigation because to the absorption maxima of Au/CuS nanocomposites at 981 nm. Additionally, there are two advantages to employing a 980 nm laser in photothermal treatment rather than an 808 nm laser. To begin, 980 nm light has a greater penetration depth into tissue than 808 nm light. Second, the safety limit for human skin exposure to 980 nm lasers is 0.726 W/cm^2, more than double that of 808 nm lasers (0.33 W/cm^2).

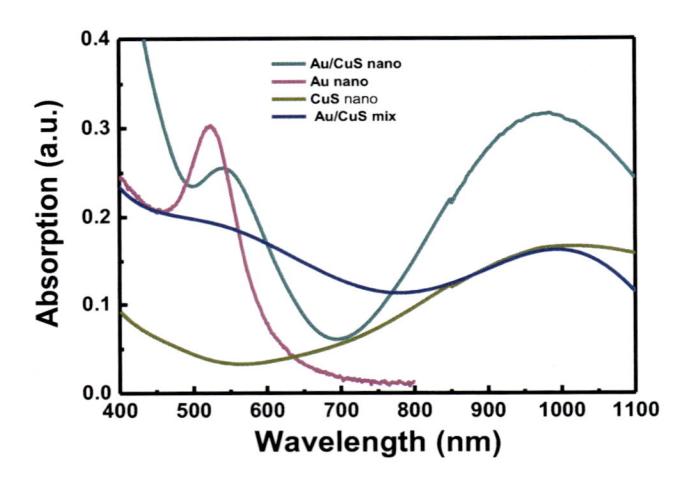

Figure 7-12. Absorption spectra of Au, CuS, Au/CuS nanocomposites and the mixtures of Au and CuS nanoparticle solutions. Enhancement is seen in the core-shell nanoparticles but not in the mixtures. **Adopted from ref. 4 with permission**

Figures 7-13 detail the findings of the cell killing tests. Calcein is used to visualise active cells, while Ethidium Homodimer-1 (EthD-1) is used to visualise dead cells, as recommended by the manufacturer (Invitrogen). As a control, Figure 3 illustrates the effects of treatment with PBS and a 980 nm laser at a power density of 5 W/cm2 for 5, 10, and 20 seconds on MCF-7 cancer cells. As demonstrated, no cancer cells were destroyed by PBS and 980 nm laser therapy. Figures 4–6 illustrate the time dependence of the treatment at a 5 W/cm2 laser power for 5, 10, and 20 seconds at various Au/Cu nanoparticle concentrations, and Figure 7-14 displays the results of photothermal treatments on MCF-7 breast cancer cells using Au/CuS nanocomposites at a 5 W/cm2 laser power. The data depicted in Figure 7-13 (top) illustrate that nanoparticles or lasers alone are incapable of killing cancer cells. However, when combined with a laser for activation, the nanoparticles can successfully kill cancer cells. At a laser power of 5 W/cm2 and a 25% concentration of the original Au/CuS nanocomposites, practically all cells were killed. The time dependence of the treatment at a 5 W/cm2 laser for 5, 10, and 20 seconds is shown in Figure 7-13 (bottom). As demonstrated by the data, for 10% concentrations, 20 seconds is sufficient to destroy nearly 100% of the cells, whereas for 25% of the original concentration, a 5-second treatment is sufficient to eradicate all cells. This suggests that the treatment requires a very low light exposure and is quite successful.

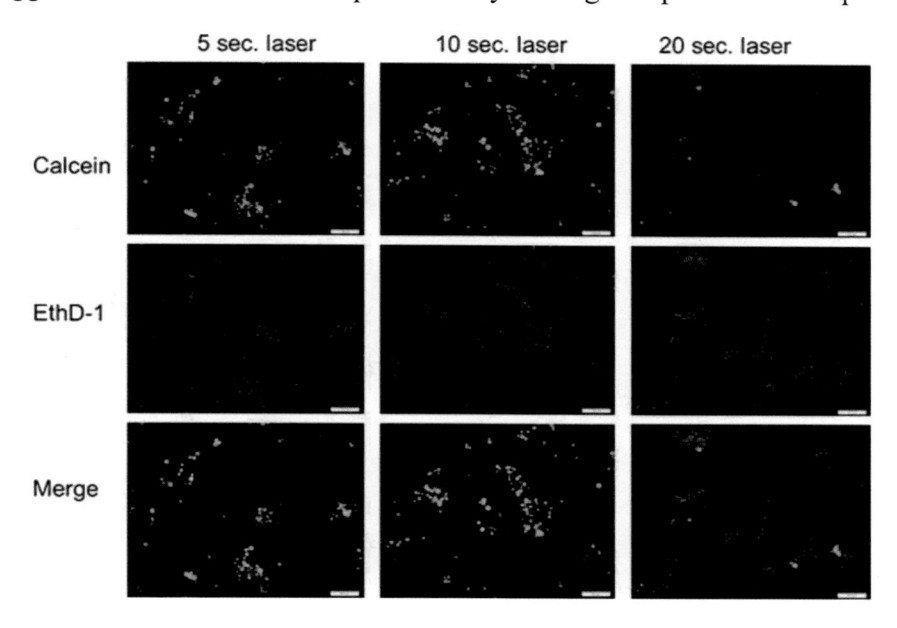

Fig. 7-13. Treatment of Michigan Cancer Foundation–7 (MCF-7) cells with Au/CuS nanocomposites (10% the original concentration of Au/CuS, 2.4 _M) and 980 nm laser at 5 W/cm2 for 5, 10 and 20 seconds. Scale bar: 100 _m **Adopted from ref. 4 with permission**

A quantitative analysis of Au/CuS nanocomposite-PTT was conducted using two distinct laser powers (0.125 and 0.2 W/cm^2) and three different concentrations (2.5, 10%, and 25% of the initial Au/CuS nanocomposites concentration, 2.4 M). To evaluate cell survival following photothermal treatment, the 3-(4,5-Dimethylthiazol-2-yl)-2,5-diphenyltetrazolium bromide (MTT) assay was utilised. Our observations indicate that the 0.125 W/cm^2 laser power is insufficient for the treatment (Fig. 7-14). However, as illustrated in Figure 9, 0.2 W/cm^2 is sufficient to activate our Au/CuS nanocomposites via PTT (right). Over 50% of cancer cells were destroyed at the 25% dosage. This laser power is far less than the safe level of exposure to human skin (0.726 W/cm^2 for a 980 nm laser). In our previously reported therapy using CuS nanoparticles, the lowest laser power required to eradicate cancer cells was 24 W/cm^2 for 5 minutes (from an 808 nm laser). 10 W/cm2 laser power is required to destroy hematopoietic stem cells and human ovarian cancer cells when hollow Au nanospheres are used. As a result, we can conclude that Au/CuS nanocomposites-based PTT is much improved when compared to CuS nanoparticles. The treatment laser power described here is also significantly less than that reported by Tian et al., who employed 0.51 W/cm^2 laser power with CuS superstructures for PTT. Indeed, to our knowledge, 0.2 W/cm^2 is the lowest documented laser power for photothermal cancer treatment.

We also examined the cytotoxicity of the Au/CuS nanocomposites, and the results are presented on the left of Figure 9 in contrast to control phosphate buffered saline. Cell viability is greater than 80% at all nanoparticle doses examined. The findings indicate that Au/CuS core–shell nanoparticles exhibit little or negligible cytotoxicity, making them ideal transducer agents for photothermal cancer treatment.

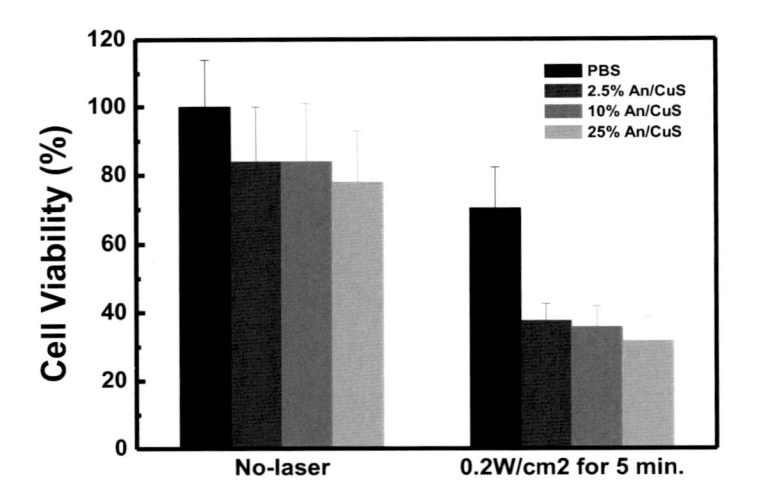

Fig. 7-14. Cell viability without laser treatment (on the left) and after 0.2 W/cm² of 980 nm laser treatment for 5 minutes (on the right). The Au/CuS nanocomposite concentrations are 2.5%, 10% and 25% of the original concentration of Au/CuS, 2.4 µM. **Adopted from ref. 4 with permission**

The Bottom Line

In summary, we have proven for the first time that surface plasmon coupling can be exploited to increase the PTT of CuS nanoparticles for cancer treatment. The same technique as described here can be utilised to improve the PTT of related nanoparticles such as CuSe and CuTe nanoparticles, or any other nanoparticle capable of PTT. Au/CuS nanocomposites with improved local field exhibit a better absorbance and PTT efficacy than both Au and CuS nanostructures. As a result, local field enhanced Au/CuS nanocomposites or core–shell nanoparticles are interesting photothermal transducer agents.

7.5 self-sensitized photothermal cancer therapy to overcome heat stress

PTT alone is not always effective in completely getting rid of tumors, especially breast tumors. One of the reasons for this is that tumor cells have protective mechanisms that activate when they are exposed to laser heat, and this makes them more resistant to the treatment as illustrated in Figure 7-15.

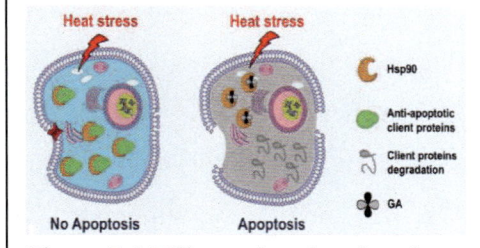

Figure 7-15 Illustration showing the use of GA-containing nanosystem to overcome thermal resistance by inhibiting HSP90. Adopted from ref. 7 with permission

Scientists have found that a group of proteins called Heat Shock Proteins (HSPs) play a role in protecting tumor cells from the heat damage caused by the laser. Among these proteins, HSP90 is particularly important because it is involved in regulating proteins related to tumor growth and progression, and it is highly expressed in tumors.

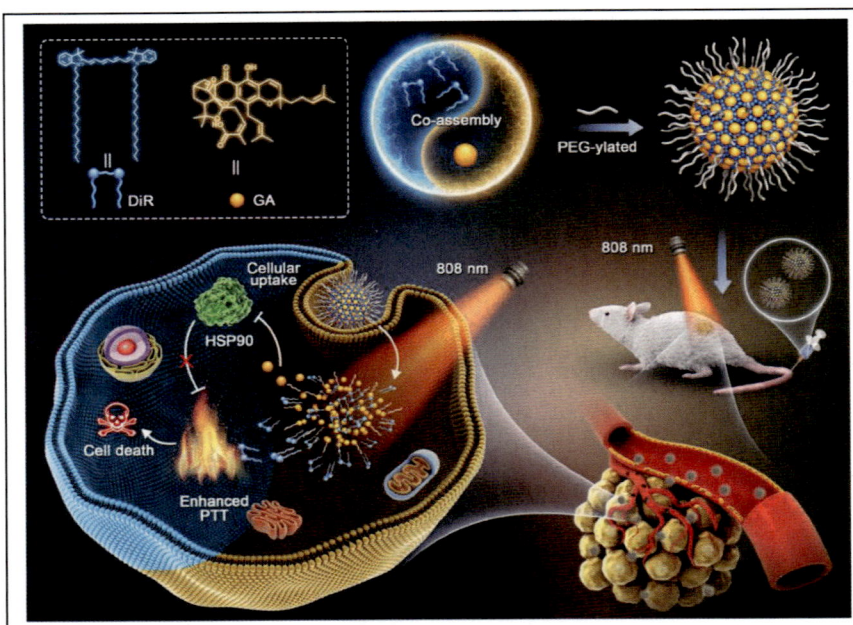

Figure 7-16 Schematic illustration of DiR/GA co-delivery nanoassembly and HSP90 inhibition-enhanced PTT by hyperthermia sensitization. adopted from ref. 6 with permission

To improve the effectiveness of PTT, researchers have looked into using substances that can inhibit HSP90. One such substance is gambogic acid (GA), which is a natural product that has been found to inhibit HSP90. Combining GA with the laser treatment could potentially make the tumor cells more sensitive to the therapy. The challenge is how to deliver both the GA and the laser-sensitive substances to the tumor at the same time. Scientists have been working on creating tiny particles called nanocarriers that can carry multiple drugs and deliver them to the tumor simultaneously. However, the conventional nanocarriers have some limitations, such as low efficiency in carrying drugs, difficulty in controlling the drug proportions, and inconsistency in drug release.

To overcome these limitations, researchers have developed a new approach. They found that GA and a commonly used laser-sensitive substance called DiR can naturally assemble together in water. Using this unique feature, they created a carrier-free nanoassembly containing both GA and DiR in the right proportion. This new nanosystem showed great potential in effectively inhibiting HSPs and enhancing the PTT treatment in mice with breast tumors. (Figure 7-16)

The researchers also investigated how the nanoassembly is taken up by tumor cells. They found that the nanoassembly was more efficiently taken up by the cells compared to the individual drugs, thanks to the mechanism of particles being engulfed by the cells. (Figure 7-17)

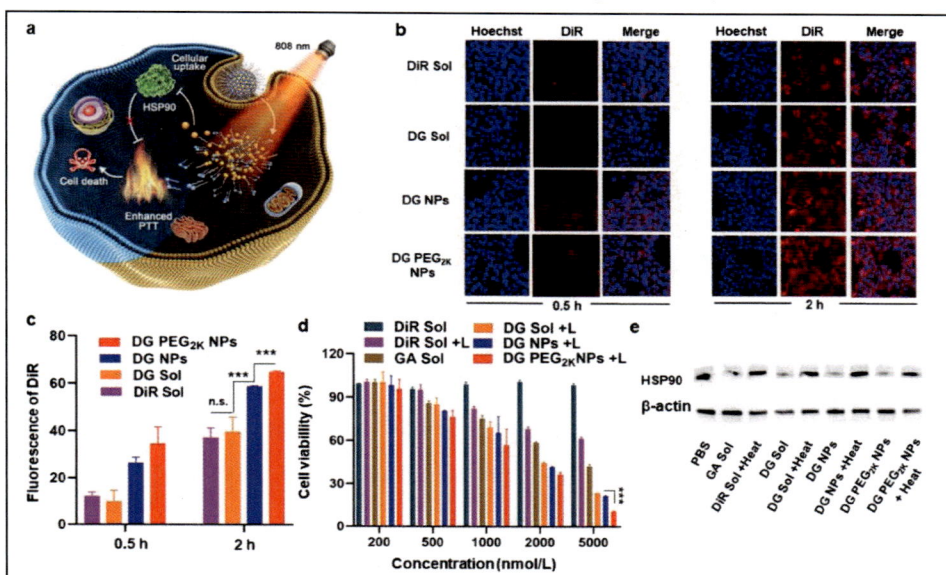

Fig. 7-17 Cellular uptake and synergistic in vitro antitumor effect of hybrid nanoassemblies. a Intracellular mechanism of HSP90 inhibition -enhanced PTT by hyperthermia sensitization; b Confocal imaging of 4T1 cells treated with DiR Sol, DG Sol, DG NPs and DG PEG2K NPs for 0.5 and 2 h, at a DiR equivalent dose of 2 μmol/L; c Quantitative results of cellular uptake in 0.5 and 2 h from flow cytometry, respectively; d Synergistic cytotoxicity against 4T1 cells with or without laser irradiation (3 W/cm2, 3 min); e Western blotting analysis of HSP90 protein expression in 4T1 cells with simulated heat treatment at 50 °C for 3 min. Scale bar = 50 μm. n.s. no significance, ***P < 0.001. adopted from ref. 6 with permission

The researchers successfully developed a new approach to combine a substance that inhibits HSPs (GA) with a laser-sensitive substance (DiR) to improve the effectiveness of Photothermal Therapy for treating tumors. The nanosystem they created showed great promise in delivering the drugs effectively to the tumor site and enhancing the therapeutic outcome. This represents a significant step towards a potential new treatment strategy for cancer.

References for this chapter

1. O'Neal, D. P., Hirsch, L. R., Halas, N. J., Payne, J. D., and West, J. L. (2004). Photo-thermal tumor ablation in mice using near infrared-absorbing nanoparticles. *Cancer Lett.* 209, 171–176. doi: 10.1016/j.canlet.2004.02.004

2. Link, S., and El-Sayed, M. A. (1999). Size and temperature dependence of the plasmon absorption of colloidal gold nanoparticles. *J. Phys. Chem. B* 103, 4212–4217. doi: 10.1021/jp984796o

3. Yuebin Li, Wei Lu, Qian Huang, Chun Li, **Wei Chen**, *In vitro* Photothermal Ablation of Tumor Cells with CuS nanoparticles, *Nanomedicine (London)*, 2010, 5(8): 1161-1171

4. Santana Bala Lakshmanan, Xiaoju Zou, Marius Hossu, Lun Ma, Chang Yang, and Wei Chen, Local Field Enhanced Au/CuS Core-Shell Nanoparticles as efficient Photothermal Transducer Agents for Cancer Treatment, *J. Biomed. Nanotechnol.*, 2012, 8(6),883-890

5. Yu Yang, Wenjun Zhu, Ziliang Dong, Yu Chao, Lai Xu, Meiwan Chen, Zhuang Liu, 1D Coordination Polymer Nanofibers for Low-Temperature Photothermal Therapy Adv. Mater. 2017, 29, 1703588

6. Shan, X., Zhang, X., Wang, C. *et al.* Molecularly engineered carrier-free co-delivery nanoassembly for self-sensitized photothermal cancer therapy. *J Nanobiotechnol* **19**, 282 (2021). https://doi.org/10.1186/s12951-021-01037-6

7. Deng X, Shao Z, Zhao Y. Solutions to the Drawbacks of Photothermal and Photodynamic Cancer Therapy. Adv Sci (Weinh). 2021 Jan 5;8(3):2002504. doi: 10.1002/advs.202002504. PMID: 33552860; PMCID: PMC7856884.

8. Zhou J, Lu Z, Zhu X, Wang X, Liao Y, Ma Z, Li F. NIR photothermal therapy using polyaniline nanoparticles. Biomaterials. 2013 Dec;34(37):9584-92.
doi: 10.1016/j.biomaterials.2013.08.075. Epub 2013 Sep 14. PMID: 24044996.

Chapter 8

Hypoxia and Therapy

8.1 Definitions - Hypoxia, hypoxia-inducible factors, and glucose metabolism

The metabolism of a solid tumour is markedly different from that of normal tissue surrounding it. Otto Warburg identified the major metabolic changes occurring within the tumour more than 70 years ago. He discovered that normal tissue generates around 10% of the cell's ATP via glycolysis, whereas mitochondria create 90%. However, in tumour sections, glycolysis accounts for more than 50% of cellular energy production, with the remaining coming from the mitochondria. Interestingly, this transition occurs even when there is sufficient oxygen available to maintain mitochondrial function; this is referred to as aerobic glycolysis. Because tumour cells rely on glycolysis for energy production, they use more glucose due to glycolysis's low efficiency at creating ATP. The mechanisms underlying this ansition are being elucidated, and they are providing new information and hypotheses about how this metabolic profile can confer a growth advantage to tumours.

One of the most well-established explanations for abnormal tumour metabolism is the tumour's specific physiological stressors. The tumour microenvironment is hypoxic (low oxygen saturation), acidic, and has an elevated interstitial fluid pressure. These microenvironmental stressors are mostly caused by abnormal tumour vascular formation. Significant portions of the tumour are located far from the supporting blood arteries, creating a gradient of diffusion-limited hypoxia, low nutrition levels, and high waste product levels. (Figure 8-1) Hypoxia is perhaps the most prevalent of these stresses, occurring when O_2 delivery falls short of the demand within tumour tissue. Tumour cells respond to these conditions by adjusting their metabolism to accommodate the limited supply of O_2. Perhaps the most critical feature of how cells respond to this distinct milieu is the activity of the transcription factor hypoxia-inducible factor 1 (HIF1).

Hypoxic HIF1 activation has the net effect of redistributing energy generation by enhancing glycolysis and lowering mitochondrial activity. Although HIF1 was initially identified in response to low O_2 levels, it is now clear that it can be regulated by other variables such as oncogene activation or loss of tumour suppressors. For example, HIF1 accumulates in tumour cells upon activation of oncogenes such as Ras, SRC, and phosphoinositide 3-kinase (PI3K), or the loss of tumour suppressors such as VHL (von Hippel–Lindau) or PTEN8. Additionally, increasing amounts of metabolites such as succinate and fumarate, or O_2 by-products such as free radicals, can stabilise HIF1α in a tumour. The total effect

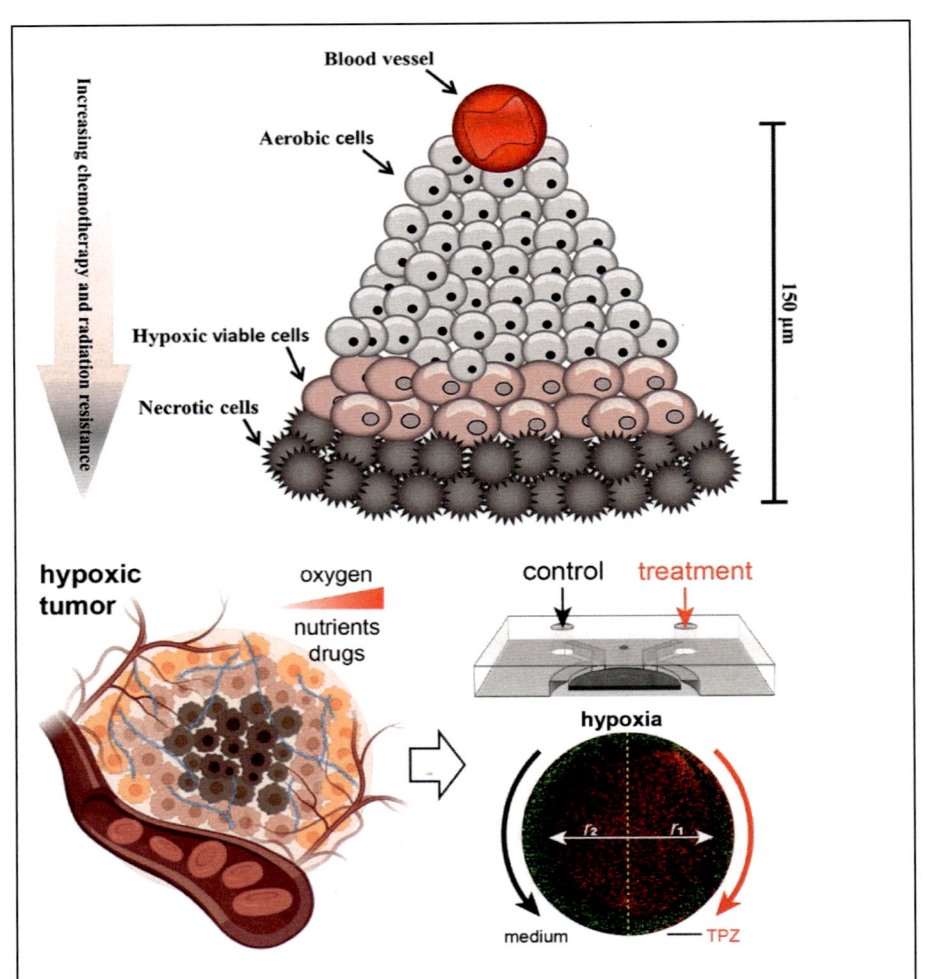

Figure 8-1 **Top**: Hypoxic regions of solid tumors. Tumors contain regions of oxygenated cells situated near to blood vessels, becoming increasingly hypoxic with increased distance from a functional blood supply. **Bottom**: Integrated microfluidic design of 2-D and 3-D tumor hypoxia models- Tumor hypoxia in vivo, Recapitulating tumor hypoxia in vitro in 2-D and 3-D models with diffusion barriers and Design of hypoxia microdevice with a polycarbonate (PC) film as the top oxygen diffusion barrier. Adopted from refs. 2 and 3 with permissions

of these genetic and physiological changes within the tumour is to increase HIF1 and actively shift energy generation away from mitochondrial to glycolytic sources in both hypoxic and oxygenated regions.

HIF1 activation and the HIF1 transcriptional programme have two significant effects on metabolism, both of which serve to balance O_2 demand and supply. To begin, HIF1 promotes glycolytic energy generation by transactivating genes involved in extracellular glucose import (such as GLUT1, also known as SLC2A1) and glycolytic enzymes responsible for internal glucose breakdown (such as phosphofructokinase 1 (PFK1) and aldolase). Glycolysis is the biological process by which glucose is converted to pyruvate and two molecules of ATP are generated. If glucose is available, this low-yield energy synthesis is sufficient to produce ATP for cellular energetics. Pyruvate can be further degraded in the mitochondria by a process called oxidative phosphorylation, which utilizes oxygen to produce CO_2, H_2O, and approximately 18 more molecules of ATP. HIF1 also inhibits oxidative phosphorylation within the mitochondria by transactivating genes such as pyruvate dehydrogenase kinase 1 (PDK1) and MAX interactor 1 (MAXI1) (MXI1). These two processes result in a decrease in the O_2 requirement of tumour cells within hypoxic tissue while maintaining enough energy to supply the cell. By achieving both of these primary impacts, HIF1 can induce the major metabolic alterations discovered by Otto Warburg within the tumour. Cancer cells with limited efficiency must take in quantitatively far more glucose than normal tissue. This disparity can be evaluated clinically by labelling the glucose tracer 2-deoxyglucose with the radioemitter ^{18}F and detecting and quantifying its uptake by the tumour (and normal tissues) using a positron-emission tomography scanner.

HIF1 regulation

The transcription factor HIF1 is so termed due to the cellular machinery that maintains HIF1α stability under hypoxia. This hypoxia response is undoubtedly the most well-characterized component of HIF1's ability to regulate metabolism. Because hypoxia is produced by a mismatch between O_2 delivery and consumption, a large number of gene expression alterations are intended to correct this mismatch. This can be accomplished by reducing consumption (through changed metabolism) or increasing supply (through erythropoietin and vascular endothelial growth factor production). Additional variables, however, have been identified that can result in the buildup of HIF1 and may potentially regulate metabolism under aerobic settings. Aspects peculiar to solid tumours, such as oncogenic mutations and the buildup of intermediate metabolites, are especially significant because they can contribute to HIF1 regulation in areas with increased oxygenation.

Hypoxia

HIF1 is a heterodimeric transcription factor composed of the O_2-responsive subunit HIF1α or HIF2α (also known as ePAS1) and the constitutively expressed subunit HIF1 (also known as

ARnT). HIF1, whether comprising HIF1α or HIF2α, recognizes equivalent hypoxia-responsive elements (HRes) in the promoters of target genes; nevertheless, the two subunits appear to activate somewhat distinct groups of genes. Notably, HIF1 appears to possess a novel transactivation domain that promotes the activation of hypoxia-responsive glycolytic genes. HIF1α and HIF2α appear to regulate hypoxia responses differently in cell types such as kidney malignancies, although our comprehension of this is limited.

Due to ubiquitin-mediated degradation, HIF1α is unstable in well-oxygenated tissues but rapidly becomes stable in hypoxic environments. Human HIF1 is degraded via hydroxylation of prolines 402 and 564. Because O_2 has a low affinity for the prolyl hydroxylases (PHDs, which give sensitivity to O_2), HIF1α is not hydroxylated and so maintained when the O_2 tension (pO_2) decreases. vHL complexed to elongins B and C recognises the hydroxylated prolines. vHL functions in conjunction with neDD8 as an e3 ubiquitin ligase, modifying and targeting HIF1 for destruction. When vHL expression in renal malignancies is eliminated, HIF1α and HIF2α become constitutively stable (even in normoxia), leading to constitutive transactivation of target genes and loss of vHL-mediated tumour suppression. The asparagine hydroxylase factor inhibiting HIF (FIH, also known as HIF1An) inhibits HIF1α activity by hydroxylating asparagine 803 in the carboxy-terminal transactivation domain of human HIF1α. Thus, hydroxylation-mediated regulation is the primary mechanism by which HIF1α is regulated in normal tissue and influences HIF1 activity in tumour cells. Several other changes, however, can also increase HIF1α protein levels in the absence of hypoxia.

Oncogenes

When it was discovered that the stability of the HIF1 protein was actively regulated, multiple genes involved in this mechanism were identified. In both normoxic and hypoxic situations, the production of oncogenes such as HRAS-v12 results in the buildup of HIF1. Due to this effect, tumour cells frequently exhibit enhanced activation of HIF1 target genes *in vitro*, and subsequent investigation revealed that activation of the Ras–MAPK (mitogen-activated protein kinase) pathway resulted in HIF1α accumulation in a variety of model systems. Additionally, in normoxic conditions, production of the oncogenes encoding SRC28 and eRBB2 can boost HIF1α protein and target gene expression. Although the specific mechanism(s) by which these oncogenes act is unknown, HIF1α is hyperphosphorylated, indicating that activated kinases reacting to oncogenic stress may be candidates.

Additionally, stimulation of the PI3K pathway in normoxia might result in HIF1α accumulation. Increased HIF1α levels and activity are induced by direct activation of PI3K or its downstream kinase Akt, or by inactivation of the inhibitory PTen tumour suppressor. Although this effect may be cancer-type-specific, there appears to be a link with cancer types that lose PTen or gain Akt during carcinogenesis (such as glioblastoma and prostate cancer cells). Notably, the method does not appear to be dependent on direct Akt30 phosphorylation of HIF1α. While HIF1α hydroxylation and degradation appear to be unaltered in these cells, HIF1α translation appears to be enhanced, which is assumed to be owing to Akt-dependent activation of mTOR (also known as FRAP1). Alternatively, oncogenes' indirect effects on cell proliferation or metabolism could also lead to HIF1 buildup.

Adverse consequences

Along with HIF1 being the primary regulator of glucose metabolism, there are glucose metabolites that can positively influence HIF1 via a feedback mechanism. The significance of this regulation was recently recognised when it was discovered that the genes encoding succinate dehydrogenase (SDH) and fumarate hydratase (FH) were indeed tumour suppressors, contributing to the transformation of malignant pheochromocytomas and leiomyomas, respectively. Normally, these enzymes of the tricarboxylic acid (TCA) cycle create reducing equivalents for the mitochondrial electron transport chain. When they are mutated, they obstruct the passage of metabolites, resulting in a buildup of succinate and/or fumarate. One impact of these elevated levels is the development of a syndrome known as 'pseudohypoxia.' Due to the fact that the HIF1 PHDs convert 2-oxoglutarate (α-ketoglutarate) and O_2 to succinate and CO_2, elevated succinate levels can inhibit this enzyme, resulting in HIF1α stabilisation. Thus, mutations in SDH or FH have been demonstrated to result in the stabilisation of HIF1 in normoxic cells. Numerous other endogenous 2-oxoacids, including pyruvate and lactate, have been shown to stabilise HIF1, establishing a novel feed-forward mechanism. By inhibiting this mechanism of HIF1α stabilisation with exogenous α-ketoglutarate derivatives, treatment options for these tumours may be developed.

Additionally, it has been postulated that reactive oxygen species (ROS) produced as a byproduct of electron transport in the mitochondria can signal to stabilise HIF1 in hypoxia. Although the interaction between mitochondrial superoxide and the HIF degradation mechanism is unknown, it has been observed that hydrogen peroxide can oxidise the Fe^{2+} necessary for PHD activity. The resultant Fe^{3+} is incapable of hydroxylation, and the loss of PHD activity results in the stabilisation of HIF1α. This, however, is debatable, as other groups have reported that HIF1α can be stabilised in hypoxia in cells lacking mitochondria.

Mechanisms of HIF1-induced glycolysis enhancement

HIF1 can accelerate glucose absorption by inducing the facultative glucose transporters GLUT1 and GLUT3 (SLC2A3). These transporters are members of a superfamily that also includes 13 facultative transporters50. However, due to their widespread expression pattern, amount of molecules per cell, and affinity for glucose, GLUT1, GLUT3, and GLUT4 (SLC2A4) regulate the bulk of glucose uptake. Due to the fact that these transporters transfer glucose down its concentration gradient from relatively high blood levels to relatively low intracellular levels, just raising the protein's quantity boosts glucose flow into the hypoxic cell. HIF1 is a significant physiological inducer of glucose transporters in tumour cells.

Once glucose is absorbed by the cell, it can take on a variety of metabolic fates. Hexokinase (HK) rapidly phosphorylates intracellular glucose to glucose-6-phosphate. While HIF1 can stimulate both HK1 and HK2, it appears that HK2 is more relevant for glucose modification in hypoxia. Due to the fact that the charged glucose molecule cannot easily move back through the plasma membrane, it becomes imprisoned within the cell. Glucose-6-phosphate is then employed in one of several ways: as a structural component in the production of glycoproteins, as a metabolite in the pentose shunt to generate ribose, as a precursor for glycogen synthesis, or, most commonly, as a pyruvate precursor in glycolysis. HIF1 can direct glucose into glycolysis by boosting the activity of the glycolysis enzymes. All 12 enzymes required for glycolysis are directly regulated — at least in part — by HIF1, implying that HIF1 coordinately stimulates the entire process. Due to the reversibility of each step, the rate of glycolysis is essentially determined by substrate and product availability; thus, one way to increase glucose breakdown is to increase the expression of enzymes within the cell. PFK1, on the other hand, catalyses an irreversible process and is allosterically regulated by the amount of fructose 2,6-bisphosphate. This metabolite is produced by PFKFB2, a member of the 6-phosphofructo-2-kinase/fructose 2,6-bisphosphatase family of enzymes (PFKFB1 to PFKFB4). PFKFB3 is likewise activated by HIF1 and can be blocked by TIGAR (C12orf5), a p53 target. However, higher glycolytic enzyme expression generally favours the usage of glucose in glycolysis. Thus, glycolysis converts glucose, two ADP, and two NAD$^+$ to two pyruvate, two ATP, and two NADH.

Pyruvate is a byproduct of glycolysis, and as glycolysis proceeds, more pyruvate is generated and must be eliminated. Although the mechanism is unknown, tumour cell proliferation can be slowed when the pyruvate elimination mechanism is genetically disrupted by short hairpin RNA directed against LDHA. It is possible that accumulation of glycolysis's end product hinders the pathway's future activity, or that LDHA is essential for recycling the cytosolic NAD+ required for further glycolysis. Pyruvate from the cytoplasm reaches the mitochondria under normoxic circumstances, and the reducing equivalents in NADH are shuttled into the mitochondria (through the malateaspartate or 3-phosphoglycerate shuttles) to serve as substrates for oxidative phosphorylation. Pyruvate is oxidised to CO_2, creating extra NADH and $FADH_2$ in the mitochondria. These mitochondrial reducing equivalents contribute electrons to the electron transport chain and mix with O_2 to form water and a proton gradient for ATP synthesis. However, as mentioned below, the mitochondria within the hypoxic cell do not appear to operate well, resulting in the accumulation of cytoplasmic pyruvate and NADH. HIF1 also activates a second mechanism for the elimination of these chemicals. HIF1 induces the expression of LDHA, which catalyses the conversion of pyruvate and nADH to lactate and NAD$^+$. After that, the lactate can be eliminated from the cell via the HIF-inducible plasma membrane monocarboxylate transporter 4. (MCT4, SLC16A4). This concurrently resolves two issues: excess pyruvate elimination and NAD$^+$ regeneration, which is required by glyceraldehyde-3-phosphate dehydrogenase (GAPDH) for subsequent glycolysis cycles.

HIF1 has an effect on mitochondrial function

Papandreou and colleagues were the first to demonstrate that HIF1 is both essential and sufficient for hypoxia downregulation of mitochondrial function (using gene deletion and knockdown cells). Additionally, these investigations demonstrated that HIF-negative cells exhibited higher mitochondrial activity, which results in increased intracellular hypoxia under specific growth conditions, such as high cell density. This consumption-driven hypoxia was most pronounced at intermediate hypoxia levels, such as 1–2% O_2. Recent research has discovered numerous methods by which HIF1α-regulated genes influence mitochondrial function, resulting in decreased O_2 consumption and intracellular hypoxia.

The mechanisms by which HIF-dependent hypoxia impairs mitochondrial function

Pyruvate, amino acids, and fatty acids can all be used as fuel to generate energy in the mitochondria. Although glutamine has been demonstrated to contribute considerably to overall energy production in tumour cells, hypoxia has not been proved to trigger these activities. As a result, the predominant carbon source in the majority of hypoxic cells is pyruvate, which is the end product of glycolysis. In hypoxic tumour cells with enhanced glycolysis and pyruvate levels, an active mechanism for excluding this increased pyruvate from the mitochondria is required. Several groups recently established that PDK1 is a direct transcriptional target of HIF1. This gene is upregulated in a variety of different types of tumour cells in response to hypoxia and HIF1 stabilisation. PDK1 is a protein kinase that has the ability to phosphorylate and inactivate the e1 component of the mitochondrial enzyme pyruvate dehydrogenase (PDH). PDH catalyses the irreversible breakdown of pyruvate in the mitochondria into acetylCoA and CO_2 while producing NADH. At citrate synthase, acetyl-CoA is metabolised and directly transfers two carbons to the TCA cycle (CS). The reducing equivalents generated by this mechanism (in the form of NADH and FADH2) are immediately utilised in the electron transport chain to generate an additional 18 ATP. By inactivating PDH, PDK isoforms prevent pyruvate from entering the mitochondria. Pyruvate is not incorporated into the TCA cycle, and hence the generation of reducing equivalents required to power the electron transport chain is reduced. This reduction in fuel leads to a reduction in oxidative phosphorylation, a reduction in total cellular O_2 consumption and ROS production.

A second way by which HIF1 decreases the demand for O_2 has been identified is through regulation of mitochondrial biogenesis. This method needs chronic HIF1 activity and appears to be more pronounced in cells that lack vHL but have constitutive HIF1 activation, such as those found in renal cell carcinoma. This method involves the stimulation of MXI1 by HIF1 resulting in a reduction in the number of mitochondria per cell. The mechanism underlying this effect is the oncogenic transcription factor MYC's function in stimulating mitochondrial biogenesis. MYC can dimerise with its activating partner MAX and transactivate the transcription factor A-encoding gene directly (TFAM). TFAM has a role in the expression of the mitochondrial genome and the genes required for DNA replication in the mitochondria. HIF has the ability to directly activate another Myc family member, the negative regulator MXI1, hence disabling MAX and inactivating MYC. As a result of the loss of vHL, TFAM expression, mitochondrial mass, and mitochondrial O_2 consumption are decreased in renal cancer cells. However, because MYC and HIF have been shown to cooperate in promoting gene expression, it is unclear why MYC promotes mitochondrial biogenesis while HIF and hypoxia impair mitochondrial function. Furthermore, oncogenic transformation typically contributes to cancer cells' glycolytic phenotype, making the contribution of a potent oncogene like MYC to mitochondrial function surprising.

The third way by which HIF1 regulates mitochondrial function under hypoxia is by modifying the activity of cytochrome c oxidase (COX) to ensure that it operates efficiently in the presence of limited substrate supply. Cytochrome c oxidase, being the final complex in the electron transport chain, utilises O_2 as the terminal electron acceptor. The model predicts an isoform switch in one of the cytochrome c oxidase complex's regulatory subunits. When HIF1 is stimulated, human kidney cells express COX4I1, COX4I2, and the mitochondrial LOn protease (LOnP1). In situ, the LOn protease is responsible for COX4I1 protein subunit turnover. The two isoforms are biochemically distinct and are thought to have a different affinity for oxygen and a different turnover rate of the catalytic COX1 and COX2 subunits. This hypothesis looks to be analogous to the way yeast Saccharomyces cerevisiae responds to anoxia, which similarly involves an isoform transition at the cytochrome c oxidase complex. In the more studied S. cerevisiae, the COX v component (which is closely linked to the mammalian COX4 protein) is expressed in two forms: COXva in normoxia and COXvb in anoxia. When COX4I2 is overexpressed ectopically in kidney epithelial cells, there is an increase in O_2 consumption in cells grown in hypoxia. In hypoxic cells, however, loss of function of COX4I2 led in decreased O_2 consumption. This regulated O_2 consumption (together with other observations) was interpreted to indicate that COX4I2 was more efficient at utilising the remaining O_2 under hypoxia.

A metabolic advantage for tumour growth

Warburg made crucial observations showing tumour cells had increased glycolysis and decreased oxidative phosphorylation compared to normal cells, but he was unable to explain how this metabolic shift resulted in a growth advantage for tumour cells *in vivo*. It has been speculated that enhanced glycolysis is responsible for the phenotypic alterations observed in tumour cells.

However, greater glycolysis is required in cells with impaired mitochondrial activity, as these are the cell's only energy producing systems. Thus, it is possible that the decreased mitochondrial activity is causing the glycolytic increase, rather than vice versa. The diminished mitochondrial function may account for the tumour cell growth advantage. I will cover two of the better established explanations for why downregulating mitochondrial function could benefit tumour cells, as well as present a third possibility. Because these three models are not mutually exclusive, they could all contribute to the aggressive tumour phenotype caused by the metabolic change.

Reduced mitochondrial function results in decreased ROS generation

ROS generated metabolically can originate in the mitochondria as a byproduct of electron transport. ROS at high concentrations can be hazardous to cells due to their corrosive effects on cellular macromolecules. During the Q cycle, a small fraction of single electrons travelling through complex 3 of the electron transport chain can 'leak' from ubisemiquinone cofactors. These free electrons are grabbed with high affinity by molecular oxygen to create the superoxide radical O_2^-. Superoxide and its breakdown products have a pleiotropic effect on normal and tumour cell signaling systems. However, the involvement of reactive oxygen species (ROS) in hypoxia-induced mortality remains debatable. To bolster this hazardous ROS idea, researchers have demonstrated higher survival in cells exposed to hypoxia that are capable of enzymatic ROS detoxification (such as superoxide dismutase). One must account for ROS produced by non-mitochondrial sources and following re-oxygenation. Additionally, there is considerable debate regarding the influence of hypoxia on ROS generation. Some findings indicate that hypoxia can enhance ROS production, whereas others indicate no increase.

Reduced mitochondrial function should also result in a decrease in the amount of reactive oxygen species (ROS) created as a by-product of respiration. HIF1 has been shown to inhibit mitochondrial function via mechanisms that result in decreased ROS generation. Reduced ROS generation has been associated with enhanced *in vitro* survival in several investigations. Certain groups, but not all, have found higher survival of HIF1-competent cells subjected to hypoxia *in vitro* compared to HIF1-deficient cells. Comparing these research is complicated by the intricacy of measuring reactive oxygen species (ROS): there are numerous different short-lived species that are normally detected indirectly by their action on reporter molecules such as fluorescein derivatives.

Mitochondrial dysfunction results in an increase in anabolic substrates

One prerequisite of fast dividing tumour cells is that each cell division must reproduce all of their elements. This biosynthetic process necessitates a huge number of precursors for proteins, nucleic acids, and lipids to be produced by the cell. In normoxia, tumour cells have been found to have enhanced metabolic turnover as a result of oncogene activation such as Akt and HRAS. Numerous precursors are generated as products of the glycolytic route (for example, ribose for nucleic acid synthesis) or the TCA cycle as a result of the increased metabolic activity (such as citrate for lipid synthesis). Increased glucose uptake in the tumour cell and lower metabolite consumption for energy in the mitochondria allow for the usage of a greater proportion of the substrates for these alternate uses.

The reduction in mitochondrial activity caused by HIF should restrict the amount of TCA cycle intermediates available for lipid production. HIF1 can regulate the availability of TCA cycle intermediates for lipid synthesis by regulating the flow of pyruvate into the mitochondria (through PDK1 expression) and the turnover of carbons in the TCA cycle (by COX4 subunit determination). Citrate is shuttled from the mitochondria to the cytoplasm during de novo lipid synthesis, where it is converted to acetyl-CoA and oxaloacetate by the enzyme ATP citrate lyase. Acetyl-CoA carboxylase is utilised to synthesise lipids from acetyl-CoA. The proliferative advantage of cells with high ATP citrate lyase activity is readily apparent when the enzyme is inhibited *in vitro*.

However, HIF1 appears to be able to regulate macromolecular synthesis and proliferation in growth factor-dependent hematopoietic cells, even under normoxia. HIF1 actually slows the growth of these cells by boosting glycolysis and creating lactate instead of citrate for lipid synthesis. This promotes survival. However, increased carbon flux into the TCA cycle occurs in glioma cells as a result of glutamine incorporation, which should not be regulated by HIF1. PDK1 inhibited the entry of pyruvate into the TCA cycle in hypoxic tumour cells. However, altering the COX4 isoforms has resulted in a decrease in the carbon flux required to power the electron transport chain. Reduced input and outflow may result in an excess of carbons available for lipid synthesis. This way, even in hypoxic tumour cells with impaired mitochondrial function, acetyl-CoA can still be produced to maintain growth.

Mitochondrial function is reduced, which conserves O_2 for alternate uses

Initially, it was believed that hypoxia increased glycolytic genes because there was insufficient oxygen to support oxidative phosphorylation in the mitochondria. However, this idea currently looks to be erroneous, as evidenced by two observations. To begin, HIF1α, HIF1 target genes, and the associated metabolic alterations are readily generated in the majority of cells examined at mild hypoxia levels of 2–3% pO$_2$, which are low enough to promote HIF1 activity but high enough to support robust oxidative phosphorylation. At concentrations less than 0.5 percent, O$_2$ has been proven to be a limiting substrate for oxidative phosphorylation 86. Second, as previously established, HIF1 actively inhibits mitochondrial activity via PDK1 induction, MXI1 induction, and COX4I2 expression. Thus, HIF1 appears to store O$_2$ when ambient availability declines but before it reaches a critical level.

Cells in human tumours were constrained to develop within approximately ten cells of a blood artery. This distance was determined to be the 'diffusion limit' of O$_2$ reaching the outermost cell. The limit is determined by the O$_2$ content of the blood artery and the rate at which O$_2$ is used by tumour cells as it diffuses out of the channel (Figure 8-1). Reduced consumption is the most efficient technique to expand this diffusion limit *in vivo*, theoretically. Cells exposed to this O$_2$ gradient are able to proliferate and are not killed by anoxia. Additionally, the preserved O$_2$ is available for cellular operations that do not need energy production. For instance, various types of enzymes either directly or indirectly employ O$_2$ as a substrate. Oxidases, hydroxylases, protein disulphide isomerases, and histone demethylases are only a few of these enzymes. This extracellular O$_2$ consumption is required for sterol production and oxidative protein folding and can contribute for up to 10%–30% of total cellular O$_2$ consumption.

The model's therapeutic implications

Tumour cells have increased glycolysis and decreased oxidative phosphorylation, whether due to HIF1 activation, alternative oncogenic alterations, or a combination of these factors. Tumour cells are believed to be 'dependent' on the energy provided by glycolysis, whilst normal cells continue to get significant energy from the mitochondria. This metabolic differential between normal and malignant tissue may constitute a target for anti-tumour therapy. Numerous organisations are developing strategies to target glycolysis, hypoxia, and HIF1 metabolically in solid tumours.

Glycolysis is inhibited directly

Historically, the majority of anticancer methods targeting metabolism have attempted to leverage the tumour's enhanced glycolytic activity rather than its decreased mitochondrial function. The non-metabolizable competitive inhibitor of glucose 2-deoxyglucose (2-DG) and the suspected hexokinase inhibitor lonidamine have advanced to clinical testing. *In vitro* studies have demonstrated that these medicines are effective at killing tumour cells, particularly when the cells are hypoxic. However, 2-DG exhibits antitumour activity as a single agent in cells *in vivo* at dosages severalfold greater than those tolerated in humans. Regrettably, even if the tumour increases glycolysis rates, some tissues, such as the brain, heart, and retina, rely on glycolysis for regular function. Patients have reported headaches as the dose-limiting effect of 2-DG.

Recent *in vitro* investigations indicate that sublethal dosages of glycolytic inhibitors may sensitise tumour cells to conventional chemotherapy or radiotherapy. It is postulated that increased glucose metabolism results in resistance to typical DNA-damaging drugs. In xenograft models or *in vitro*, combining 2-DG with doxorubicin or paclitaxel resulted in additive toxicity. Mechanistic studies in a variety of cancer cell lines indicate that elevated glycolysis levels may protect cells from apoptotic triggers. Perhaps this effect is due not to increased glycolysis in these cells, but to impaired mitochondrial activity, which changes apoptotic signaling via the mitochondria. If this is one method by which altered metabolism protects against chemotherapeutic death, then inhibiting glycolysis via pharmacological inhibition may be of limited use in sensitising tumour cells to chemotherapy or radiation-induced apoptosis. However, given the numerous functions of glucose within the cell, it is vital to keep in mind that the anti-tumour actions of 2-DG may be mediated by non-glycolytic mechanisms.

Inhibitors of HIF1 with metabolic effects

Additionally, researchers are seeking to disrupt the HIF1 transcription factor in order to prevent the metabolic effects of HIF1 in solid tumours as well as other physiological pathways regulated by HIF1 (such as angiogenesis). HIF1 is an interesting target for anticancer therapy since it is expected to be inactive in normal, well-oxygenated tissues, implying that side effects from suppression should be limited. Numerous drugs and natural items have been reported to inhibit HIF1 activity via a variety of pathways, although their therapeutic usefulness has not been established. Additionally, while many glucose-metabolising enzymes are expressed at a basal level, inhibiting HIF1 effectively may not totally stop glycolysis. Glycolysis should be inhibited more effectively with direct glycolytic inhibitors or competitors such as 2-DG.

Recognizing these limitations regarding the potential to inhibit glycolysis in tumours, our laboratory has concentrated on the HIF1 pathway, which regulates mitochondrial O_2 consumption. We demonstrated that echinomycin, a small molecule inhibitor of HIF1, and dichloroacetate (DCA), a small molecule inhibitor of PDK1, can increase O_2 consumption within the xenografted tumour. Treatment with either echinomycin or DCA increased mitochondrial activity and O_2 consumption in tumours harbouring wild-type HIF1.

Due to the fact that the supply of O_2 to the tumour is restricted, this increase in demand causes the tumour to become increasingly hypoxic. However, these medications do not promote hypoxia in tumours generated from HIF1-deficient cells, indicating that hypoxia and HIF1 have a targeted specificity. While increasing hypoxia makes cells more resistant to radiation and chemotherapy, it also renders them more susceptible to hypoxic cytotoxins such as tirapazamine. These findings corroborate prior publications demonstrating that hypoxic tumours are more susceptible to tirapazamine-containing therapy in xenografted mouse tumours and clinical trials. While it appears that transcription factors such as HIF1 can be targeted to exert anticancer effects, it is worth noting that targeting downstream genes may be a more controlled and/or specific strategy.

Both of Warburg's first results — an increase in aerobic glycolysis and a loss in mitochondrial function — can be linked to tumour-induced activation of the HIF1 transcription factor. This does not preclude the possibility that other oncogenic alterations play a role in modifying the metabolic profile of the tumour. Perhaps oncogenic alterations, like increased glycolysis, contribute to impaired mitochondrial function. When activated, the p53 tumour suppressor can either decrease glycolysis or decrease O_2 consumption when altered.

With the fluorodeoxyglucose-uptake positron- emission tomography scan, the glycolytic tumour phenotype has been used diagnostically. This functional imaging provides additional information not available from anatomical imaging alone. However, metabolic changes within the tumour do not appear to represent the Achilles heel that was envisioned. The use of glycolytic inhibitors may be insufficiently selective to kill tumour cells without generating side effects in normal organs that rely on glycolysis as well. The first attribute of a next-generation glucose-targeting' metabolic medication' would be decreased blood–brain barrier penetration, given that organ appears to be the most sensitive. Second, a well-defined modulation of metabolic processes must be established for such medications in order to logically choose certain combinations. Third, inhibiting glycolysis alone may not be sufficient to kill the tumour cell directly; therefore, combining inhibitors targeting other metabolic processes may be more successful. For instance, a glycolytic inhibitor might enhance the action of a fatty acid synthase inhibitor by reducing the available acetyl-CoA for lipid synthesis. Alternatively, a non-metabolizable glucose analogue may enhance the effectiveness of a glycosylation inhibitor.

Cancer Cell Metabolism is Modified by Hypoxia

Hypoxic zones, or areas of decreased tissue oxygen saturation, are observed in a large number of solid tumours as a result of the disordered vasculature generated to feed oxygen to the fast developing tumour. Tumour hypoxia has been associated with a poor prognosis in cancer patients, owing to the possibility of increased malignancy, resistance to chemotherapy and radiation treatment, and an increased risk of metastasis. In contrast to normal human tissues, where the oxygen tension is typically greater than 40 mmHg, tumours may retain an oxygen tension of 0–20 mmHg. Hypoxia often manifests itself in solid tumours roughly 100 metres from a viable blood artery.

Due to the fact that tumour cells are exposed to a range of oxygen concentrations, solid tumours are classified into three tissue regions: normoxic, hypoxic, and necrotic (Figure 8-1). Normoxic cells are normally viable and proliferating when they are located near working blood arteries. At 150 metres from patent blood arteries, cells may become anoxic, resulting in necrosis patches. Typically, peri-necrotic cells are hypoxic and capable of surviving at extremely low oxygen concentrations ($PO_2 \leq 1\%$). Hypoxia often results in cell death in normal cells. Contrary to popular belief, hypoxia can cause genetic alterations in tumour cells that enable them to adapt to insufficient nutrition and a hostile microenvironment and so remain viable. As a result of this selection pressure, hypoxia promotes the survival of subpopulations of viable cells that have the genetic machinery for malignant development. Tumours can circumvent the proliferation constraints imposed by the stressful microenvironment by encouraging the formation of new blood vessels through the release of hypoxia-inducible angiogenic factors such as vascular endothelial growth factor (VEGF). Contrary to popular belief, even after neovascularization of solid tumour tissue, which consists of poorly organised, elongated, dilated, twisted, and blind-ended blood vessels, the tumour's oxygen supply may remain inadequate.

According to the usual categorization used in research and medical oncology, hypoxia manifests itself in human cancers as either chronic or acute forms. The structural and functional abnormalities associated with a tumour's chaotic vasculature and structure, such as dilated, elongated, and twisted blood vessels, poor endothelium, reduced functional cell receptors, and an absence of blood flow regulation, which results in spontaneous stasis, leads to inadequate oxygen delivery as a result of insufficient blood flow. Ischemic hypoxia is a type of hypoxia that is typically transitory. Chronic, diffusion-limited hypoxia develops from an imbalance of oxygen supply and demand caused by tumour growth, when tumour tissue located more than 70–150 μm from patent blood arteries receives insufficient oxygen. Occasionally, anemic hypoxia can occur as a result of a diminished capacity of the blood to carry oxygen as a result of chemotherapy-induced anaemia. Both acute and chronic hypoxia are associated with a poor patient outcome and a tumour phenotype that is aggressive.

Cellular Responses & Hypoxia Adaptations

Hypoxia alters both the proteome and genomic profiles of tumour cells (Figure 8-2). Proteomic alterations can result in the arrest of the cell cycle, differentiation, necrosis, and apoptosis. Additionally, hypoxia-induced proteome alterations may promote tumour growth, invasion, and metastasis by enabling adaptation and survival in a hostile, nutrient-deficient environment. At the molecular level, hypoxia-inducible factor (HIF) regulates the adaptation of tumour cells to hypoxic stress. HIF is a transcription factor that accumulates in response to decreased cellular oxygen levels.

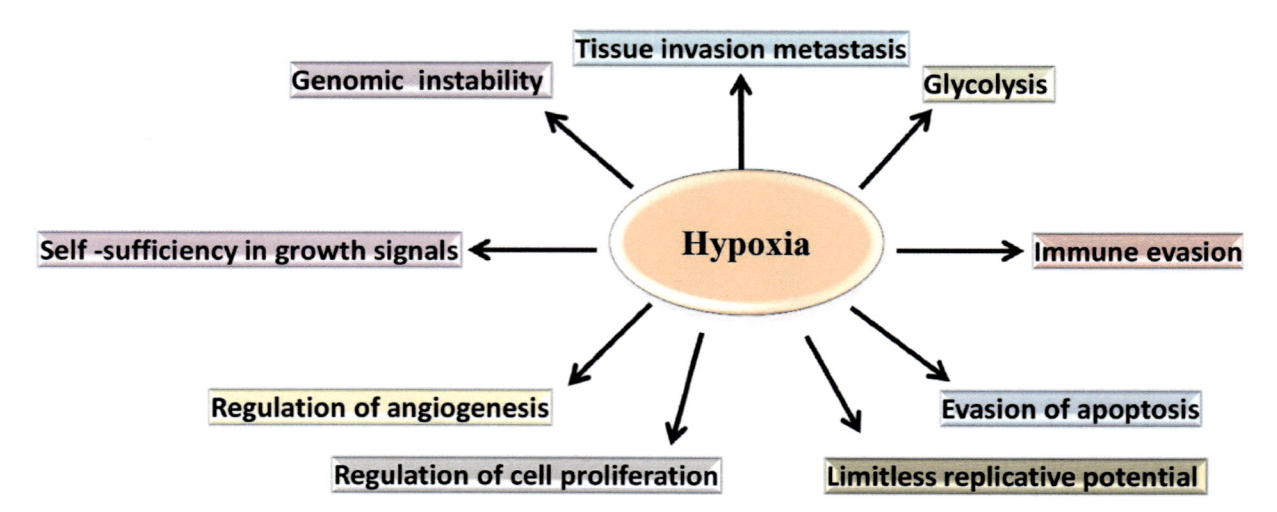

FIGURE 8-2 | The role of hypoxia in the cancer-specific biological pathways. In hypoxic conditions, cancer cell metabolism undergoes a shift from oxidative phosphorylation to aerobic glycolysis. Additionally, hypoxia regulates cell proliferation and supports evasion of apoptosis by the tumor cells. Furthermore, hypoxia contributes to the changes that confer limitless replicative potential and to the expression of genes, allowing invasion, and metastasis. Adopted from ref. 3 with permission

HYPOXIA-INDUCIBLE FACTORS (HIFs) ARE AN ESSENTIAL PART OF HYPOXIA SIGNALING

Three members of the human HIF family have been identified: HIF-1α, HIF-2α, and HIF-3α. These heterodimers are composed of subunits that dissociate under normoxic circumstances (Figure 8-3). HIF-1α is frequently overexpressed in tumour cells, whereas HIF-2α [endothelial PAS domain protein 1 (EPAS1)] is highly expressed in subsets of tumour-associated macrophages, and HIF-3α is expressed in pulmonary alveolar epithelial cells and the human kidney (Yang e HIF-1α has been the most thoroughly characterised. Although the DNA binding and dimerization domains of HIF-1α and HIF-2α are structurally similar, their transactivation domains are distinct. This may explain why a genome-wide screen detected both forms binding to identical (hypoxia-response elements) HRE consensus sites, but activating distinct transcriptional responses. Another distinction is that HIF-1α is ubiquitously expressed, whereas HIF-2α is expressed in a subset of tissues. On the whole, the two types respond differently to hypoxia. It was discovered that HIF-1α alone regulates the transcription of genes encoding glycolysis enzymes. In comparison, HIF-2α is thought to contribute to adaptation to high elevations. In late stage colon cancers, HIF-1α labelling was prominent and HIF-2α staining was modest, whereas the opposite was observed in early stage tumours. It may deduce that HIF-1α and HIF-2α were not equally involved in human colon cancer. On the other hand, HIF-3α lacks the transactivation domain, implying that this version acts as a suppressor, preventing HIF-1α from beginning transcription by binding. HIF-3α is often referred to as the 'inhibitory Per-Arnt-Sim PAS domain' (IPAS) due to this effect.

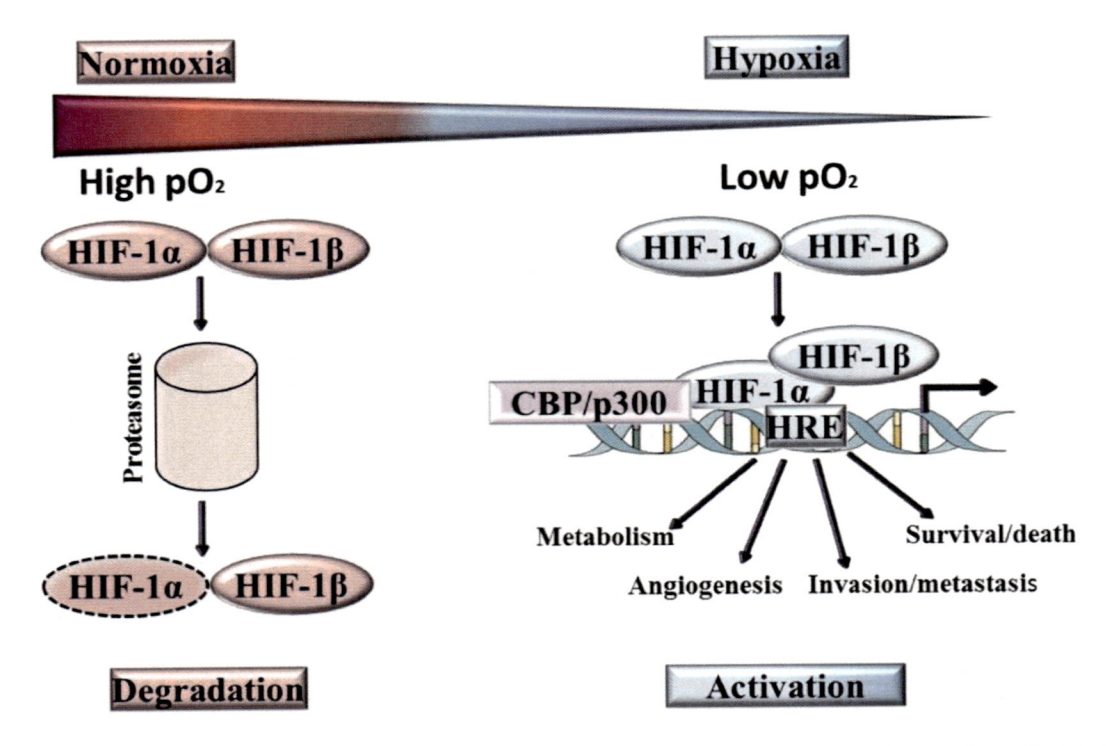

FIGURE 8-3 | Activation and degradation of the hypoxia inducible factor-1a (HIF-1a). In normoxia HIF-1a is rapidly degraded, while it accumulates in hypoxic conditions. HIF-1a associates with HIF-1b and the resulting heterodimer binds to the hypoxia response element (HRE) of target genes. Adopted from ref. 3 with permission

METABOLIC ADAPTATIONS CAUSED BY HIF-1

Metabolic changes were one of the first biochemical characteristics of cancer cells to be identified, and a better understanding of tumour metabolism permits the discovery of novel targets and the creation of new anticancer medicines. The distinction between normal tissue and cancer metabolism was first recognized in the 1920s; in healthy cells, glucose is broken down into pyruvate, which is then further metabolized in the mitochondria via the tricarboxylic acid cycle and oxidative phosphorylation. In normal cells, the presence of oxygen inhibits glycolysis (Pasteur effect). Mitochondrial activity maintains elevated ATP levels, which results in allosteric regulation of the glycolysis enzyme phosphofructokinase. Under hypoxic conditions, anaerobic glycolysis produces pyruvate, which is ultimately converted to lactate. In comparison to non-malignant tissue, tumours rely substantially on enhanced glycolysis to meet their energy demands even when oxygen is abundant, a process known as aerobic glycolysis or the Warburg Effect. (Figure 8-4).

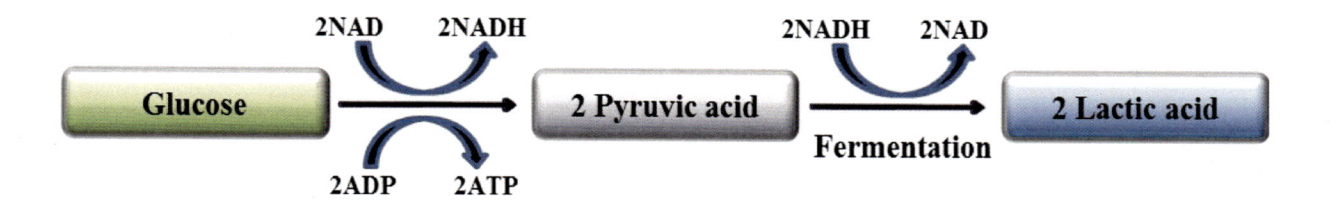

FIGURE 8-4 | Anaerobic glycolysis. Glycolysis provides two ATP molecules and does not require oxygen. One glucose molecule is converted into two pyruvate molecules, which are subsequently fermented to two lactic acid molecules. Adopted from ref. 3 with permission

Warburg observed that tumour cells, in comparison to normal cells, had a faster rate of glucose metabolism and preferred glycolysis to oxidative phosphorylation, even when oxygen levels were adequate. (figure 8-5) Since then, a wide variety of tumour forms have been discovered to exhibit aerobic glycolysis, and evidence has accumulated indicating cancer growth is accompanied by a reorganization of the metabolic landscape.

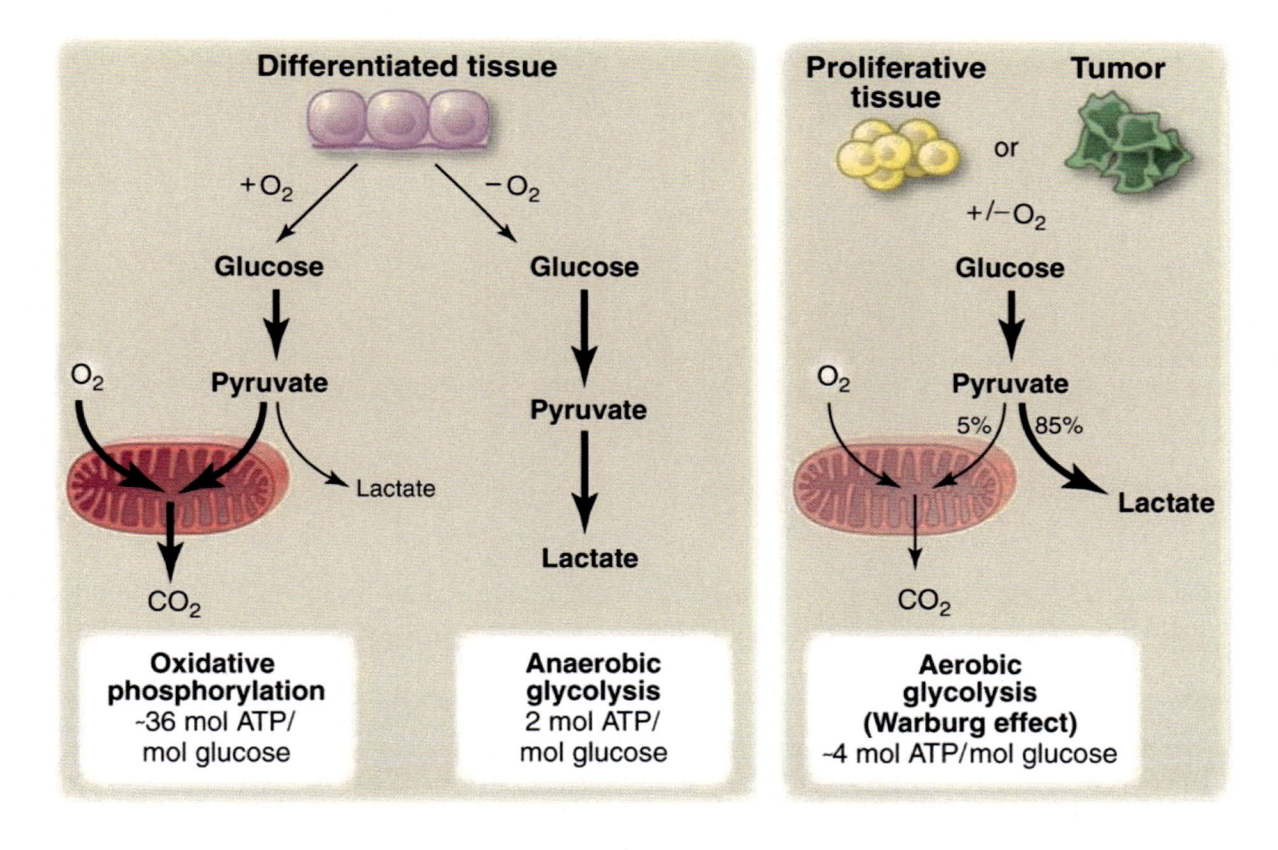

Figure 8-5 Schematic representation of the differences between oxidative phosphorylation, anaerobic glycolysis, and aerobic glycolysis (Warburg effect). In the presence of oxygen, nonproliferating (differentiated) tissues first metabolize glucose to pyruvate via glycolysis and then completely oxidize most of that pyruvate in the mitochondria to CO_2 during the process of oxidative phosphorylation. Because oxygen is required as the final electron acceptor to completely oxidize the glucose, oxygen is essential for this process. When oxygen is limiting, cells can redirect the pyruvate generated by glycolysis away from mitochondrial oxidative phosphorylation by generating lactate (anaerobic glycolysis). This generation of lactate during anaerobic glycolysis allows glycolysis to continue (by cycling NADH back to NAD^+), but results in minimal ATP production when compared with oxidative phosphorylation. Adopted from ref. 1 with permission

The effect of HIF-1α on glycolytic metabolism is well recognized; glycolysis in tumours may be facilitated by HIF-1α stability, regardless of the hypoxic environment. According to a previous assessment of cancer cell lines, around 50% of HIF-1α stabilization occurred under normoxic conditions in malignancies. Additionally, HIF-1α regulates the enzymes responsible for the metabolic shift caused by the suppression of oxidative phosphorylation and the promotion of anaerobic glycolysis. HIF-1α promotes tumour cell overexpression and increases the activity of a number of glycolytic protein isoforms that are not present in non-malignant cells. Adenylate kinase-3; aldolase-A,C (ALDA,C); carbonic anhydrase-9; enolase-1 (ENO1); glucose transporter-1,3 (Glut-1,3); glyceraldehyde phosphate dehydrogenase (GAPDH); hexokinase 1,2 (HK1,2); lactate dehydrogenase-A (LDHA); phosphofructokinase (PFK).

Hypoxia-inducible factor directly regulates the expression of genes encoding glucose transporters such as Glut-1 and glycolytic enzymes. HIF-1α promotes the production of pyruvate dehydrogenase kinase 1 (PDK1), which phosphorylates and so inhibits pyruvate dehydrogenase (PDH), the enzyme responsible for the conversion of pyruvate to acetyl-CoA. Reduced PDH activity under hypoxic conditions reduces acetyl-CoA entrance into the Krebs cycle, hence limiting the amount of substrate available for downstream mitochondrial respiration and, consequently, oxygen consumption. Additionally, HIF-1α enables cells to adapt to the decreased intracellular pH caused by increased anaerobic glycolysis and lactic acid generation.

The synthesis of ATP via less effective anaerobic glycolysis and a deficiency of substrates such as acetyl-CoA and O_2 to the mitochondria results in significant structural, functional, and dynamical alterations. The structural and dynamical changes are characterized by an impairment of the fusion process, which results in mitochondrial depolarization, mitochondrial DNA (mtDNA) loss, which may be associated with altered respiration rates, and an uneven distribution of mitochondria within cells. Under chronic hypoxia, neurons exhibit decreased mitochondrial size and changed mitochondrial shape, possibly in response to changes in nitric oxide synthase activity. Numerous changes in mitochondrial expression and function are connected with an enhanced rate of glycolysis in quickly growing malignancies. Along with the decrease in the number of mitochondria in cells, there is a drop in the expression of oxidative enzymes and transporters, and an increase in a protein (IF1) that inhibits mitochondrial ATP synthesis. Additionally, activating glycolysis decreases oxidative phosphorylation. Aerobic glycolysis significantly increases the rate of glucose metabolism, with lactate generation from glucose being between 10 and 100 times faster than total glucose oxidation in mitochondria. However, regardless of the type of glucose metabolism used, the amount of ATP generated during a particular time period is similar.

THE ROLE OF HYPOXIA IN CONVENTIONAL CHEMO- AND RADIATION THERAPY RESISTANCE

Hypoxia-induced treatment resistance is well established. This link may be partly explained by the fact that many anticancer medications are big molecules that cannot diffuse into target tissue due to poorly developed vasculature. Furthermore, because hypoxic tumour cells are not connected to the blood supply, only a subset of them may be exposed to a deadly dose of a cytotoxic chemical.

Hypoxia in tumours has been found to enhance drug resistance, specifically by increased expression and amplification of the P-glycoprotein (P-gp) membrane exporter genes. Increased P-gp expression results in decreased cellular sequestration of numerous anti-cancer medications, and this pathway is believed to be associated with tumour resistance to topoisomerase II-targeted therapies. Radioresistance is a side effect of tumour hypoxia that impairs radiotherapy's ability to treat malignancies. When the local pO_2 is less than 25–30 mmHg (3.3–3.9 percent), the tumour's sensitivity to radiation exposure rapidly decreases.

The term "oxygen enhancement" refers to the process through which hypoxia confers radioresistance on a tumour. Tumour cell DNA is destroyed as a result of radiation, either as a result of ionisation or as a result of oxygen-favoring radicals, such as the hydroxyl radical and superoxide, produced by the ionisation of water around DNA. In summary, radiation damages the DNA, and the cell's inability to repair the damage typically leads to cell death. When cells are exposed to hypoxia, they have a greater capacity to repair disrupted DNA than when they are exposed to oxygen; stable peroxides form between oxygen and free DNA ends, which are significantly more resistant to cellular repair. After therapy, resistant tumour cells can remain alive, resulting in resistant subpopulations of cells and poor local control for the patient. Additionally, there is a correlation between HIF-1, the tumour blood vascular network, and radiation resistance, because radiation affects HIF-1 activity. HIF-1 activity in a tumour can nearly quadruple 24–28 hours after radiation treatment. This process is only observed *in vivo*, as it is dependent on critical input from the tumour microenvironment. Tumours may have a brief increase in oxygen tension, or reoxygenation, following radiation, as a result of the reduction in diffusion-limited (chronic) hypoxia caused by cytoreduction. Following that, radiation-induced reoxygenation of hypoxic tumour cells generates reactive oxygen species (ROS), which promotes the synthesis of cytokines such as VEGF and basic fibroblast growth factor (bFGF), which confer radioprotective effects on surrounding endothelial cells. Finally, this results in the prevention of endothelial apoptosis via the production of anti-apoptotic signals in tumour blood vessels, so boosting another mechanism of radiation resistance

Innovative Hypoxic-Tumour Photodynamic Therapy Strategies

Photodynamic therapy (PDT) is a promising cancer treatment method. As a result of its unique characteristics, such as low systemic toxicity, absence of starting resistance, and little invasiveness, PDT has gained growing interest. PDT generates reactive oxygen species (ROS) using a light-excited photosensitizer (PS), often via a type II mechanism involving the transformation of triplet ground state molecular oxygen ($^3O_2$) into its highly reactive singlet oxygen ($^1O_2$) analogue (Figure 8-6). The ensuing reactive oxygen species (ROS) cause cell death or necrosis, microvascular damage, and immunological responses.

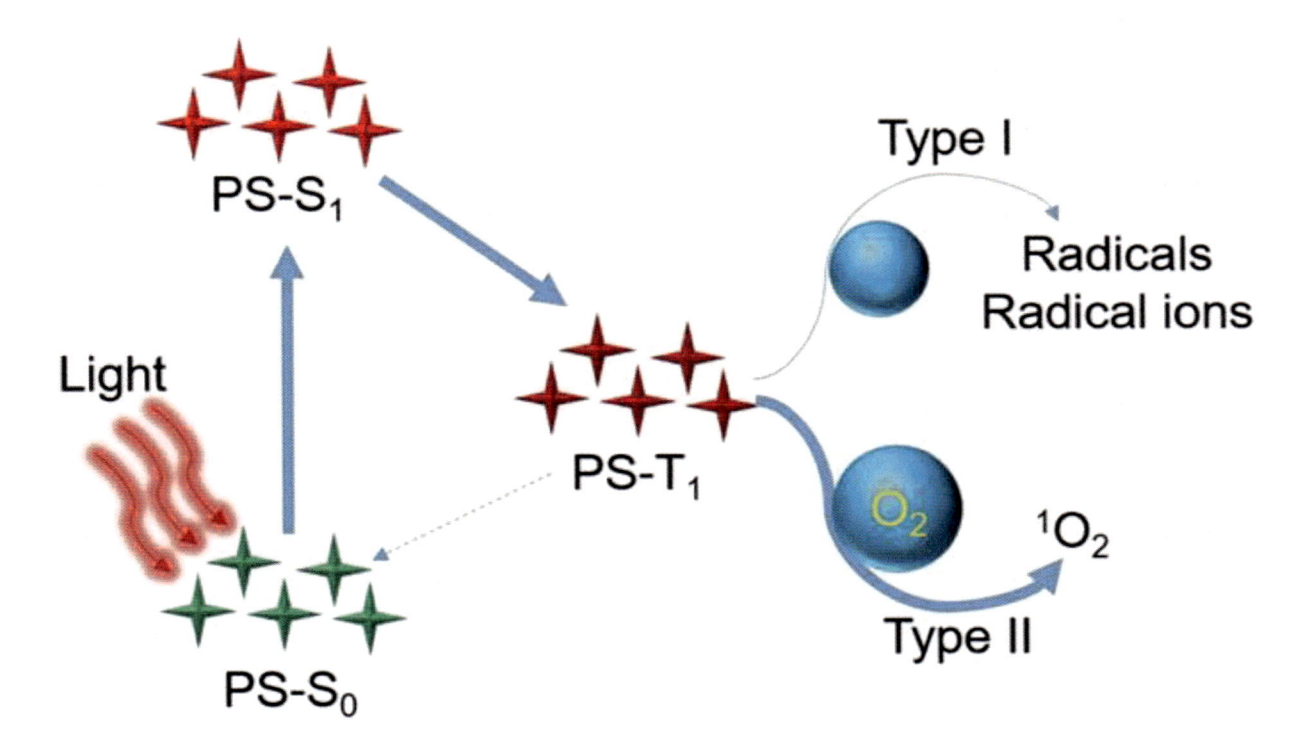

Fig. 8-6 Schematic of the photophysical and photochemical basis of PDT. Type I, electron or hydrogen atom abstraction. Type II, direct energy transfer. Adopted from Ref. 4 with permission

As a result of the more prevalent operation of the type II pathway, the majority of present PDT systems are highly O_2-dependent and consume a significant amount of O_2. Unfortunately, O_2 concentrations in solid tumours vary by location, with certain internal regions having extremely low levels (partial pressure of O_2<5 mmHg, equivalent to 7 mm). This is due to cancer cells' aggressive proliferation and an insufficient blood supply in tumours. Due to the lack of O_2 in tumours, PDT's anticancer efficacy is greatly diminished, especially in situations requiring continuous treatment. As a result, hypoxia is the Achilles heel of this strategy.

Recently, considerable effort has been made to overcome the limitations of PDT imposed by hypoxia. These investigations have resulted in the development of numerous novel solutions for resolving this issue. According to the mechanics underlying the PDT process, the techniques described thus far can be categorized into three types. These approaches include the following: 1) O_2-replenishing strategies that can be used to directly or indirectly increase tumour O_2

concentrations prior to and/or during PDT; 2) new PDT paradigms that reduce the reliance on O_2; and 3) combining PDT with other hypoxia-activated or O_2-independent therapeutic modalities. Here we introduce these tactics in greater detail below by illustrating the design of systems, their operation, and examples of their application. Finally, the Minireview discusses the future prospects and concerns connected with these methodologies, particularly in terms of clinical applications.

PDT for O_2-Replenishing

Delivery of O_2 into Tumours

Direct O_2 administration into tumours using an O_2 carrier like as haemoglobin or perfluorocarbons is one of the most often used strategies for overcoming tumour hypoxia during PDT. Haemoglobin is made up of four heme groups (an iron ion ligated in the centre of a porphyrin ring) to which O_2 has a strong affinity. Haemoglobin contained within red blood cells transports oxygen from the lungs to various tissues in the body. However, due to its low stability and short circulation half-life, free hemoglobin is not a strong option for O_2 delivery to tumours. As a result, a technique suitable for practical application must be developed to "hide" haemoglobin by inserting it into composites, sometimes referred to as fake red blood cells. Various nanotechnology-based techniques have been developed to date for this goal. In this regard, systems composed of artificial red blood cells with internalised PSs have a great deal of potential for increasing the efficacy of PDTs.

Artificial red blood cells were synthesized using a biomimetic lipid-polymer with indocyanine green as the PS and haemoglobin as the O_2 carrier. The close proximity of indocyanine green and haemoglobin in this nanosystem, which is held together by hydrophobic and electrostatic interactions (Figure 8-7), enables O_2 self-enrichment for effective ROS generation during PDT. Additionally, ROS stimulate the oxidation of ferrous-haemoglobin to the deadly ferric form, which has a synergistic effect on tumour eradication. Additionally, dynamic self-monitoring during treatment is enabled by the fact that this combination generates fluorescence and photoacoustic signals. In general, this type of biomimetic technology is an efficient method of replenishing the O_2 depleted during the PDT process. As a result, it has significant therapeutic potential for hypoxic malignancies. Other haemoglobin-related O_2 carrier systems have been investigated recently (for example, polymeric micelles and liposomes). These systems, however, have low O_2 loading efficiency due to the fact that each haemoglobin molecule can only bind four O_2 molecules.

In comparison to its low loading efficiency on haemoglobin, O₂ has a very high solubility in perfluorocarbons (about 40–50 mL O₂ per 100 mL liquid, equivalent to the solubility of around 200 mL blood at 25-88 °C under 1 atm). As a result, these compounds have been incorporated into critical components of O₂ delivery systems. The near-infrared PS IR780 is disseminated uniformly in a lipid monolayer (DSPE-PEG2000, lecithin, and cholesterol) in a 200 nm nanodroplet together with the perfluorocarbon. Due to the perfluorocarbon's high O₂ capacity, a sufficient O₂ concentration is maintained in the nanodroplet to enable efficient and enhanced PDT. Additionally, the prolonged lifespan of $^1O_2$ in perfluorocarbons boosts the efficacy of the PDT.

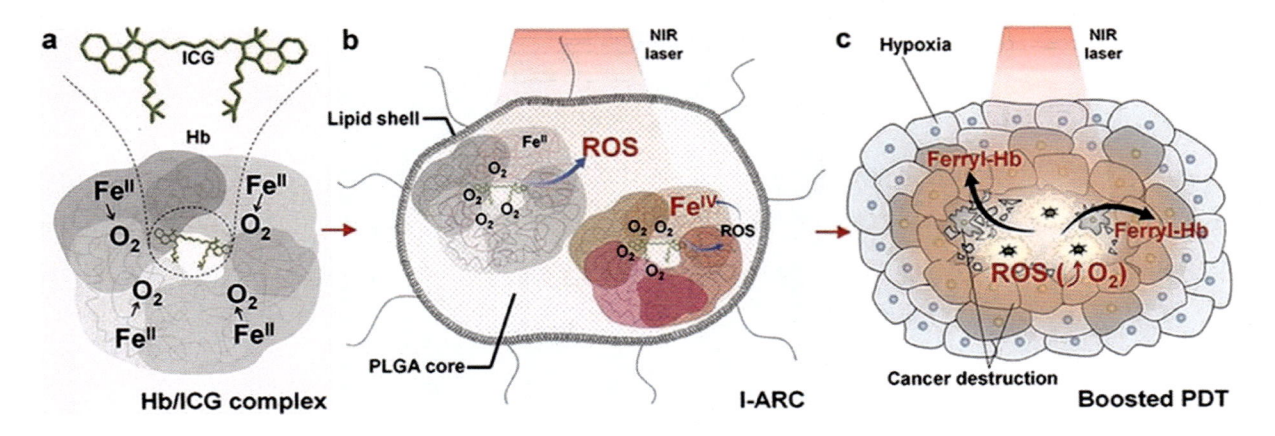

Fig. 8-7 Schematic of an artificial red blood cell internalized PS system for tumor-boosted PDT. ICG=indocyanine green. Hb=hemoglobin. I-ARC=ICG-loaded artificial red cells. Adopted from ref. 5 with permission

While perfluorocarbons have a high O₂ capacity, straightforward diffusion controlled by an O₂ concentration gradient is typically not practicable. Recently, Song et al. used concurrent ultrasonic treatment to adjust tumour-specific O₂ supply using a method based on a perfluorocarbon nanodroplet stabilised with human serum albumin. After intravenous injection of the nanodroplet (containing 30 mL of perfluorocarbon) into 4T1 tumour-bearing mice, the mice were treated to 30 minutes of pure O₂ breathing followed by 30 minutes of tumour therapy with ultrasound (1 MHz, 3.5 W). The nanodroplet adsorbs O₂ in the lungs, transports it to the tumour via blood circulation, and efficiently releases it within the tumour via an ultrasound-guided mechanism. O₂ levels in the tumour were shown to rapidly increase from roughly 17% to 49%, significantly increasing the anticancer efficacy of this PDT treatment.

Enhancing Tumour Blood Flow

Because hypoxia in tumours is primarily caused by changes in the microvasculature and chaotic blood flow, increasing blood flow has proven to be an efficient method of increasing O_2 concentrations in tumours. It has been established that mild heating (about 43-88 °C) increases tumour blood flow and increases the O_2 level inside tumours. As a result, photothermal treatment (PTT), which typically involves the use of photothermal agents to convert light energy to heat, is a well-studied therapeutic method for tumour hyperthermia ablation. Thus, preparation of a tumour with modest photothermal heating is a beneficial strategy for minimising hypoxia and increasing tumour susceptibility to PDT.

New PDT Concepts with Reduced O_2 Dependence

PDT fractional

Along with those that focus on replenishing O_2 in tumours, novel paradigms that reduce O_2 reliance have gained popularity in PDT research recently. It has been suggested that fractional (i.e., intermittent) light treatment may be a superior strategy for achieving more effective PDT effects due to the lower short-term O_2 consumption throughout the PDT process.

Boron-dipyrromethene (BODIPY)-based PS was used to increase fractional PDT. BODIPY is combined with 2-pyrdidone to form a single bifunctional molecule in this system (PYR6). The concept is based on the fact that 2-pyridone and its endoperoxide derivative conduct a reversible recovery reaction that yields extremely large amounts of $^1O_2$ (Figure 8-8). As a result, the upon process is used in the majority of existing PDT systems. In contrast to the type II process, which involves direct energy transfer from excited PS to O_2, the type I process involves either electron or hydrogen atom abstraction from substrates by the electrically excited PS. This reaction generates the corresponding radical ions or radicals. Although the details of how type I mechanisms work are unresolved, particularly how O_2 is involved, numerous studies have demonstrated that type I PDT performs well even under low O_2 conditions and, thus, that it may serve as the basis for developing new approaches to overcome the limitations of type II PDT due to hypoxia.

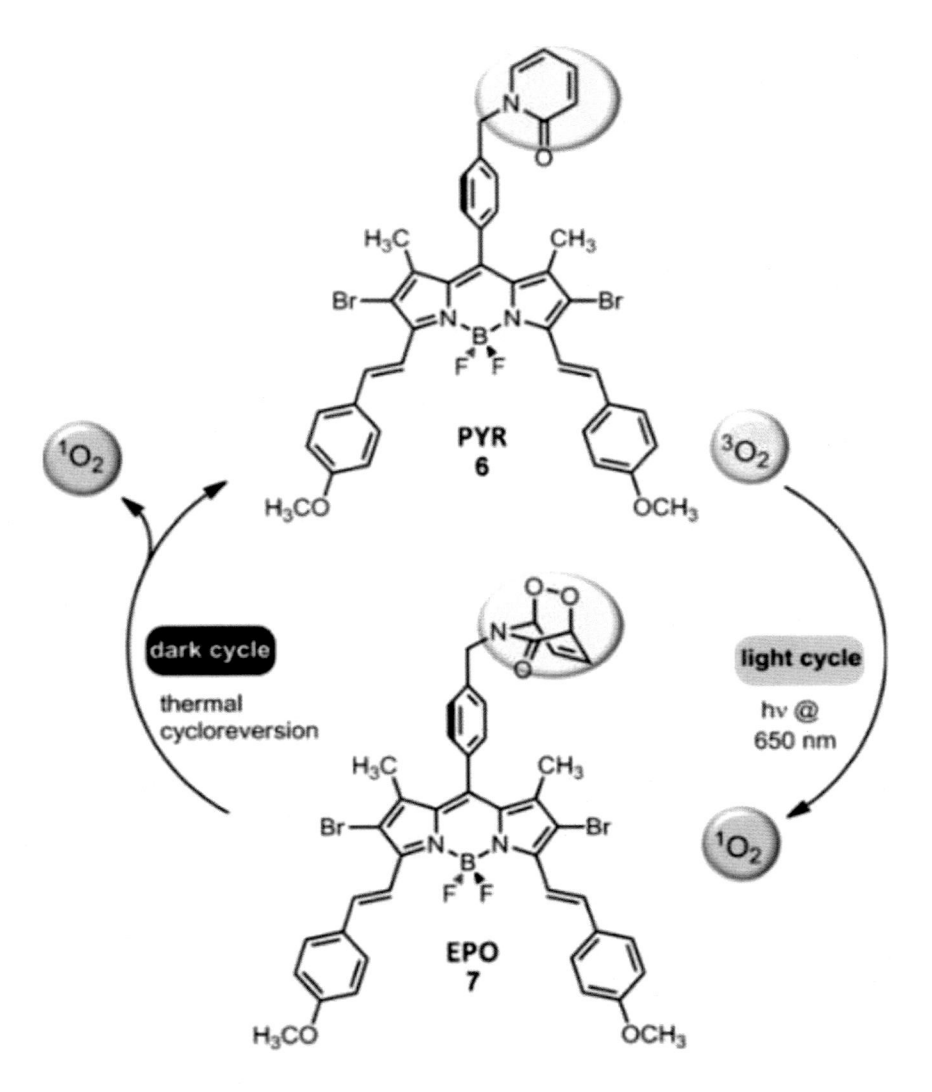

Figure 8-8. The basic principle of a fractional PDT utilising a 2-pydidone conjugated BODIPY is depicted schematically. Adopted from ref. 6 with permission

PDT Type I

As noted in the introduction (Figure 8-7), the primary photophysical and photochemical process in the majority of existing PDT systems is the type II mechanism. In contrast to the type II process, which involves direct energy transfer from excited PS to O₂, the type I process involves either electron or hydrogen atom abstraction from substrates by the electrically excited PS. This reaction generates the corresponding radical ions or radicals. Although the details of how type I mechanisms work are unresolved, particularly how O_2 is involved, numerous studies have demonstrated that type I PDT performs well even under low O_2 conditions and, thus, that it may serve as the basis for developing new approaches to overcome the limitations of type II PDT due to hypoxia.

Immunotherapy has recently been a prominent topic in the realm of cancer treatment. Numerous studies have been conducted to determine the efficacy of combining immunotherapy and PDT to achieve synergistic effects in the treatment of hypoxic tumours. Notably, the combined immunotherapy/PDT approach had an abscopal effect on metastasis inhibition. Additionally, the PDT agent used in this work is noteworthy for its pH-responsive tumour homing, mitochondrial targeting, and O_2 self-enrichment.

The Bottom Line

PDT has advanced dramatically over the last three decades as a result of its feasibility and efficacy in cancer treatment. Although dozens of PDT drugs have been licenced for clinical trials or clinical usage, they are not currently considered first-line therapy choices. Recent advancements in nanotechnology have created extremely promising avenues for approaching the creation of novel PDT systems and for providing diverse solutions to the difficulties associated with present PDT paradigms. Recent efforts have focused on developing 1) O_2-replenishing strategies, such as systems for O_2 delivery into tumours via haemoglobin and perfluorocarbon carriers, improving tumour blood flow via mild heating or antiangiogenic agents, enhancing O_2 generation via catalase or catalase-like materials, and other tumour microenvironment-regulating strategies; and 2) new PDT paradigms with decreased O_2 dependence, such as fractional PDT, type I PDT, and rPDT and remote control of $^1O_2$ release; and 3) systems combining PDT with hypoxia-activated chemotherapy or O_2-independent PTT and immunotherapy.

References for this chapter

1. Vander Heiden MG, Cantley LC, Thompson CB. Understanding the Warburg effect: the metabolic requirements of cell proliferation. Science. 2009 May 22;324(5930):1029-33. doi: 10.1126/science.1160809. PMID: 19460998; PMCID: PMC2849637.

2. Oh JM, Begum HM, Liu YL, Ren Y, Shen K. Recapitulating Tumor Hypoxia in a Cleanroom-Free, Liquid-Pinning-Based Microfluidic Tumor Model. ACS Biomater Sci Eng. 2022 Jul 11;8(7):3107-3121. doi: 10.1021/acsbiomaterials.2c00207. Epub 2022 Jun 9. PMID: 35678715; PMCID: PMC9299272.

3. Al Tameemi W, Dale TP, Al-Jumaily RMK, Forsyth NR. Hypoxia-Modified Cancer Cell Metabolism. Front Cell Dev Biol. 2019 Jan 29;7:4. doi: 10.3389/fcell.2019.00004. PMID: 30761299; PMCID: PMC6362613.

4. Li X, Kwon N, Guo T, Liu Z, Yoon J. Innovative Strategies for Hypoxic-Tumor Photodynamic Therapy. Angew Chem Int Ed Engl. 2018 Sep 3;57(36):11522-11531. doi: 10.1002/anie.201805138. Epub 2018 Aug 7. PMID: 29808948.

5. Luo, Z., Zheng, M., Zhao, P. *et al.* Self-Monitoring Artificial Red Cells with Sufficient Oxygen Supply for Enhanced Photodynamic Therapy. *Sci Rep* **6**, 23393 (2016). https://doi.org/10.1038/srep23393

6. Lv Z, Wei H, Li Q, Su X, Liu S, Zhang KY, Lv W, Zhao Q, Li X, Huang W. Achieving efficient photodynamic therapy under both normoxia and hypoxia using cyclometalated Ru(ii) photosensitizer through type I photochemical process. Chem Sci. 2017 Oct 31;9(2):502-512. doi: 10.1039/c7sc03765a. PMID: 29619206; PMCID: PMC5868078.

Chapter 9

Cancer Resistance and Therapeutic Strategies

How does Radiation cause cell death?

Irradiation generates both single- and double-stranded breaks (dsbs) in DNA, and the occurrence of dsbs is typically regarded as fatal. Radiation also affects the cell membrane, initiating or contributing to cell death pathways. Radiation-induced damage results in cell death via two mechanisms: apoptosis (or programmed cell death), an active process of cellular suicide, and necrosis, a generally considered passive process that occurs when cells with unrepaired DNA breaks and lethal chromosomal aberrations pass through mitosis. Here we address the targets of radiation damage and the signals that follow from this damage, ultimately leading to death.

Radiation targets cause DNA damage

The fact that ^{125}I incorporation into DNA induces a high rate of apoptosis in multiple cell lines provided evidence that DNA is an excellent target for cell death induction. Apoptosis occurred shortly following cell division and was associated with mitosis, but it also happened during interphase (the portion of the cell cycle between mitoses). The incorporation of 5-bromedeoxyuridine (BrdU) into DNA gave additional evidence that DNA is a target of cell death. When BrdU is replaced for the natural DNA precursor thymidine, the damage to DNA caused by irradiation is amplified. This modification increased apoptosis significantly in a mouse T cell hybridoma cell line. These investigations established that radiation-induced cell death occurs as a result of DNA damage.

Membrane of the cell

Recent investigations have demonstrated that irradiation also damages the cell membrane and that this damage triggers signaling processes critical for the apoptotic response. The most well-characterized membrane signaling pathway is triggered by radiation-induced sphingomyelin cleavage by acidic or neutral sphingomyelinases, which results in the production of ceramide, a lipid second messenger. Ceramide production by activation of sphingomyelinases occurs prior to apoptosis in response to a variety of various stimuli, including tumour necrosis factor, Fas ligand, and glucocorticoid exposure. Santana et al. demonstrated that tissues and cells from mice lacking acidic sphingomyelinases are more resistant to apoptosis in the presence of ionizing radiation. Additionally, following irradiation, numerous Burkitt's lymphoma cell lines (which are resistant to radiation-induced death) failed to accumulate ceramide. Haimovitz–Friedman et al. demonstrated that ionizing radiation induces ceramide formation in nucleated membrane preparations by increasing sphingomyelin hydrolysis via a neutral sphingomyelinase. This shows that ionizing radiation initiates sphingomyelin hydrolysis directly on the cell membrane, without requiring any nuclear components.

Subsequent events

Additional insights about the signaling events underlying radiation-induced apoptosis have emerged. Ceramide, for instance, has been demonstrated to activate the c-Jun amino-terminal kinase (JNK) pathway, which has been involved in the induction of apoptosis in response to ionising radiation and H_2O_2 damage.

Ceramide synthesis can be suppressed by Bcl-2, a 26 kDa integral membrane protein with anti-apoptotic properties, including the maintenance of the mitochrondrial membrane potential. Ceramide has been involved in the down-regulation of Bcl-2, implying that there may be a feedback inhibition between the activity of these two apoptotic regulators. Bcl-2 expression has been shown to be inhibited by the tumour suppressor protein p53, which is a positive regulator of apoptosis (see Figure 9-1 and discussion below), but overexpression of Bcl-2 has been related with greater cellular resistance to ionizing radiation-induced apoptosis. Additionally, it has been demonstrated that protein kinase C (PKC), a signalling protein that can be activated by growth hormones, calcium, and diacylglycerol, adversely regulates the ceramide pathway. The PKC inhibitor chelerytine increases neutral sphingomyelinase activity and accelerates radiation-induced apoptosis in the radioresistant cell line SQ-20B [13•], but basic fibroblast growth factor, which activates PKC, protects endothelial cells from radiation-induced apoptosis. PKC probably functions by inhibiting sphingomyelin hydrolysis to ceramide.

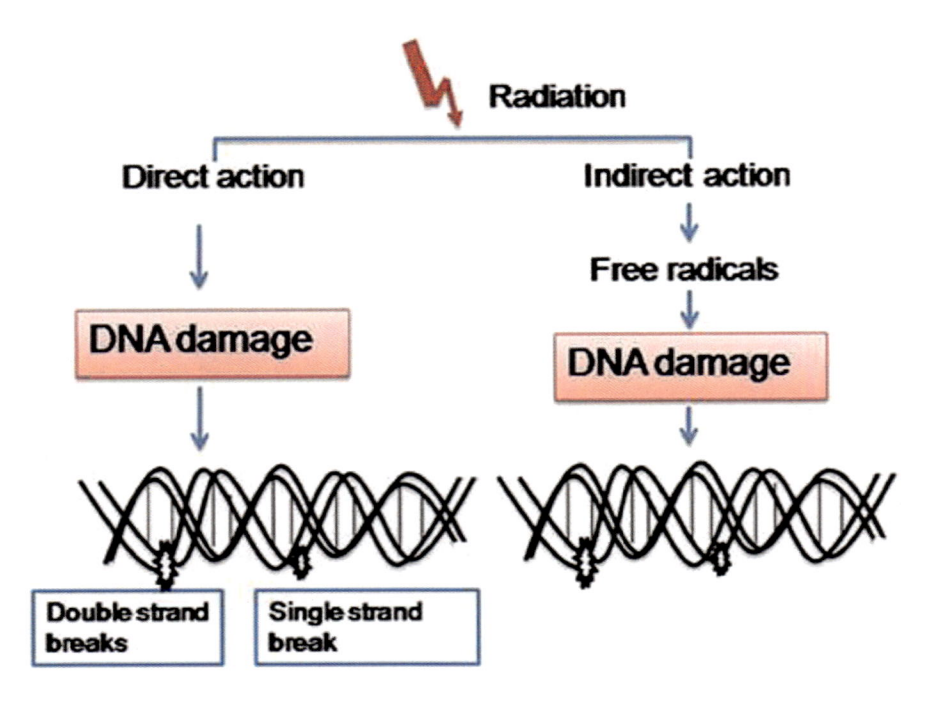

Figure 9-1. **Radiation mainly acts in two ways**. (1) Induces ionizations directly on the cellular molecules and cause damage. (2) Also acts indirectly, producing free radicals which are derived from the ionization or excitation of the water component of the cells. Adopted from ref. 2 with permission

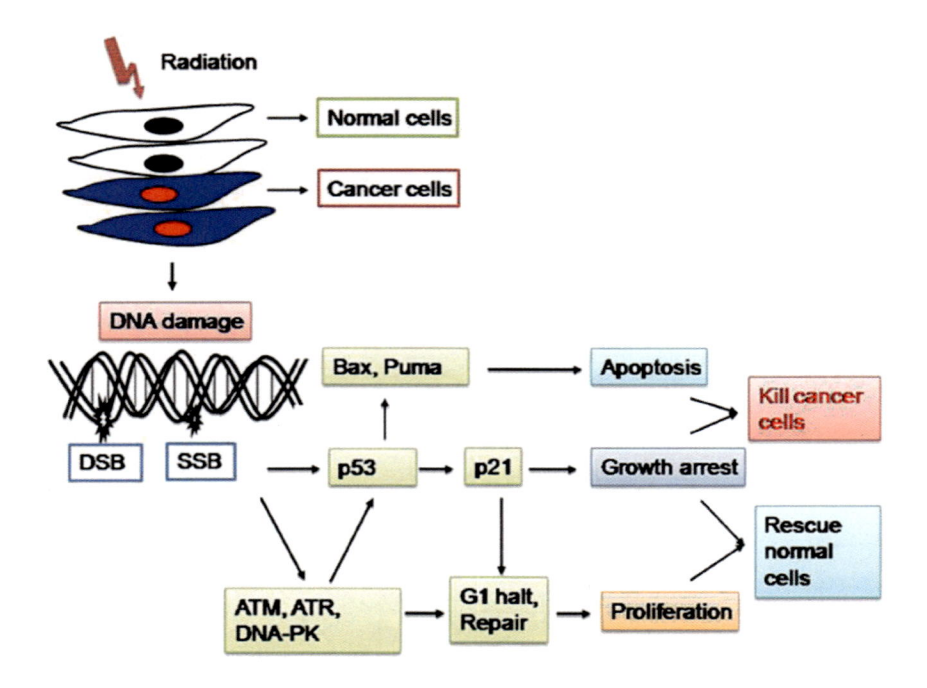

Figure 9-2. **Radiation damages the genetic material (DNA) causing single strand breaks (SSB) or double strand breaks (DSB) in the cells, thus blocking their ability to divide and proliferate further.** Mechanisms involved in the decrease of radiosensitivity of the fast doubling cancer cells, while increasing radioresistant of the slow doubling normal cells benefits the cancer patients. Adopted from ref. 2 with permission

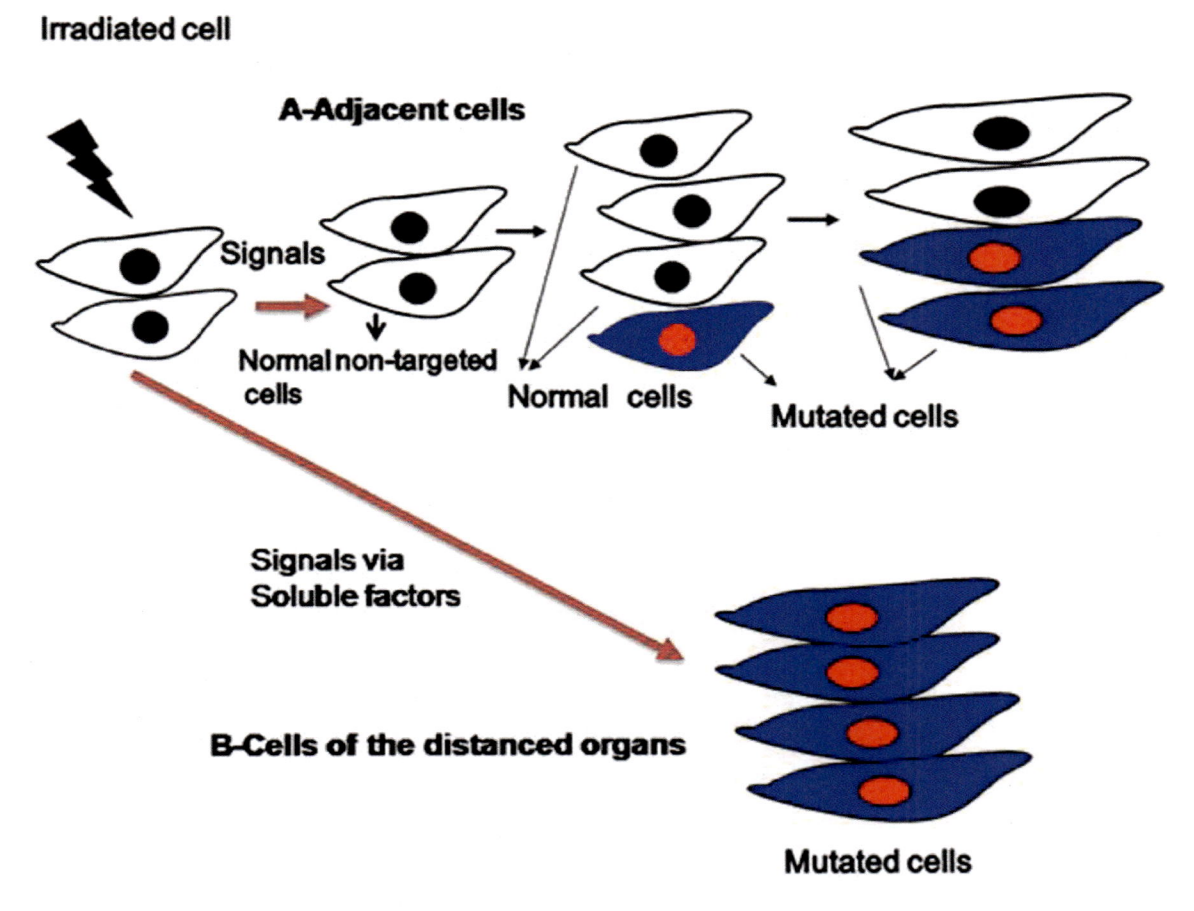

Figure 9-3. **Schematic representation of bystander effects induced by radiation to the adjacent cells and distanced organs.** Adopted from ref. 2 with permission

While DNA damages caused by irradiation are fatal if not repaired appropriately, it is obvious that membrane events contribute to radiation-induced apoptosis as well. However, it is unclear whether membrane processes triggered by radiation are capable of inducing apoptosis in all cells. Whereas early apoptosis, as exhibited by lymphocytes, is more likely to be caused by the propagation and amplification of radiation-induced DNA damage following passage through one or more mitoses, the delayed onset or late apoptosis exhibited by many other cell types that are more resistant to apoptosis induction is more likely to be caused by the propagation and amplification of radiation-induced DNA damage following passage through one or more mitoses.

Cell death mechanisms

Radiation-induced death is associated with mitosis

The most common cause of cell death following irradiation is mitosis-linked death, in which cells with chromosomal abnormalities during division divide to create nonclonogenic daughter cells with micronuclei (MN). The DNA double-strand break (dsb) is widely accepted as the molecular lesion responsible for chromosome abnormalities. Necrosis is frequently the result of mitotic cell death. Necrotic cells exhibit a breakdown of membrane integrity, resulting in cell enlargement, vesicle dilation, and subsequent random DNA destruction. This procedure frequently leads in local inflammation in individuals undergoing radiation therapy.

Radiation-induced cellular senescence: a putative function for telomeres in DNA double-stranded break stabilization

Along with necrosis, certain irradiation cells will undergo a process comparable to senescence, in which they retain metabolic activity but are unable to divide. Due to the similarity between this type of DNA damage-induced reaction and senescence, it has been hypothesized that insertion of telomeric sequences at the site of the dsb via telomorase activity may prevent the dsb from reuniting, thereby establishing stable chromosome breaks. Telomeres are short, highly repetitive DNA sequences found at the chromosome ends. Telomeres shorten with each cell division in normal cells. Cells experience G_1 arrest and senesce when their telomeres reach a certain length (about 4 kb). If senescent cells are forced to divide further, their telomeres shorten until they reach a length of 1 kb, at which point division ends and a necrotic-like death occurs. DNA dsbs may also acquire telomeres via telomere capture (and hence be stabilized), a process that involves the transfer of telomeres from normal chromosomes to damaged chromosomes in a non-telomerase-dependent way. Slijepcevic et al. demonstrated that up to 5% of radiation-induced chromatid breaks in mammalian cell lines can be modified by telomere capture using fluorescence in situ hybridization (FISH) with telomeric probes (i.e. fluorescent peptide–nucleic acid telomere oligonucleotides that hybridize with telomeres in cells). Sister chromatids are sister chromosomes that have not yet separated from one another during the G_2 phase following DNA replication. Sister chromatid telomeres frequently pair. The telomere transferred at the chromatid break will associate with the telomere of its intact sister chromatid. Thus, a daughter cell holding the repaired chromosome may be viable if the deleted portion lacks critical genes, whereas a daughter cell containing the donor chromosome may not be viable. Because the FISH technique cannot detect all minor chromosomal rearrangements, the value of 5% may be underestimated. DNA double-strand breaks that are not stabilized by telomere capture are rejoined to other DNA ends, resulting in their disappearance over time (post-irradiation); however, improper rejoining (resulting in dicentric, acentric, or ring chromosomes) can result in additional chromosomal damage in subsequent mitoses, ultimately leading to the death of the daughter cells.

The other resemblance between the radiation reaction and senescence is the induction of cell cycle arrest, which is permanent in senescence but usually transient following irradiation. Protein dimers consisting of catalytic cyclin-dependent kinases (cdks) and regulatory cyclin subunits closely govern cell cycle progression. Through the expression of inhibitory molecules such as $p^{21Waf-1}$ and $p^{16INK4A}$, the cdks that govern the G_1/S transition are blocked. After irradiation, the transistory G_1 arrest is dependent on a signalling cascade (Figure 1) including ATM and p^{53} that results in the induction of $p^{21Waf-1}$. Recent research has demonstrated that the G_1 arrest that occurs upon irradiation can be maintained in cells that retain metabolic activity but are unable to divide. Senescence is induced molecularly via upregulation of the cdk inhibitors $p^{21Waf-1}$ and $p^{16INK4A}$. It appears as though $p^{21Waf-1}$ is induced first, most likely independently of p53, and is involved in initiating senescent G1 arrest. The expression of p^{21Waf1} then decreases, but the expression of $p^{16INK4A}$ is stimulated, thereby preserving this arrest.

Apoptosis triggered by radiation

Proteolytic cascade and morphology

Apoptosis is characterised morphologically by nuclear chromatin condensation, blebbing of the nuclear and cytoplasmic membranes, and finally disintegration of nuclear structures, resulting in the creation of membrane-bound apoptotic bodies. The molecular steps involved in this type of cell death include the activation of proteolytic caspases, a family of cysteine proteases linked to the Caenorhabditis elegans cell death protein CED-3, and mitochondrial permeability changes. Caspases cleave a variety of proteins, including the DNA repair enzyme poly(ADP-ribose) polymerase (PARP), heteronuclear ribonucleoproteins C1 and C2, nuclear lamins, retinoblastoma protein, DNA fragmentation factor DFF, Bcl-2, mitogen-activated protein kinase family When these and other caspase targets are cleaved, the cytoskeleton is disrupted and DNA fragmentation begins. Caspase-3 is one of the caspases that has been linked to radiation-induced apoptosis.

Apoptotic cell death

Although apoptosis is a stochastic process within a population of cells, the initiation of apoptosis varies between cell types. Apoptosis can occur quickly after irradiation (referred to as interphase death, or rapid apoptosis), after G_2 arrest, or after one or more cell divisions (known as late apoptosis). Following irradiation, certain radiosensitive cells, such as thymocytes, lymphocytes, and intestinal crypt cells, experience rapid death, without cell division. Umansky showed that radiation-induced apoptosis occurred only after thymoma cells passed through the G_2 stage and entered mitosis. Additionally, Tauchi and Sawada irradiated mouse leukaemia cells, resulting in a G_2 block, and found that the apoptotic fraction increases upon liberation from the G_2 block.

In contrast to these faster types of apoptosis, Yanagihara et al. identified a late radiation-induced apoptosis in human gastric epithelial tumour cells, where apoptosis began to increase 12 hours after irradiation upon liberation from G_2 arrest and peaked between 72–96 hours (i.e. at the G_1 phase subsequent to irradiation). These findings establish a relationship between apoptosis and mitotic cell death, as the highest level of apoptosis occurred immediately following the first mitotic cell death following irradiation, and suggest that apoptosis may be the final step in some forms of mitotic cell death.

Irradiation is known to cause cell cycle arrests, which allow cells to repair some of the DNA damage caused by the radiation. These occur in G_1 just prior to DNA replication in S phase, as well as in G_2 just prior to mitosis. Both of these arrests are mediated by suppression of cdk–cyclin complexes, which regulate the G_1/S and G_2/M checkpoints, respectively. The G_2/M checkpoint is regulated by a complex composed of cyclin B and serine/threonine kinase $p34^{cdc2}$ (cdk1). The arrest in G_2 following irradiation has been associated with a decrease in cyclin B accumulation.

Numerous studies indicate that the G_2/M checkpoint may alter the extent of radiation-induced apoptosis: McKenna et al. demonstrated that transfecting fibroblasts with Myc increases radiation-induced apoptosis by immortalising these cells and reducing their capacity to arrest in G_1. These cells undergo a relatively brief G_2 delay following irradiation and display just a little decrease in cyclin B1 mRNA accumulation following irradiation. By contrast, transfection of fibroblasts with

Myc plus the transforming oncogene H-Ras results in a significant G_2 delay, which is related with decreased cyclin B1 mRNA expression and prevention of radiation-induced apoptosis. These findings imply that the G_2 delay is a critical step in determining whether or not a cell will undergo apoptosis. Additional support for this comes from research with coffee and staurosporine, both of which increase apoptosis in response to irradiation and inhibit the radiation-induced G_2 arrest. Additionally, in some conditions, activation of the mitotic cdk $p34^{cdc2}$ results in apoptotic cell death. Premature $p34^{cdc2}$ activation may contribute to apoptosis by phosphorylating substrates that are normally not phosphorylated until mitosis. Delia et al. also demonstrated that 24 hours after irradiation, the activity of the $p34^{cdc2}$ kinase remained unchanged in lymphoblastoid cells expressing mutated p53 that are resistant to radiation-induced apoptosis, but had an increased in radiosensitive cell lines that undergo apoptosis following irradiation. These findings imply that $p34^{cdc2}$ is implicated in radiation-induced apoptosis and may be used to radiosensitise malignancies via apoptosis induction.

Apoptosis mediated by p53

The tumour suppressor protein p53 is required for radiation-damaged cells to undergo apoptosis. Radiation and other kinds of DNA damage do not induce apoptosis in thymocytes generated from mice homozygously deficient in p53. Merritt et al. demonstrated that small intestinal epithelial cells from p53 null mice are radioresistant, with no apoptotic death observed between 4 and 8 hours after 8 Gy irradiation (a dose and time window at which apoptosis is readily observed in normal crypt cells), a finding that was confirmed by Clarke et al. using different $p53^{-/-}$ mice. Delia et al. compared two immortalized Epstein–Barr virus lymphoblastoid cell lines derived from individuals with the cancer-predisposing Li–Fraumeni syndrome and carrying a germ line heterozygous for p53 missense mutations. They found that both lines were resistant to apoptosis 48 hours after irradiation, with a level of radio resistance greater than that of cells expressing wild type p53, while only Similarly, Deng et al. demonstrated that $p21^{Waf1}$ was required for the induction of a G_1 arrest following irradiation, but not for the induction of apoptosis, employing $p21^{Waf1-/-}$ mice. These results demonstrate that p53-induced apoptosis is unrelated to G1 arrest induction.

Apoptosis in the absence of p53

Whereas p53 is required for apoptosis caused by irradiation and other stimuli, apoptosis can also occur in the absence of p53 under specific circumstances; for example, while p53$^{-/-}$ thymocytes are resistant to radiation-induced apoptosis, they remain susceptible to dexamethasone-induced apoptosis. Merritt et al. recently revealed that irradiation-induced delayed G$_2$/M-associated p53-independent apoptosis occurred in small intestine epithelial cells generated from p53$^{-/-}$ mice. Although the absence of p53 fully abolished the early wave of apoptosis in these mice, there was a wave of apoptosis in the small intestine at 24 and 40 hours after 8 Gy irradiation. Early apoptosis was demonstrated to be p53-dependent, but late apoptosis was demonstrated to be p53-independent in this model. Along with apoptotic cells, the appearance of some dying cells resembled that of multinucleated cells during mitotic death at later time periods.

ATM's function in irradiation-induced apoptosis

The Atm gene product has been linked to a signal transduction system that uses p53 to trigger a G$_1$ arrest in response to irradiation. Numerous studies have demonstrated that cells derived from ataxia telangectasia patients failed to induce p53 following irradiation (p53 is normally overexpressed and stabilised in these conditions by an unknown mechanism), implying that normal ATM function is required for optimal signal transduction from initial DNA damage to the modulators of this increase in p53 level. ATM has also been implicated in the induction of apoptosis in specific tissues by radiation. Numerous recent studies have examined the link between ATM and p53 in the apoptotic response generated by radiation. Barlow et al. demonstrated that after whole-animal irradiation, apoptosis in the thymus was promoted in a p53-dependent but not ATM-dependent way, implying that ATM is essential for normal cell cycle checkpoint function but not for the apoptotic response to irradiation in this paradigm. Similarly, Westphal et al. demonstrated that removal of ATM renders thymocytes somewhat resistant to irradiation-induced apoptosis, whereas loss of p53 confers total resistance, implying that the irradiation-induced apoptotic pathways involving ATM and p53 are not completely consistent. Even if radiation-induced apoptosis in the thymus is not ATM-dependent, it has been proven that ATM is essential for irradiation-induced apoptosis in the developing central nervous system, which is mediated by p53. These diverse investigations demonstrate that radiation-induced apoptosis occurs via a p53-dependent, ATM-independent route in some tissues, whereas both functions appear to be required in others.

Apoptotic cell death and radiosensitivity

Numerous studies have attempted to establish a correlation between the degree of apoptosis following irradiation and radiosensitivity. Certain studies indicate that an increased apoptotic response resulted in increased radiosensitivity; however, the increase in radiosensitivity generated by transfection with genes regulating apoptosis has never exceeded threefold. McKenna and colleagues demonstrated that radiation resistance induced by Ras oncogene transfection was related with resistance to irradiation-induced apoptosis using rat embryo fibroblasts. Aldridge et al. recently demonstrated that in five human hematopoietic cell lines with varying degrees of radiosensitivity, there was a clear correlation between the rate at which irradiation induced apoptosis and the cell line's clonogenic survival, and that this correlation was related to post-irradiation cell cycle checkpoint function. After equitoxic doses of irradiation, the rate of induction of apoptosis differed significantly between the five cell lines studied, and the relative ordering of the responses reflected the clonogenic survival dosage responses. HSB-2, the most radiosensitive cell line, demonstrated the quickest induction of apoptosis, which occurred at various stages of the cell cycle. The most radioresistant cell line, HL-60, exhibited the greatest G_2 delay prior to the commencement of apoptosis induction, which happened following the radiation-induced G_2 arrest. These findings imply that the overall amount of time available for DNA damage repair before apoptosis is a major factor of radiosensitivity in hematopoietic cell lines. On the other hand, Kyprianou et al. demonstrated that overexpression of Bcl-2 significantly delayed radiation-induced apoptosis but had no effect on clonogenic survival in human prostate cancer cell lines. These seemingly contradicting findings may reflect differences in the contribution of apoptosis to total cell death in various cell types.

The Bottom Line

Ionizing radiation-induced cellular death results in both apoptosis and mitosis-related mortality, as well as loss of reproductive ability. Apoptosis can occur during interphase, prior to division following radiation-induced G_2 block, or after division. Apoptosis is triggered by components found in the nucleus and the cell membrane, where the sphingomyelin pathway is launched by the hydrolysis of sphingomyelin to become ceramide. Apoptosis is regulated at multiple levels by a number of proteins that have been extensively studied in recent years, including ATM, p53, Bcl-2, Bax, Cdc2, and JNK; however, cell death in response to irradiation occurs more frequently as a result of mitotic death due to irreversible chromosome damage. This damage is now believed to be repaired via telomere capture, a process in which telomeres are transferred from normal chromosomes to damaged chromosomes.

Hypoxia within the tumour, radiation resistance, and HIF-1

Cancer biology has undergone a paradigm shift with the recognition that malignancies are not simply clonal collections of cells gone awry, but rather complex multicellular tissues in which individual cells respond to intercellular signals, the microenvironment, and the therapies aimed against them. The emergence of angiogenesis as a critical factor in cancer progression has been a driving force behind this shift, from the initial development of a vascularized primary tumour, which is no longer constrained by O_2 diffusion from host vessels, to the establishment of metastases, which define the terminal stage of the disease.

It was demonstrated the critical role of the tumour microenvironment in affecting therapeutic outcome by proposing that hypoxic cancer cells are resistant to radiation therapy. Hypoxia was interpreted as indicating a requirement for O_2 as a source of radiation-induced radicals involved in tumour cell death. The broader premise, which was overlooked at the time, is that hypoxia plays a significant role in the course of many malignancies.

The discovery of hypoxic cells' radiation resistance was followed decades later by the demonstration that hypoxia is the primary physiological stimulus for angiogenesis and, later, by the identification of hypoxia-inducible factor 1 (HIF-1) as the major transcriptional regulator of hypoxia-induced angiogenesis via transactivation of multiple angiogenic growth factors, including vascular endothelial growth factor (VEGF). The showing that the tumour vasculature is a significant target of radiation therapy and a significant predictor of clinical response established a critical link between radiation and angiogenesis.

HIF-1 has also been implicated in radiation resistance in clinical and preclinical research. Overexpression of HIF-1 in tumour biopsy samples from patients with oropharyngeal cancer is associated with an increased chance of failing to achieve complete remission following radiation therapy. On the other hand, tumour xenografts of HIF-1-deficient mouse embryo fibroblasts exhibit higher radiation sensitivity.

It was revealed that there is a link between HIF-1, tumour vasculature, and radiation resistance in this issue of Cancer Cell. Irradiation of tumour xenografts activates HIF-1, resulting in the expression of VEGF and basic fibroblast growth factor (bFGF), both of which work to protect endothelial cells (ECs) from radiation-induced mortality (Figure 9-4). Surprisingly, induction of HIF-1 does not begin until 12 hr after radiation and peaks at 48 hr. Moeller et al. (2004) demonstrate that radiation-induced reoxygenation of hypoxic tumour cells results in the production of reactive oxygen species (ROS) that induce HIF-1 activity, as determined by the expression of green fluorescent protein (GFP) driven by a hypoxia response element-containing promoter (HRE).

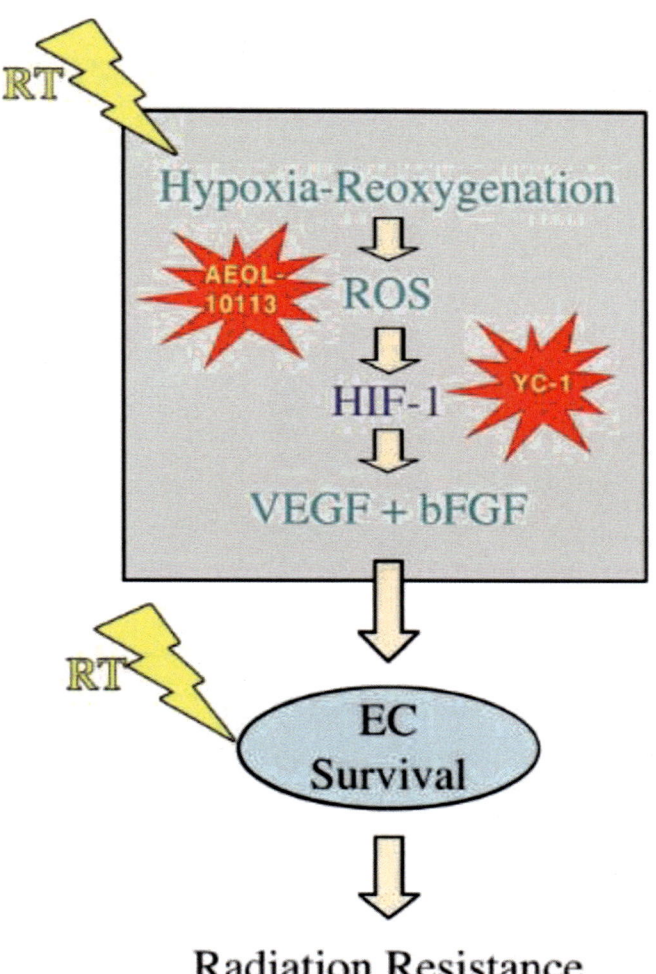

Fig. 9-4 Radiation increases HIF-1 activity and the generation of survival factors (Figure 1). Radiation therapy (RT) reoxygenates hypoxic tumour cells and generates reactive oxygen species (ROS), which activates hypoxia-inducible factor 1 (HIF-1), which directly promotes transcription of the VEGF gene, which encodes vascular endothelial growth factor. Unknown mechanisms also promote basic fibroblast growth factor (bFGF) expression in an HIF-1-dependent way. Tumor cells secrete VEGF and bFGF, which increase endothelial cell (EC) survival. Maintaining a functioning vascular promotes tumour cell survival. Thus, to the extent that radiation-induced EC death aids in the killing of new tumour cells, activation of the HIF-1 response pathway may aid in radiation resistance. AEOL-10113, a superoxide dismutase mimic, or YC-1, a small molecule inhibitor of HIF-1, can be used to inhibit the reaction. Adopted from ref. 3 with permission

How Can Tumor Hypoxia Be Overcome in Radiation Therapy?

Wilhelm Conrad Röntgen's 1895 discovery of X-rays paved the way for radiation therapy, one of the three major therapeutic options for cancer. Radiation therapy has evolved and improved as a result of the combination of engineering, physics, biology, and chemistry technologies and understanding. Additionally, interactions between scientists and clinicians have aided development significantly; for example, basic scientists have offered novel concepts in radiation treatment, while radiation oncologists have evaluated their therapeutic benefits and encouraged improvement. Even the most novel strategies, however, have failed to achieve complete remission, and patients frequently have tumour recurrence and/or distant metastases following radiation therapy. To address these issues, it is vital to understand how cancer cells survive, recur, and metastasis following radiation therapy.

It is well established that the presence or absence of molecular oxygen has an effect on the biological effect of ionising radiation; cells develop radioresistance in hypoxic environments. Since Thomlinson and Gray demonstrated that malignant tumours contain both hypoxic and well-oxygenated cancer cells, this phenomenon, dubbed the "oxygen effect," has garnered substantial attention in radiation oncology. Radiation chemistry investigations have established that a lack of oxygen results in an inefficient creation of DNA strand breaks when ionising radiation is used, and additionally hinders the damage from being repaired. Meanwhile, radiation biology research have demonstrated that hypoxic stimuli alter both the "DNA damage repair route" and the "cell death/survival signalling pathway," increasing the radioresistant phenotype of cells. Additionally, it was established that a transcription factor called hypoxia-inducible factor 1 (HIF-1) is critical for hypoxia-induced tumour radioresistance.

Numerous therapeutic techniques have been developed to address the difficulties associated with tumour hypoxia. Treatment using hyperbaric oxygen tries to deliver radiation to tumour tissues that are well-oxygenated and less hypoxic. Fractionated radiation therapy is used to specifically target hypoxic tumour cells that have just been reoxygenated following ex-irradiation. Additionally, radiation oncologists have recently acquired two highly effective new tools: "simultaneous integrated boost intensity-modulated radiation therapy (SIB-IMRT)," which enables the delivery of a booster dose of radiation to specific subpopulations of cells in a malignant tumour, and "hypoxia-selective cytotoxins/drugs." To fully utilize these novel and interdisciplinary radiation therapy options, it is necessary to understand the features, location, and dynamics of hypoxic tumour cells throughout tumour growth and after radiation therapy.

HYPOXIA, A TUMOR-SPECIFIC MICROENVIRONMENT

Proliferation that is abnormally accelerated as a result of oncogene activation and/or loss of tumour suppressor genes is a characteristic of cancer cells and results in an imbalance between oxygen supply and consumption in a malignant solid tumour. This imbalance, combined with insufficient diffusion of molecular oxygen within a tumour, is a primary contributor to cancers being very diverse and having substantially impaired oxygenation (Fig. 9-5). Tumor cells multiply and expand actively only when oxygen and nutrients are provided by tumour blood vessels (normoxic zones), and they will inevitably perish in places less than 100 μm from tumour blood vessels (necrotic regions). Between these two locations are so-called chronic hypoxic patches, where cancer cells receive the bare minimum amount of oxygen required for life.

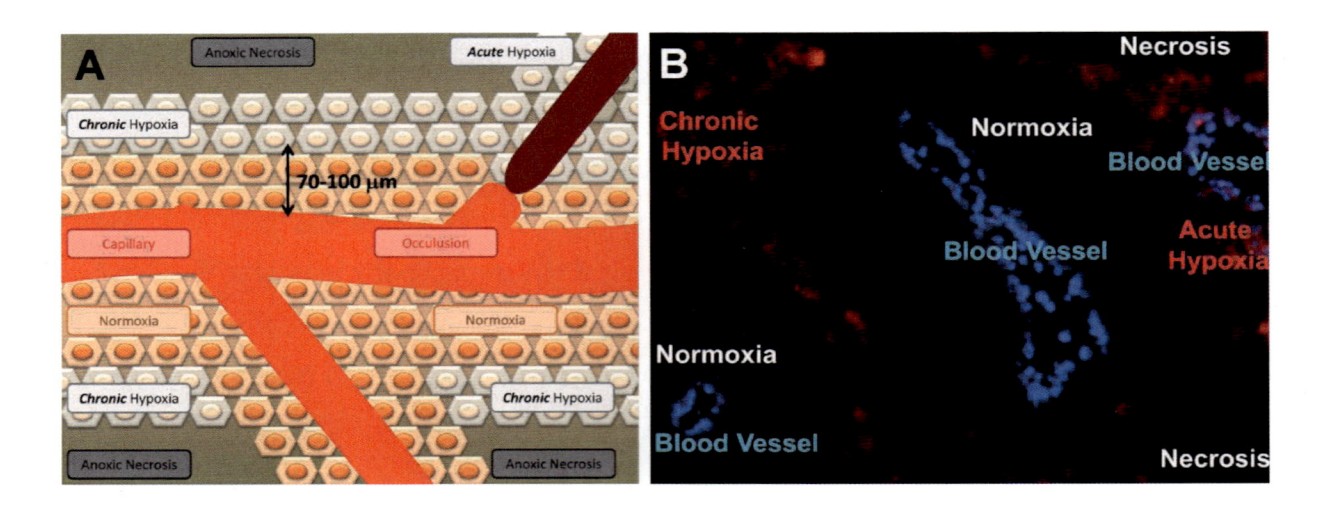

Fig. 9-5 Spatial relationship between blood vessels and hypoxia in a malignant solid tumor. Chronic hypoxia exists 70 - 100 μm from tumor blood vessels. Acute/cycling hypoxia caused by fluctuations in tumor blood flow occurs proximal to tumor blood vessels. A) Schematic diagram of tumor microenvironments. B) Frozen section of a tumor xenograft was stained with anti-HIF-1α antibody (red fluorescence). Tumor blood vessels can be seen as blue fluorescence (Hoechst33342 perfusion marker) adopted from ref. 4 with permission

Along with chronic hypoxia, acute/intermittent/cycling hypoxia has garnered considerable attention because to its association with cancer and radioresistance. Brown et al. discovered acute hypoxia for the first time in 1979, stating that a defective tumour vasculature results in transient blood vessel opening and closing, variations in blood flow, fluctuations in tumour perfusion, and eventually transitory hypoxia even within 70 μm tumour blood arteries. Subsequent investigations revealed that at least 20% of cancer cells in malignant solid tumours experience acute hypoxia, confirming the hypothesis that both acute and chronic hypoxia is a prevalent hallmark of solid tumours. Furthermore, it is widely accepted that hypoxia is unique to malignant solid tumours and hence can be exploited to differentiate cancer from normal cells and to build highly tumor-specific therapeutic methods.

TUMOR RADIO-RESISTANCE MECHANISMS UNDER HYPOXIA: RADIOCHEMICAL AND RADIOBIOLOGICAL MECHANISMS

The oxygen effect: cancer cells' radio resistance in hypoxic environments

The presence or lack of molecular oxygen has an effect on how x-rays act biologically. This phenomenon, dubbed the oxygen effect, was originally seen in 1912 when a radium applicator was pressed tightly against the skin, reducing blood flow there. It was postulated that oxygen levels in a solid tumour are decreased through successive layers of cancer cells distal to blood vessels, and that cancer cells distal to blood vessels are alive but radioresistant. Although there is no direct proof in vivo that this population survives radiation therapy better than well-oxygenated cancer cells and causes local tumour recurrence, many in vitro research, such as clonogenic assays, corroborate this notion. As a result, hypoxia tumour cells have been identified as a significant impediment to radiation therapy.

The molecular mechanics underlying the oxygen effect in radiation

Although the structure of the oxygen impact is not completely known, it is widely considered that oxygen works on free radicals. Ionizing radiation promotes ionisation in or near target cells' genomic DNA, generating different radicals that cause DNA strand breaks. Oxygen oxidizes the DNA radicals, which is known to cause lasting damage. In the absence of oxygen, on the other hand, DNA radicals are reduced by molecules containing sulfhydryl groups (SH groups), which restore/repair the DNA to its original state. Taken together, DNA damage, particularly irreversible double stranded breaks, is substantially less severe in the absence of molecular oxygen, resulting in cancer cells developing hypoxia-induced radioresistance.

The biological mechanisms underlying the oxygen effect are based on radiation

Along with radiochemical mechanisms, radiobiological mechanisms are critical as well. Hypoxic stimuli have been shown to alter both the "DNA damage repair route" and the "cell death/survival signaling pathway," increasing the radioresistant phenotype. Additionally, data from molecular biology and radiation oncology demonstrated a critical role for a transcription factor called hypoxia-inducible factor 1. (HIF-1). After radiation therapy, it has been found that expression of the HIF-1 alpha subunit and the intratumor hypoxic fraction associated with a poor prognosis, local tumour recurrence, and distant tumour metastases. Inhibition of intratumor HIF-1 activity with a pharmacological HIF-1 inhibitor, YC-1, or a dominant negative HIF-1α, or knockdown of HIF-1α expression with short hairpin RNA or short interfering RNA, respectively, resulted in a delay in tumour development following radiation. I will concentrate on recent improvements in our understanding of how HIF-1 produces tumour radioresistance in the sections that follow.

Managing HIF-1 movement

HIF-1 is a heterodimeric transcription factor that consists of a α-subunit (HIF-1) and a -subunit (HIF-1 β/ARNT). Its hypoxia-dependent activity is regulated at a number of different levels, including translational start and posttranslational modification.

The mechanism that is most understood is the one that affects the stability of HIF-1. Under normoxic conditions, prolyl hydroxylases hydroxylate the oxygen-dependent degradation (ODD) domain of HIF-1, which is then ubiquitinated by a pVHL-containing E3 ubiquitin ligase, resulting in fast destruction of the HIF-1α protein. On the other hand, hypoxic circumstances stabilise and activate HIF-1α, which interacts with its binding partner, HIF-1β. The resulting HIF-1 binds to its cognate transcriptional enhancer sequence, the hypoxia-responsive element (HRE), and promotes the expression of a variety of genes involved in angiogenesis, glycolysis, as well as cancer cell invasion and metastasis. Along with the PHDs-VHL-dependent process, it is known that HIF-1 is destroyed via the receptor of activated protein kinase C (RACK1, also known as GNB2L1). RACK1 competes with heat shock protein 90 for binding to HIF-1, hence stabilising the HIF-1 protein. As a result of the interaction with RACK1, HIF-1α is degraded in an oxygen-independent manner.

It was recently discovered that the HIF-1 protein is produced via a signalling cascade involving phosphatidylinositol 3-kinase (PI3K)-Akt-mammalian target of rapamycin (mTOR). The 5'-untranslated region of HIF-1α mRNA has a 5'-terminal oligopolypyrimidine tract that modulates HIF-1 translational initiation in response to mTOR and its downstream factors, p70 S6 kinase and eukaryotic initiation factor-4E activation (eIF-4E). Thus, the Akt-mTOR signalling pathway promotes HIF-1α translation even in normoxic conditions in response to certain growth factors, cytokines, and signalling molecules, including epidermal growth factor (EGF), fibroblast growth factor 2 (FGF-2), heregulin, insulin, insulin-like growth factor (IGF)-1 and IGF-2, and interleukin 1β (IL2β).

HIF-1α post-translational alteration also contributes significantly to its transactivational action. Factor inhibiting HIF-1 (FIH-1) becomes active in normoxic circumstances and hydroxylates an asparagine residue (N803) in HIF-1. The hydroxylation inhibits HIF-1α association with transcriptional cofactors p300 and CBP, hence inhibiting HIF-1α transactivational activity. Because oxygen is a substrate for FIH-1 hydroxylation of asparagine, hypoxic environments depleted of oxygen restore HIF-1α transactivational activity. Additionally, HIF-1α transactivation activity is enhanced by phosphorylation via the ERK (p42 and p44) and p38 MAP kinase pathways.

HIF-1 plays a role in hypoxic tumour cell radioresistance

Recently, an intriguing model of HIF-1's role in cellular radioresistance to hypoxia was proposed: 1) radiation activates HIF-1 in a solid tumour, 2) HIF-1 induces the expression of VEGF, 3) VEGF protects endothelial cells from the cytotoxic effects of radiation, and 4) radio-protected tumour blood vessels ensure the supply of oxygen and nutrients to tumour cells and promote tumour growth. The following results corroborate this concept. Optical real-time imaging investigations with an HIF-1-dependent reporter gene demonstrated that radiation therapy significantly increases intratumor HIF-1 activity, corroborating the first phase of the model. In vitro, hypoxia-conditioned media supplemented with a high concentration of VEGF dramatically reduced the incidence of radiation-induced apoptosis in human umbilical vein endothelial cells (HUVECs). After radiation therapy, an HIF-1 inhibitor, YC-1, or a neutralizing antibody against VEGF significantly increased endothelial cell death and decreased micro vessel density, resulting in a radio sensitizing effect in a tumour growth delay experiment.

HYPOXIC AND HIF-1 ACTIVE CELL INTRATUMORAL DYNAMICS

As indicated previously, cancer cells' radioresistance is controlled by both oxygen concentrations and HIF-1 activity; thus, it is critical to increase our fundamental understanding of their intratumor location and dynamics in order to design novel therapeutic techniques.

Hypoxic zones' spatiotemporal dynamics

Because persistent hypoxia resides essentially 70–100 μm from tumour blood veins, its intratumoral distribution and volume are easily predicted histologically. On the other hand, acute/cycling hypoxia is more difficult since it is impacted by a variety of factors, including erythrocyte flux, neoangiogenesis, temporary arterial blockage, variations in blood flow, and tumour perfusion oscillations. A twofold labelling technique utilizing two different types of hypoxia tracers indicated that acute/cycling hypoxia is prevalent in human malignancies as well as tumour xenografts in experimental animals, and that 8–20% of tumour cells suffer acute/cycling hypoxia. Cycle frequency varies considerably, ranging from one cycle per minute (with an average cycle period of 20–30 minutes) to one cycle every several hours, and even one cycle per day (24 hours). A clinical report indicates that PET imaging for tumour hypoxia utilising 18F-misonidazole (18F-MISO) at 3-day intervals revealed changes in the signal's position, shape, size, and intensity.

The evolution of hypoxic regions during and following radiation therapy

The oxygen-dependent differential in radiosensitivity is connected with changes in the tumour microenvironment following irradiation. Specifically, it has been hypothesised that radiotherapy significantly improves oxygen distribution from tumour blood arteries to hypoxic tumour cells as a result of the death of well-oxygenated tumour cells and the subsequent decrease in oxygen consumption there. This is referred to as tumour reoxygenation. My colleagues and I validated the phenomena in immunohistochemical analyses employing tumour xenografts: hypoxic cells that were first detected with the hypoxia marker pimonidazole at the border between normoxic and necrotic regions were not stained 6–24 hours after 5 Gy of X-irradiation.

HIF-1-active cell dynamics/HIF-1 activity

To study the dynamics of HIF-1-active cells/HIF-1 activity in a malignant solid tumour, molecular imaging with HIF-1-dependent reporter genes is the optimal way. My colleagues and I created a series of reporter plasmids that express fluorescent proteins such as enhanced green fluorescent protein (EGFP) and DsRed2, as well as bioluminescent proteins such as firefly luciferase. The reporter gene was stably transfected into cancer cells and put into immune-deficient nude mice. The resulting tumor-bearing mice were exposed to real-time optical imaging tests with the reporter gene expressed in their xenograft.

During tumour progression, the dynamics of HIF-1-positive tumour cells

Bioluminescent imaging, which allows for quantitative analysis, demonstrated a progressive increase in intratumoral HIF-1 activity as the xenograft expanded. On the other hand, fluorescence imaging, which enables spatiotemporal study at the micron scale, revealed that the distribution of HIF-1-activated cancer cells altered drastically from day to day due to neovascularization. Tumor cells expressing HIF-1 were found far from tumour blood arteries. The distance between HIF-1-active areas and the nearest blood artery and the width of the vessel in the tumour xenograft model are highly correlated: Distance equals 1.38 diameter multiplied by 19.4 (r = 0.801, n = 25).

Changes in the activity of HIF-1 following radiation therapy

Bioluminescent imaging of a tumour xenograft expressing the HIF-1-dependent promoter revealed that intratumor HIF-1 activity declined rapidly and reached a minimum after 6 hours following 5 Gy of local ionising radiation (early phase). Following that, HIF-1 activity increased and reached a plateau at 18–24 hours postirradiation (late phase), although the timing and duration of activation appear to be dose- and cell-line-dependent. Immunohistochemical research with an anti-HIF-1α antibody demonstrated that the two phases of intratumor HIF-1 activity are reliant on the drop and increase in HIF-1α protein in the border between normoxic/viable and necrotic regions, respectively, after 6 and 24 hours after radiation. Radiation-induced alterations in the tumour microenvironment, particularly in glucose and oxygen availability (reoxygenation) in border regions, are critical for the down-regulation and subsequent up-regulation of HIF-1α expression during both stages. Immunostaining with the hypoxia marker pimonidazole demonstrated that in the early phase, the border regions were well-oxygenated (reoxygenated). In reoxygenated regions, PHD(s)-VHL-dependent degradation of HIF-1α predominates over neo-synthesis of HIF-1α, resulting in low HIF-1α activity. On the other hand, during the late phase, not only reoxygenation but also enhanced glucose availability in border regions significantly increases Akt-mTOR-dependent HIF-1α translation. Additionally, reoxygenation results in the generation of ROS, which results in the stability of the HIF-1α protein via the inhibition of PHD activity. Additionally, reoxygenation elevates NO levels in tumor-associated macrophages, resulting in S-nitrosylation and subsequent HIF-1α stabilization. In general, neo-synthesis of HIF-1 outpaced degradation in the late phase, resulting in up-regulation of HIF-1 activity even under reoxygenated conditions.

METHODS FOR OVERCOMING HYPOXIC TUMOR CELLS' RADIORESISTANCE

Given the critical role of hypoxic/HIF-1-positive tumour cells in radioresistance, techniques targeting them should be capable of overcoming the obstacles. This section discusses advancements in the development of hypoxia-targeted radiation oncology methods (Table 1).

Increased oxygenation

To begin, radiation oncologists attempted to increase the amount of oxygen delivered directly to locally progressed solid tumours during radiation. To improve tumour oxygenation, hyperbaric oxygenation, red blood cell transfusions, and erythropoietin administration were attempted. Additionally, normobaric oxygen or carbogen has been utilised in combination with nicotinamide, which has been shown to compensate for acute hypoxia. Although these techniques shown therapeutic effects in preclinical investigations, they have not been widely adopted due to inconsistent clinical trial findings.

Radiosensitizers

In the 1970s, it was discovered that nitroimidazole derivatives, such as misonidazole, mimicked the function of oxygen in radiochemical reactions and were investigated to determine whether they enhanced the lethal effect of ionizing radiation under hypoxic settings. In preclinical in vitro and in vivo tests, the theoretically projected oxygen enhancement ratio was verified to be approximately 1.5–2.0 at a clinically tolerable dose. Clinical investigations with nitroimidazole derivatives, on the other hand, have showed only a small therapeutic advantage and remain equivocal. Misonidazole trials conducted by the Radiation Therapy Oncology Group (RTOG) revealed no benefit. Misonidazole was likewise found to have no overall benefit in a Danish trial. Meanwhile, favorable results were seen in a subset of 304 patients with pharyngeal cancer, in ENT tumours treated with brachytherapy, and in big ENT tumours treated with hypo fractionated external radiation therapy. Additionally, a Danish experiment using another radiosensitizer, nimorazole, indicated an overall survival improvement in addition to local control. Misonidazole inconclusive outcome was partly owing to its dose-limiting toxicity. Effective levels of the medicine were discovered to cause peripheral neuropathy, which is the primary reason for the drug's withdrawal from routine clinical use. Due to misonidazole limited solubility, additional nitroimidazole derivatives with a higher solubility, such as etanidazole and doranidazole, have been created. Etanidazole is poorly absorbed into nervous system tissues and does not cross the blood-brain barrier, indicating that it is less harmful than misonidazole. Thus, an increased dose of etanidazole is approximately three times as effective as misonidazole. Then, in a subset of patients with early nodal illness, beneficial treatment results were identified.

Cytotoxins produced in hypoxia

Although tumour hypoxia is a significant impediment to radiation therapy, we can use it as a tumor-specific therapeutic target and a substitute for oxygenation of tumour hypoxia. Tirapazamine is a model hypoxia-activated prodrug that was first described more than two decades ago. Tirapazamine hypoxic selectivity is a result of its intracellular one-electron reduction to a radical anion, which can be reversibly oxidized to the parent harmless molecule in the presence of molecular oxygen. In the absence of oxygen, on the other hand, the radical anion can be further transformed to a deadly hydroxyl radical or an oxidizing radical by evaporating water. Both of the ensuing radicals cause DNA double-strand breaks (DSBs), single-strand breaks, and base damage, all of which result in cytotoxicity. Additionally, Tirapazamine is cytotoxic in part via poisoning topoisomerase II. Tirapazamine in combination with radiation has been shown to benefit patients with lung cancer or head and neck cancer in clinical trials.

HIF-1 inhibitor

Due to its crucial role in hypoxic tumour cell radioresistance, HIF-1 has been identified as an excellent molecular target for sensitising the therapeutic action of radiation. YC-1, which was initially created to activate soluble guanylate cyclase and reduce platelet aggregation, has been shown to lower HIF-1 accumulation and HIF-1 target gene expression under hypoxic environments, thereby limiting tumour development and spread. Recently, it was revealed that when combined with radiation therapy alone, YC-1 administration with proper timing inhibits radiation-induced activation of HIF-1 considerably delays tumour growth.

Inhibiting HIF-1α dimerization with HIF-1β should also have a radiosensitizing effect, as dimerization is essential for HIF-1 DNA binding and transcriptional activity. Lee et al. discovered that acriflavine directly binds to HIF-1α and suppresses its dimerization and transcriptional activity. They found that acriflavine administration decreased intratumoral expression of angiogenic cytokines, angiogenic cell mobility into peripheral circulation, and tumour vascularization, resulting in tumour growth inhibition and arrest. Although it has not been determined whether this medicine has a radiosensitizing effect, we can anticipate positive findings.

Another strategy for inhibiting HIF-1 is to inhibit the action of critical components that promote HIF-1 expression or activity. To begin, the PI3K-Akt-mTOR and Ras signalling pathways must be regulated. Mutations in these pathways are frequently observed in human malignancies, and both are known to increase HIF-1α protein expression. In a mouse model of prostate cancer with strong oncogenic Akt activity, a mTOR inhibitor, RAD001, actually lowered the quantity of HIF-1α protein and its downstream gene products. This suppressive impact adds to the radiosensitizing action of the PI3K-Akt-mTOR signalling pathway inhibitors RAD-001, LY294002, rapamycin, and wortmannin, at least in part. The second is HSP90 activity control. As previously stated, HSP90 competes with RACK1 for binding to HIF-1α and inhibits its oxygen-independent breakdown. Inhibition of Hsp90 activity with 17-allylamino-17-demethoxygeldanamycin or deguelin, a new natural Hsp90 inhibitor, reduced an increase in HIF-1α-Hsp90 association in cancer cells. Additionally, when radiation and deguelin were combined, radioresistant lung cancer cells' survival and angiogenic capacity were drastically diminished in vitro.

Approaches to gene therapy

Due to the low specificity of current gene therapy technologies, there has been no alternative to directly administering therapeutic genes into tumours. Harris and colleagues hypothesised that HIF-1/HRE-mediated transcriptional initiation may be used to specifically promote therapeutic gene expression in hypoxic regions of solid tumours in order to develop a gene therapy technique targeting hypoxic/HIF-1-active cancer cells. Then, much effort was made to build artificial HIF-1-dependent promoters, and finally, the most successful one, dubbed the 5HRE promoter (5HREp), was developed, in which five copies of the HRE boost transcription from a cytomegalovirus (CMV) minimum promoter. The 5HRE promoter was placed upstream of a suicide gene that converts a non-toxic prodrug to a harmful drug, with the assumption that suicide gene production would be promoted only in HIF-1-active cancer cells. The suicide genes herpes simplex virus thymidine kinase (HSV-TK)/ganciclovir (GCV), bacterial cytosine deaminase (BCD)/5-fluorocytosine (5-FC), and bacterial nitroreductase (NTR)/CB1954 were employed in these research. These techniques were shown to enhance radiosensitivity and retard tumour growth in an experimental tumour model employing a stable transfectant of the 5HREp-suicide gene. Additionally, suicide gene therapy utilising adenoviral vectors encoding 5HREp-BCD and 5-FC increased the impact of fractionated radiation therapy, paving the way for practical application.

Radiation therapy that is fractionated

Fractionated radiation therapy for cancer has several advantages over conventional radiation therapy in that it can enhance therapeutic effect while minimizing severe adverse effects in normal tissues. By and large, these benefits are attributable to the total of four parameters: recovery/repair of radiation-induced cell damage, redistribution of cell cycle status, reoxygenation of hypoxic cells, and repopulation of surviving cells. These factors are referred to as "four Rs (4Rs)" in radiation biology. Reoxygenation should be prioritized among these four strategies in order to fight hypoxic tumour cells. It has been reported that following radiotherapy, the distribution of oxygen from tumour blood arteries to hypoxic tumour cells improves considerably as a result of the death of well-oxygenated tumour cells and the consequent decrease in oxygen consumption in those cells.

The most standard fractionated radiation therapy regimens deliver 1.8–2.0 Gy of radiation per day, around 9.0–10 Gy each week, and up to approximately 60 Gy over a six-week period. However, because this strategy is insufficient for controlling locally advanced malignancies, other schedules have been developed. Hyperfractionation, in which a lower dose of radiation, such as 1.1–1.2 Gy, is delivered twice daily with an interval of approximately 6 hours, provides for an increase in the total dose of radiation while maintaining therapeutic effectiveness and minimising side effects. Accelerated fractionation, in which a relatively high dose of radiation, 1.5–1.6 Gy, is delivered twice daily but the total dose remains the same as the usual dose, has an advantage in cases of rapid tumour growth because the total length of therapy is shorter than the other two. Apart from these three, numerous types of fractionation have been investigated in clinical studies and have been shown to result in a considerable increase in local control rates. However, from a reoxygenation standpoint, it is vital to understand when and how reoxygenation happens, since this information should aid in further optimising fractionated radiation therapy regimens.

IMRT

Intensity-modulated radiation therapy (IMRT) is a cutting-edge cancer treatment method that enables radiation oncologists to accurately adjust the distribution of radiation doses based on the overall form of tumours. Tumor-specificity is achieved with the development of two critical technologies. The first is a radiological image generated using computed tomography (CT) or magnetic resonance imaging (MRI), both of which provide detailed anatomical information and enable the location of malignant tumours relative to normal tissues to be determined. Second is the creation of multileaf collimators, each of which moves independently during radiation therapy under the control of a computer, allowing for intensity modification of the photon beam. Additionally, the combination of numerous external beams enables a complicated three-dimensional dose distribution design that corresponds to the patients' anatomy. Thus, IMRT enables significantly greater doses to be delivered to tumours without increasing harmful effects on neighboring normal tissue. This technological advancement has resulted in an increase in the local control rates of a variety of advanced malignancies. With the development of IMRT, it is now possible to provide a non-homogeneous radiation dose within a tumour. Specifically, attempts have been made to utilise this advantageous technique to overcome tumour hypoxia, known as Hypo-IGRT, by administering a booster dosage of radiation to hypoxic fractions in a malignant tumour. To that end, numerous imaging probes for tumour hypoxia have been developed, including CuATSM, ^{18}F-FRP170, and ^{18}F-MISO.

The Bottom Line

On the basis of accumulating evidence in radiation biology and oncology, there is no doubt that hypoxic tumour cells and HIF-1 active cells are good targets for reducing the incidence of both local and distant tumour recurrence, as well as patient mortality. Significant effort has been made to create hypoxia-selective cytotoxins/drugs and HIF-1 inhibitors, among other things. Additionally, hypoxia image-guided radiation treatment (Hypo-IGRT) is being developed with the goal of administering a booster dose of radiation to radioresistant fractions. To maximize the effect of radiation therapy in combination, it is necessary to monitor changes in the localization and volume of radioresistant zones. Due to the fact that some growth factors and reactive oxygen species (ROS) are known to elicit HIF-1 activity even in normoxic conditions, imaging techniques for hypoxia (low oxygen levels) miss cells that are in normoxia yet HIF-1-active. As a result, it is critical to create imaging methods that can detect both hypoxia and HIF-1 activity. Additionally, populations identified by both methods should be targeted during radiation therapy.

References for this chapter

1. Cohen–Jonathan, Elizabeth Bernhard, Eric J. McKenna, W. Gillies, How does radiation kill cells? Current Opinion in Chemical Biology, 1999, 3, 77-83

2. Baskar R, Dai J, Wenlong N, Yeo R, Yeoh KW. Biological response of cancer cells to radiation treatment. Front Mol Biosci. 2014 Nov 17;1:24. doi: 10.3389/fmolb.2014.00024. PMID: 25988165; PMCID: PMC4429645.

3. Semenza GL. Intratumoral hypoxia, radiation resistance, and HIF-1. Cancer Cell. 2004 May;5(5):405-6. doi: 10.1016/s1535-6108(04)00118-7. PMID: 15144945.

4. Harada H. How can we overcome tumor hypoxia in radiation therapy? J Radiat Res. 2011;52(5):545-56. doi: 10.1269/jrr.11056. PMID: 21952313.

Chapter 10

Targeting and delivery

A. Targeting as a concept: acceptable usage of the terms "target" and "targeting"

In this chapter, we would like to first discuss the concept of targeting and the proper use and context for the terms targeting and target. To begin, it is necessary to recognize that pharmacological therapy is really about the interaction of two molecules. A substance delivered exogenously to a patient and the molecule within the patient with which the administered molecule interacts to elicit a physiological response. In an ideal world, the injected molecule interacts with only one physiological molecule, eliciting a physiological response beneficial to the patient's condition. In this context, it is evident that the term "target" refers to the physiological molecule, whereas "drug" refers to the delivered molecule. On the other hand, the concept of targeting has numerous definitions and can frequently cause misunderstanding if not stated effectively.

Current drug therapy problems revolve around the treatment of diseases caused by abnormalities of normal human biochemical pathways in specific tissues. Even dosage dependent selectivity is frequently difficult to obtain. As a result, the term "targeted" is becoming more connected with selective delivery. The term 'targeting' should ideally suggest that the molecule is capable of selectively accumulating at the desired site of action and that this selective accumulation is related with the molecule's selective action. This distinction is critical when designing targeted therapies for diseases such as cancer. Unless and until distinct molecular targets are discovered that are located exclusively (or at sufficiently greater levels) in the diseased state and not in the normal state, selective accumulation at the disease location is critical for therapeutic improvement. In summary, there appear to be two separate ways to pharmacological therapy targeting. The first type entails selective action on the target, whereas the second type entails selective accumulation on the target. The most, if not all, cases of targeting appear to involve a mix of selective action on the target and selective accumulation at the target site. Enhancing selective accumulation offers the extra benefit of lowering the needed dose, even for compounds with a high degree of target selectivity, and should thus be a key emphasis of all targeting efforts.

In the context of therapeutic molecules, the concept of selective accumulation is linked to the concepts of bioavailability and biodistribution, which are related to the molecule's physicochemical qualities. To circumvent the constraints imposed by a compound's physical chemical properties on its potential pharmaceutical application, the method of large-scale screening of chemical libraries has been extended beyond the identification of desired bioactivity. Selection for physico-chemical qualities known to impart high bioavailability is commonly incorporated into screening procedures. Regrettably, this method frequently results in the exclusion of numerous highly potent compounds from further research. These compounds frequently exert a significant pharmacological effect on a desired molecular target yet are unable to localize exclusively to that target. It is almost clear that there is a growing list of such compounds that are in essence potential medications if only a delivery mechanism for them to reach their molecular target in the human body can be found.

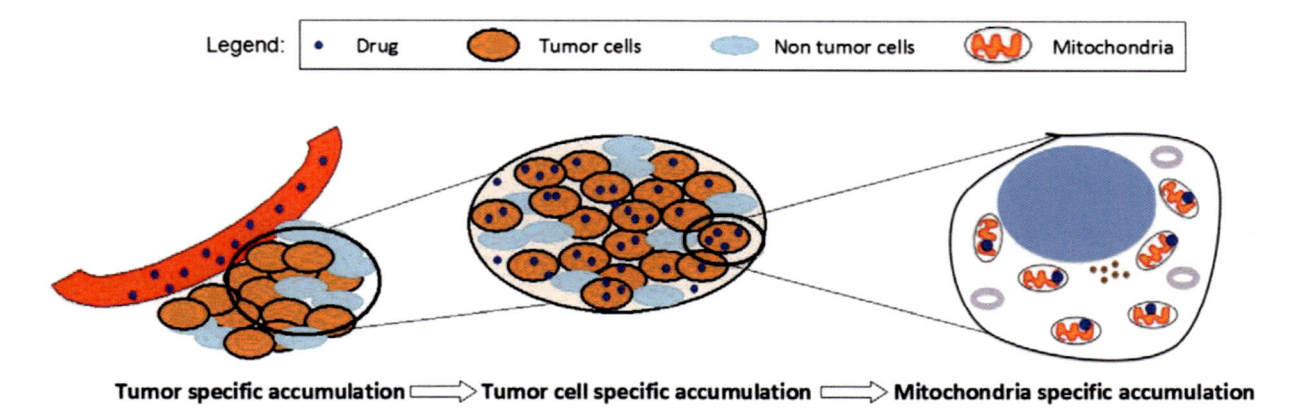

Fig. 10-1. A schematic representation of the levels of selective accumulation required in a mitochondria-specific targeting strategy. Adopted from ref. 1 with permission

Fig. 10-1 illustrates the many levels of targeting that may be required in the treatment of cancer using a targeted strategy. The medicine must reach the tumour mass, which is composed of tumour cells and supportive stroma, following systemic injection. The stroma, on the other hand, consists of connective tissue, blood vessels, and other benign cells. As a result, medication accumulation in a solid tumour is only the first step toward specific cancer therapy. The medicine must still enter the tumour cell and, once inside, reach its final subcellular target. The subcellular target may be a cytosolic molecule or, more frequently, a membrane-bound organelle-bound molecule. Additionally, the medicine must be able to enter the organelle and then locate its molecular target in the latter situation. At the moment, drug targeting is widely recognised down to the cellular level, as indicated by the enormous variety of techniques being investigated to generate drug accumulation in certain cells. However, targeting at the sub-cellular level has not been widely pursued until lately, either due to technological constraints or the argument that once a medicine enters a cell, it will eventually reach the sub-cellular target.

B. Mitochondrial cancer therapeutic targets

The mitochondrion is a crucial organelle in eukaryotic cells because it mediates various critical functions. The involvement of mitochondria in energy metabolism and cell cycle regulation is critical in the physiology of cancer. There is compelling evidence to promote the development of anticancer therapies that target mitochondria. Mitochondria are recognised to play a critical part in the complicated apoptotic pathway, causing cell death by a variety of ways, including interrupting electron transport and energy metabolism, releasing or activating apoptotic proteins, and altering cellular redox potential. The permeabilization of the mitochondrial membrane, a crucial process leading to programmed cell death, is regulated by the permeability transition pore complex (mPTPC), a multiprotein complex generated at the interface between the mitochondrial inner and outer membranes. Apoptosis is critical for tissue homeostasis, and it is well accepted that inhibiting apoptosis contributes to the process by which normal cells convert into cancer cells. The malfunction of the majority of apoptosis-regulating mechanisms has been related to a variety of different forms of cancer. For more than a decade, the critical significance of mitochondrial malfunction and altered apoptotic regulating pathways has been recognised. The changed role of mitochondria in the energy metabolism of malignant cells is closely related to the dysregulation of mitochondrial involvement in the apoptotic process. Cancer cells, even under aerobic conditions, are known to prefer the glycolytic pathway as a source of ATP. These adaptations are thought to confer invasive and adaptive advantages and are frequently the result of alterations in mitochondrial function, including mitochondrial DNA mutations (mtDNA). As a result, this organelle is increasingly being referred to as a "primary target" for pharmacological intervention, and interest in the molecular interactions of xenobiotics with cellular components situated on or within the mitochondrion is expanding. Numerous groups of researchers have found a variety of molecular targets for bioactive chemicals linked with mitochondria. To mention a few, these targets include mitochondrial DNA, the mitochondrial respiratory chain, the mitochondrial permeability transition pore complex (mPTPC), potassium channels on the mitochondria, and other anti- and pro-apoptotic molecules linked with the mitochondria. Two distinct strategies for targeting mitochondria in cancer cells are envisaged. The first strategy involves the use of medicines that act only on molecular targets in cancer cells' mitochondria without a clear preference for mitochondrial accumulation. The second strategy entails introducing chemicals capable of interfering with mitochondrial activity exclusively to cancer cells' mitochondria.

C. The selective accumulation strategy for cancer cell mitochondrial targeting

As demonstrated in Figure 10-1, the selective accumulation strategy for targeting tumour mitochondria requires two stages of accumulation: drug accumulation within the tumour and subsequently drug accumulation within the mitochondria of cancer cells. In general, drug distribution can be regulated by subtly altering the chemical structure of the drug to alter its physicochemical qualities, which are known to influence its accumulation in specific compartments. Naturally, such change must be carried out without impairing the molecular target's action. The second strategy includes conjugating ligands that are bigger than simple organic functional groups in order to alter the active molecule's biodistribution. Again, this technique is effective as long as the conjugation does not impair the molecule's targeted pharmacological action. These strategies have been extremely effective in altering medication distribution in the body and increasing drug accumulation in target tissues by employing ligands with known affinity for the target tissue. There are ligands that have been demonstrated to mediate drug accumulation in tumours and ligands that are known as mitochondriotropic. However, it is unknown if a ligand possesses both qualities to a sufficient degree to allow for high amounts of the desired accumulation. Thus, it is safe to conclude that, for the time being, a dual strategy is the most practicable option. Such a dual strategy would necessitate the employment of one targeted delivery route to generate substantial tumour accumulation, followed by another to ensure that the medication accumulates in the mitochondria, where it will have its effect. While there is much study into tissue-specific delivery targeted at raising anticancer medication levels in tumours, research into subcellular delivery is only beginning to gain traction. Nonetheless, there are some novel strategies for mitochondrial delivery that hold the promise of enhanced cancer therapy.

D. Bioactive chemical delivery to mitochondria in vivo

Mitochondria are critical for cell survival and death; thus, it is unsurprising that mitochondrial damage contributes to a wide variety of diseases, including Friedreich's ataxia, Parkinson's disease, diabetes, Huntington's disease, disorders associated with mitochondrial DNA mutations, cancer and degenerative diseases, and the pathophysiology of ageing. Despite the widespread occurrence of mitochondrial malfunction, mitochondria-specific medicines have remained undeveloped, in part due to the difficulties of delivering therapeutic compounds to mitochondria in vivo. As a first step toward developing such medicines, we established a technique for covalently attaching bioactive compounds to the triphenylphosphonium cation via an alkyl chain (Fig.10-2). Due to the substantial membrane potential (150 to 170 mV, negative inside; Fig. 10-2), these lipophilic cations rapidly permeate lipid bilayers and accumulate several hundredfold within mitochondria. The plasma membrane potential (30–60 mV, negative on the inside; Fig. 8-2) also promotes the accumulation of these molecules from extracellular fluid into isolated cells, where they are concentrated further within mitochondria, with mitochondria accounting for 90% of intracellular lipophilic cations. This selective absorption by mitochondria could significantly improve the efficacy and specificity of compounds designed to interact with mitochondria while simultaneously reducing unwanted side effects.

To have therapeutic promise, these mitochondria-targeted compounds must be taken up preferentially by mitochondria in vivo. They should accumulate to therapeutically effective levels within mitochondria in the organs most affected by mitochondrial dysfunction, including the heart, skeletal muscle, and brain. Due to the ease with which alkyl-triphenyl phosphonium cations pass through lipid bilayers via non-carrier-mediated transport, they should be taken up by the mitochondria of all tissues, in contrast to hydrophilic substances that require the expression of tissue-specific carriers for uptake. The methyl-triphenyl phosphonium cation (TPMP) is taken up by mitochondria in the perfused heart, liver, and skeletal muscle, corroborating this idea. As a result, once these mitochondria-targeted compounds enter the bloodstream, they should bind to the mitochondria in all tissues. Direct flow of lipophilic cations via lipid bilayers should enable these compounds to pass the blood–brain barrier and concentrate in brain mitochondria, which is particularly relevant for neurodegenerative disorders. However, little is known about alkyl-triphenylphosphonium cations' absorption, tissue distribution, and metabolism in vivo, or whether they can pass the blood–brain barrier. Additionally, accessible regimens for their long-term administration must be created to evaluate their efficacy in mouse models of chronic degenerative illnesses.

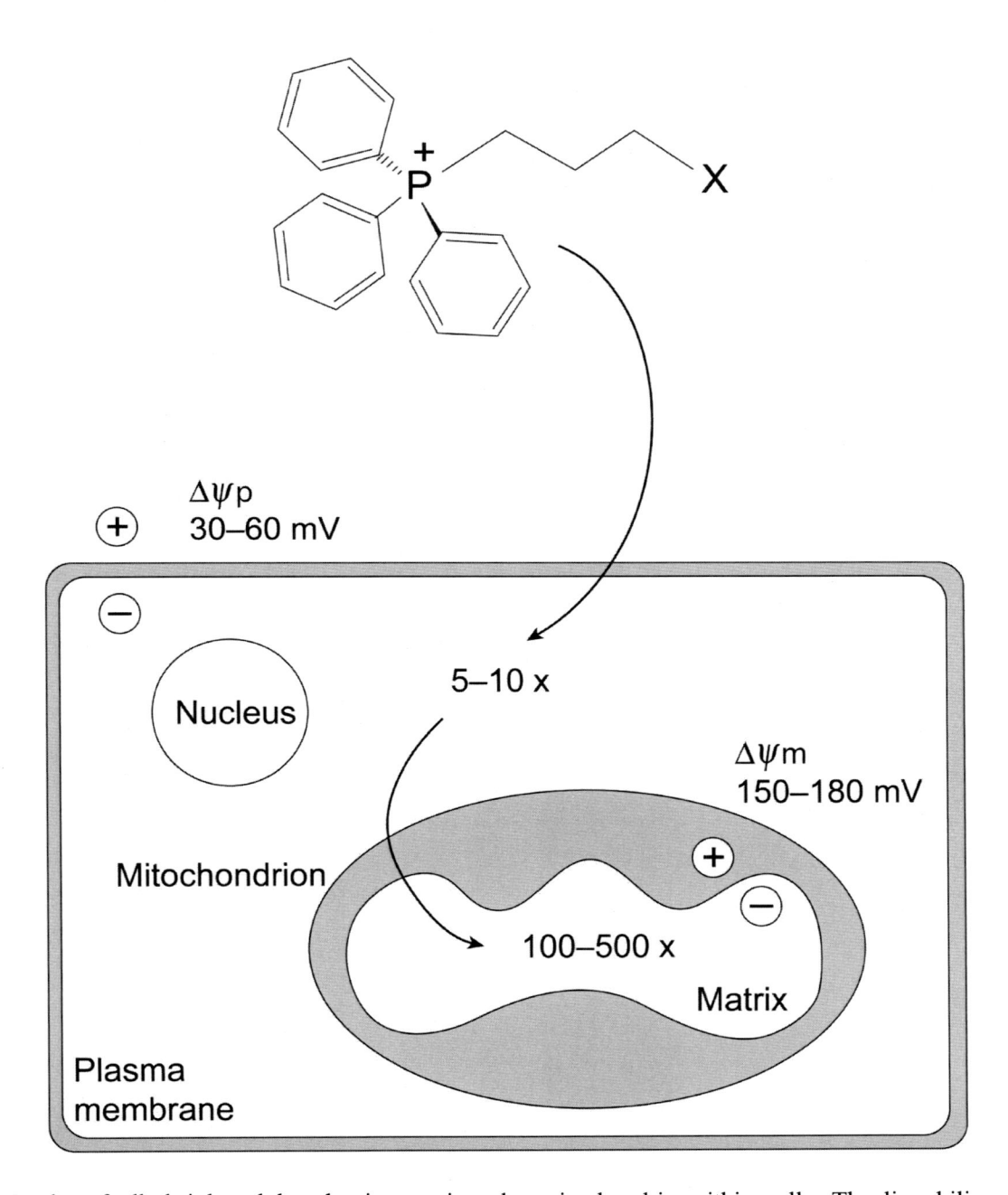

Fig. 10-2 Uptake of alkyltriphenylphosphonium cations by mitochondria within cells. The lipophilic triphenylphosphonium cation is covalently attached to a biologically active molecule (X) such as an antioxidant or pharmacophore. The lipophilic cation is accumulated 5- to 10-fold into the cytoplasm from

the extracellular space by the plasma membrane potential ($\Delta\psi_p$) and then further accumulated 100- to 500-fold into the mitochondrial matrix by the mitochondrial membrane potential ($\Delta\psi_m$). As these lipophilic cations pass directly through the lipid bilayer they do not utilize specific uptake systems and have the potential to distribute to mitochondria in all organs, including the brain. Adopted from ref. 2 with permission

This approach for mitochondrial targeting can be used for any neutral, bioactive chemical. As a first step, we chose to develop antioxidants that target the mitochondria, as the respiratory chain is the primary source of reactive oxygen species in vivo, and mitochondrial oxidative damage is thought to be a proximal cause of pathology in a number of the diseases listed in the previous section. Given that vitamin E and coenzyme Q are believed to protect mitochondria from oxidative damage in vivo, we produced mitochondria-targeted analogues of these compounds (Fig. 10-3). Experiments in vitro demonstrated that [2-(3,4-dihydro-6-hydroxy-2,5,7,8-tetramethyl-2H-1-benzopyran-2-yl) ethyl] triphenyl phosphonium bromide (MitoVit E) and a mixture of mitoquinol [10-(3,6-dihydroxy-4,5-dimethoxy-2-methyl-2-methylphenyl) decyl] triphenylphosponium. Isolated mitochondria and mitochondria within isolated cells accumulated triphenylphosphonium bromide (MitoQ) fast and selectively. Notably, mitochondrial accumulation of these antioxidants protected them against oxidative damage significantly more efficiently than untargeted antioxidants, implying that accumulation of bioactive compounds within mitochondria does boost their efficacy.

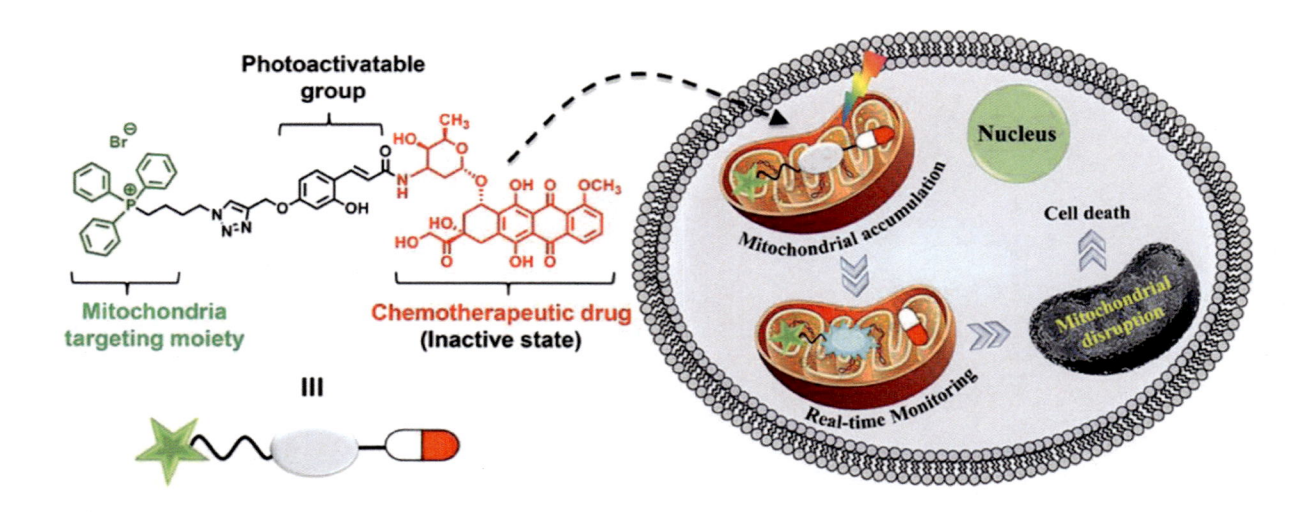

Fig. 10-3 The system is comprised of a model anticancer drug doxorubicin, an alkyltriphenylphosphonium moiety to target mitochondria in cancer cells, and a hydroxycinnamate photoactivatable linker that is covalently attached to the drug and mitochondria-targeting moieties such that it can be phototriggered by either UV (one-photon) or NIR (two-photon) light to form a fluorescent coumarin product and facilitate the release of drug payload. Adopted from ref. 3 with permission.

E. Folic acid based targeting strategy

Background

Folic acid has emerged as an optimal targeting ligand for selective delivery of attached imaging and therapeutic agents to cancer tissues and sites of inflammation. The utility of folic acid in these applications has arisen primarily from (1) its ease of conjugation to both therapeutic and diagnostic agents, (2) its high affinity for the folate receptor ($K_d = 10^{-10}$ M), even after conjugation to its therapeutic/diagnostic cargo, and (3) the limited distribution of its receptor (FR) in normal tissues, despite its upregulation on both cancer cells (primarily FR-α isoform) and activated macrophages (FR-β isoform). Cancers found to overexpress FR include cancers of the ovary, lung, breast, kidney, brain, endometrium, colon, and hematopoietic cells of myelogenous origin. Because activated macrophages are implicated in such pathologies as rheumatoid arthritis, psoriasis, Crohn's disease, systemic lupus erythematosus, atherosclerosis, diabetes, ulcerative colitis,

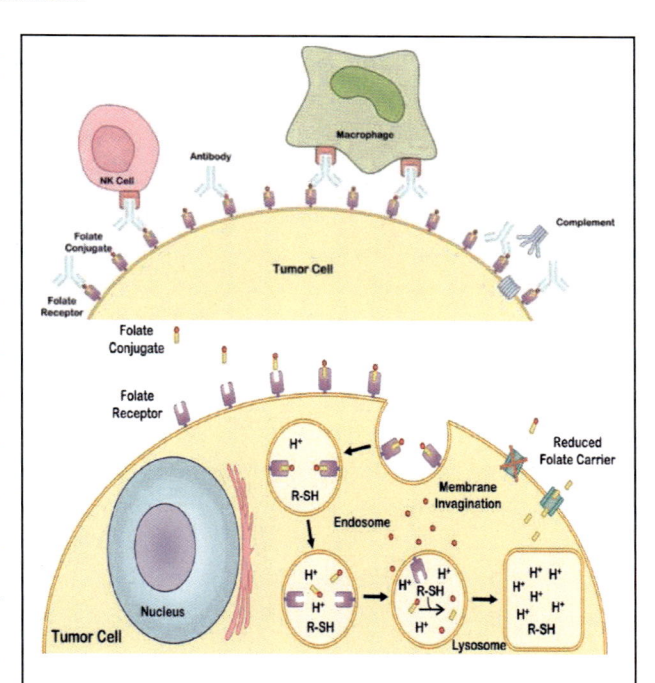

Figure 10-4 **Top:** Illustration of folate–hapten-mediated immunotherapy. Mice previously immunized against the hapten (fluorescein) are treated with folate–fluorescein. Folate targeting decorates the cancer cell surface with large numbers of foreign haptens (>106), leading to antihapten (antifluorescein) antibody binding and destruction of the marked tumor cell by macrophages, natural killer cells, and complement. **Bottom:** FR-mediated endocytosis of a folic acid drug conjugate. Folate conjugates bind FR with high affinity and are subsequently internalized into endosomes that can reduce disulfide bonds. Within the endosome, a folate–disulfide–drug conjugate is released from the FR and the prodrug is reduced to liberate the parent drug cargo. Because the pH of FR-containing endosomes is only mildly acidic, acid-labile linkers do not release the attached drug as efficiently. Adopted from ref. 4 with permission

osteoarthritis, glomerulonephritis, and sarcoidosis, applications for folate targeting now also include most inflammatory diseases. While FR-directed antifolates have proven useful in the treatment of some of the above diseases (Figure 10-4)

One additional aspect that is important for folic-acid-mediated drug delivery concerns the rate of FR recycling between the cell surface and its intracellular compartments. Net accumulation of folate conjugates in tumor tissues will depend upon not only the number and accessibility of FR on the malignant cell surfaces but also the time required for unoccupied receptors to recycle back to the cell surface for additional drug uptake. Using radioactive conjugates, we found empty FR+ to unload their cargo and return to the cell surface in ~8–12 h. Given that

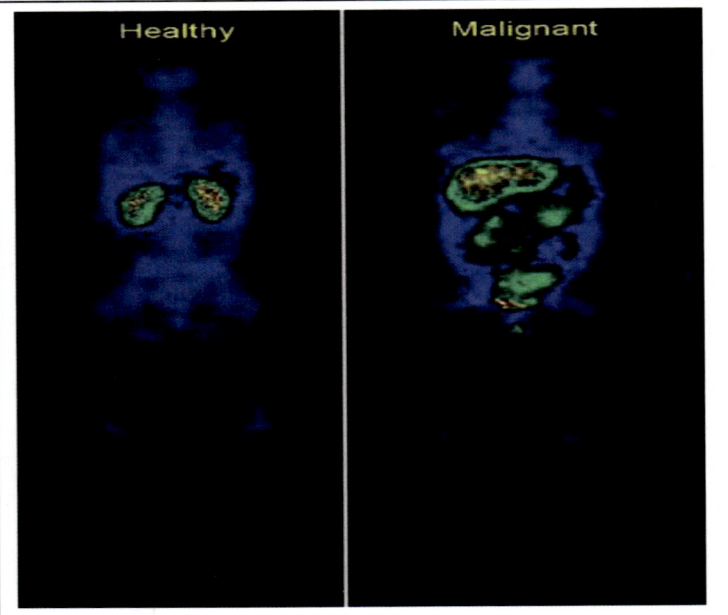

Figure 10-5 ^{111}In–DTPA–folate whole body scintigraphic images of a healthy volunteer and an ovarian cancer patient. Uptake in the cancer patient is seen in both the malignant tissue and kidneys, whereas only kidney uptake is observed in the healthy individual. Adopted from ref. 4 with permission

an average cancer cell will express anywhere from ~0 to 10^7 FR/cell, this recycling time constraint suggested that only very potent chemotherapeutic agents could succeed as folate conjugates for the treatment of cancer. In our experience, agents possessing low nanomolar range IC$_{50}$ values in their unconjugated forms have the highest potential for *in vivo* efficacy. (Figure 10-5)

Concern about folate conjugate distribution in humans, however, would not be allayed until images of cancer patients were obtained. ^{111}In–DTPA–folate was moved rapidly into the clinic, and images similar to those shown in Figure 10-5 were collected. As seen, the absence of a significant uptake in liver, spleen, bone marrow, heart, lungs, brain, muscle, etc. argued that the tumor/kidney selectivity seen in animals was also realized in humans. Also of importance was the observation that the ^{111}In–DTPA–folate would clear from FR-negative tissues in less than 1 h, suggesting that isotopes with shorter half-lives than ^{111}In could be developed for tumor imaging. Motivated by this realization, Endocyte, a company founded to develop folate-targeted imaging and therapeutic agents, designed EC20, a [99mTc]-based folate-linked chelator. Because of its shorter half-life and the consequent lower radiation exposure, EC20 has proven to be the γ-emitter of choice for cancer and inflammation imaging.

Folic acid-quantum dots for tumor targeting

As an example, here we describe the preparation, luminescence, and cancer targeting properties of folic acid-CdTe quantum dot conjugates. Water-soluble CdTe quantum dots were synthesized and conjugated with folic acid using 1-ethyl-3-(3-dimethylaminopropyl) carbodiimide-N-hydroxysuccinimide chemistry. The influence of folic acid on the luminescence properties of CdTe quantum dots was investigated, and no energy transfer between them was observed. To investigate the efficiency of folic acid-CdTe nanoconjugates for tumor targeting, pure CdTe quantum dots and folic acid-coated CdTe quantum dots were incubated with human nasopharyngeal epidermal carcinoma cell line with positive expressing folic acid receptors (KB cells) and lung cancer cells without expression of folic acid receptors (A549 cells). For the cancer cells with positive folate receptors (KB cells), the uptake for CdTe quantum dots is very low, but for folic acid-CdTe nanoconjugates, the uptake is very high. For the lung cancer cells without folate receptors (A549 cells), the uptake for folic acid-CdTe nanoconjugates is also very low. The results indicate that folic acid is an effective targeting molecule for tumor cells with overexpressed folate receptors.

To synthesize CdTe quantum dots, 1.463 g (4.70 mmol) $Cd(ClO_4)_2 \cdot H_2O$ was dissolved in 125 ml deionized (DI) water, and 0.793 ml (11.4 mmol) thioglyocolic acid was added to the aforementioned solution while stirring. The pH of the solution was adjusted to 11.5 by adding 0.5 M NaOH dropwise. Transferring the solution to a three-necked flask and degassing it with Ar gas for ten minutes; 0.4 g of Al_2Te_3 was charged into a tiny three-necked flask. H_2Te_3 gas was bubbled through the solution for 5 minutes following the addition of 3 ml of 0.5 M H_2SO_4 to Al_2Te_3. Due to the production of CdTe precursors, the solution turned orange. To stimulate the formation of nanocrystals, the CdTe precursor solution was refluxed at 100°C in open air with a condenser attached. EDC-NHS chemistry was used to conjugate folic acid to TGA-coated CdTe quantum dots (Hermanson 1996; Wang et al. 2002); 0.05 M EDC-NHS (EDC/NHS=1:10) and 0.05 M QDs were combined for 5 minutes. The aforementioned solution was then added in an equal molar ratio of 0.05 M folic acid and gently stirred at room temperature overnight. The unreacted compounds

(EDC, NHS, folic acid, and QDs) were removed for 1 day through dialysis against pH-adjusted de-ionized water (pH 11–12). The dialysis membrane had a molecular weight cutoff of 12,000 Da.

The addition of EDC and NHS to the QD solution resulted in the creation of a highly reactive intermediate (NHS-carboxylate). This activated ester was then reacted with the free amino group of folic acid to form the folic acid nanoconjugates containing CdTe quantum dots seen in Fig. 10-6. The effective conjugation of folic acid to CdTe quantum dots was confirmed using FTIR and HPLC. The IR spectra of CdTe QDs and CdTe-folic acid nanoconjugates are shown in Figure 10-7. The FTIR spectra of CdTe quantum dots reveals no absorption band at 2,570 cm^{-1}, indicating that the thioglycolic molecules were bonded to the CdTe nanoparticles' surface via the sulphur atom in the mercapto group. CdTe-folic acid nanoconjugates exhibit an OH stretching band at 3,368 cm1 and an asymmetric CO2 stretching band at 2,356 cm^{-1}. At 1,655 and 1,558 cm^{-1}, respectively, the complex bands –CO-NH2 and –CO-NH define the amide bond. The –CO-NH mode is composed of contributions from the C-N stretching vibration and the –NH bending vibration, which are caused by the carboxyl groups of the TGA-capped QDs connecting with the amide groups of the folic acid. Within the region of 1,476–1,695 cm^{-1}, the aromatic ring stretching of the pteridine ring and the p-amino benzoic acid groups of folic acid show. The symmetric vibrations of the carboxylic group at 1,556 and 1,377 cm^{-1} in the CdTe-folic acid nanoconjugate spectrum obscure the bending vibrations of the NH group in folic acid in the region of 1,500–1,600 cm^{-1}. Thus, the infrared spectrum clearly indicates that folic acid was successfully coupled to the CdTe quantum dots.

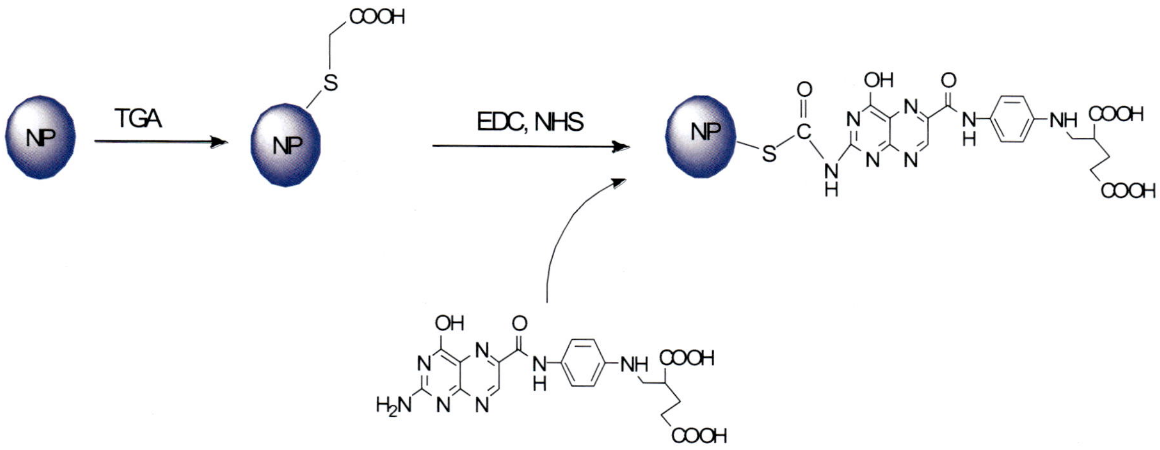

Figure 10-6. A schematic illustration depicting the conjugation chemistry of folic acid to TGA-coated CdTe quatum dots via EDC-NHS reactions. Adopted from ref. 5 with permission

The retention period of folic acid on the SEC-HPLC column was 12.7 minutes with a peak UV absorbance of 281.6 nm when eluted with 0.1 M phosphate buffer containing 0.15 M NaCl (pH 7.4) at a flow rate of 1.0 mL/min. Intriguingly, the QDs exhibited extremely weak UV signals devoid of typical absorption peaks. A fluorescence detector would be more suitable for detecting QDs. As expected, the folate-conjugated QDs exhibited a UV peak at 10.4 minutes and a UV–VIS spectrum comparable to that of folic acid, demonstrating the production of folate-QD nanoconjugates.

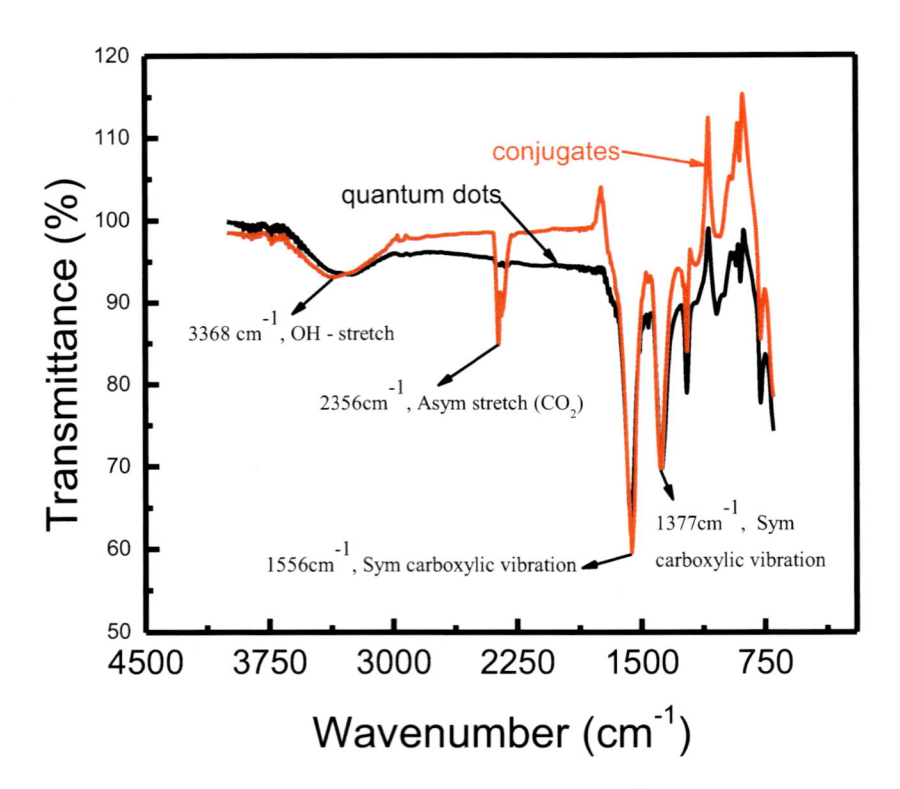

Figure 10-7: FTIR spectra of CdTe quantum dots and CdTe quantum dots conjugated to folic acid. Adopted from ref. 5 with permission

Luminescence characteristics

Fig. 10-8 illustrates the luminescence spectra of CdTe quantum dots, folic acid, and CdTe-folic acid nanoconjugates. TGA-coated CdTe QDs exhibit a small, symmetric emission peak at 631 nm, which has been extensively documented. Folic acid exhibits an emission band peaking at around 458 nm, which is consistent with previous reports. CdTe-folic acid nanoconjugates have two emission lines at 460 and 630 nm, respectively. The emission at 460 nm is assigned to folic acid, while the emission at 630 nm is due to CdTe quantum dots.

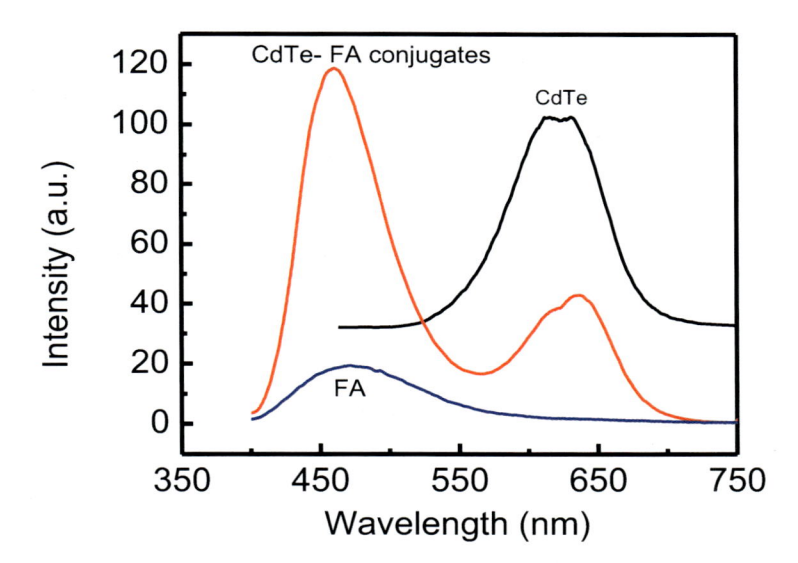

Figure 10-8: Photoluminescence spectra of CdTe quantum dots excited at 450 nm (black), CdTe quantum dot- folic acid conjugates excited at 380 nm (red), and folic acid excited at 380 nm (FA, blue). Adopted from ref. 5 with permission

As illustrated in Fig. 10-8, the emission peaks of folic acid overlap with the absorption band of CdTe quantum dots. Energy transfer from folic acid to CdTe quantum dots might theoretically occur in CdTe-folic acid nanoconjugates. The emission spectra of CdTe quantum dots, CdTe-folic acid nanoconjugates, and a CdTe-folic acid mixture stimulated at 380 and 285 nm, respectively. The concentration of CdTe quantum dots is identical in all three samples. The emission of CdTe quantum dots in CdTe-folic acid conjugates and mixtures is weaker than in CdTe quantum dot solution when excited at 380 nm. Folic acid emits two wavelengths at 360 and 450 nm in response to stimulation at 285 nm. Both of the above-mentioned emissions have been documented in the scientific literature. For excitation at 285 nm, the emission of CdTe quantum dots in the CdTe-folic acid combination is slightly stronger than that of CdTe quantum dots in solution, but it is still weaker than that of CdTe quantum dots in conjugates. It was anticipated that energy transfer from folic acid would improve the emission of CdTe quantum dots in CdTe-folic acid nanoconjugates. In comparison to pure CdTe quantum dots, the luminosity of CdTe quantum dots in CdTe-folic acid nanoconjugates is quenched. This suggests that no energy transfer occurs between folic acid and CdTe quantum dots in the nanoconjugates. To further study the possibility of energy transfer from folic acid to CdTe quantum dots, we evaluated the folic acid luminescence lifetimes at 450 nm in solution and CdTe-folic acid nanoconjugates. The energy transfer from the folic acid to the CdTe would be manifested by a decrease in the lifespan of the folic acid in the nanoconjugates. As a result, this system exhibits no signs of energy transfer.

Even though the quantum dot luminescence is quenched somewhat by folic acid, the conjugates still have fairly intense luminescence after conjugation, which allows for cell imaging or labeling. To investigate the efficiency of folic acid-CdTe nanoconjugates for tumor targeting, pure CdTe quantum dots and folic acid coated CdTe quantum dots were incubated with human nasopharyngeal epidermal carcinoma cell line with positive folic acid receptors (KB cells) and lung cancer cells with negative folic acid receptors (A549 cells). Figure 10-9 displays the results of the uptake of the CdTe quantum dots (on the left) and the CdTe-folic acid nanoconjugates (one the right) by the KB cells after incubation for 2, 4 and 8 hours, respectively. It is noted that the colors in the images are arbitary and the green emission from the cells is probably from proteins or other molecules attached to the cells. Only the red or yellowish emissions are from the CdTe quantum dots. Clearly, the uptake of the CdTe-folic acid nanoconjugates by the KB cells is very high, while the uptake of the KB cells to the pure TGA-coated CdTe quantum dots is negligeable. Figure 10-10 shows the the uptake of the CdTe quantum dots (on the left) and the CdTe-folic acid nanoconjugates (one the right) by the A549 cells after incubation for 2, 4 and 8 hours, respectively. The results show that almost no CdTe quantum dots or CdTe-folic acid conjugates were uptaken by the A549 cells. Figure 10-11 shows the uptake of CdTe-folic acid nanoconjugates by KB cells and A549 cells after incubation for 2, 4 and 8 hours, respectively. As expected, the uptake of the CdTe-folic acid conjugates by KB cells is very high, but by A549 cells is almost nonexistent. Our observations demonstrate clearly the affinity and selectivity of folic acid as a targeting ligand for tumor cells with positive folate receptors.

KB cells with QDs   KB cells with QD-FA

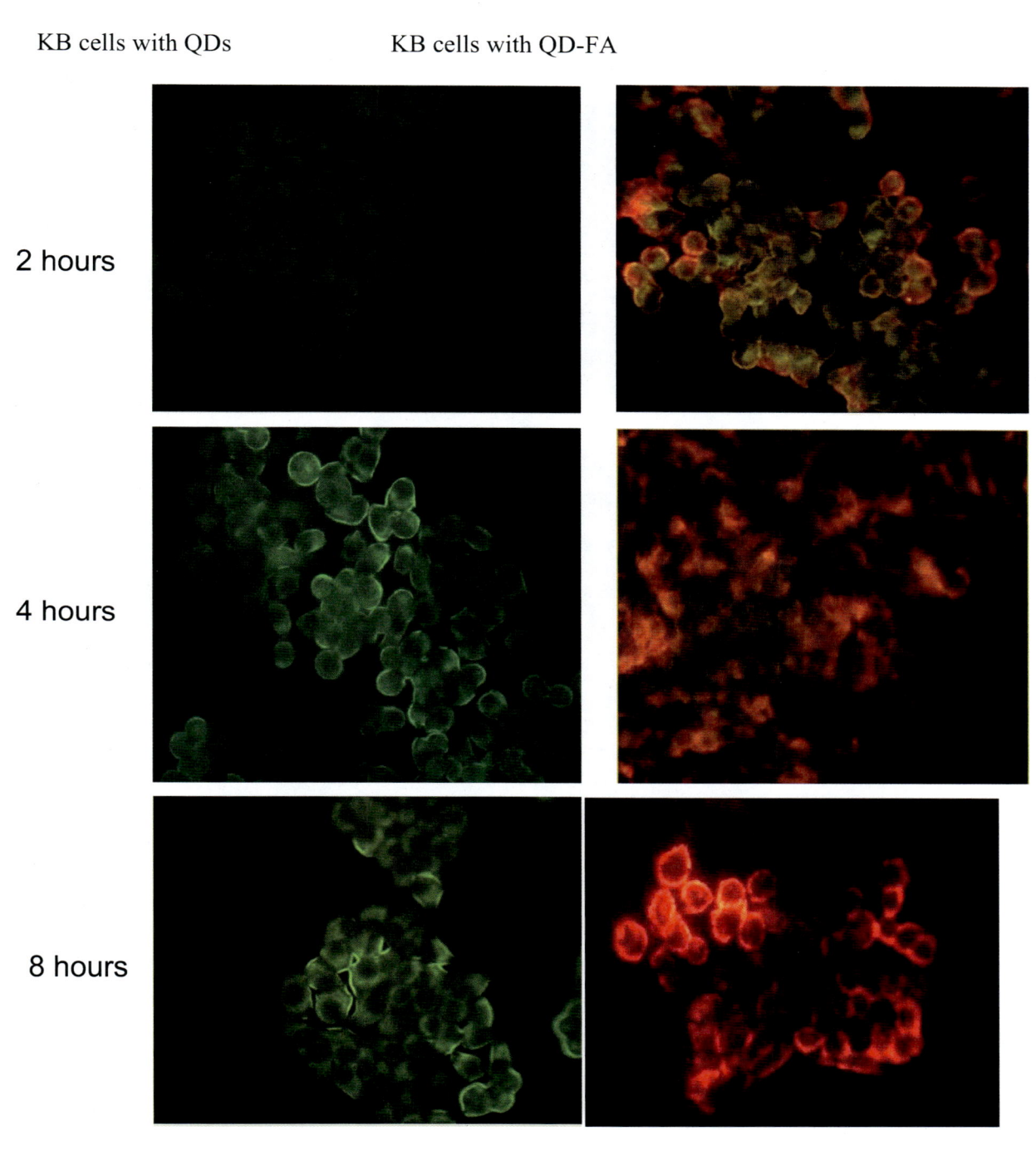

2 hours

4 hours

8 hours

Figure 10-9. Micrographs of KB cells incubated with QD/QDFA obtained through fluorescence microscopy as observed under the 20X objective. Green = Unlabeled human nasopharyngeal epidermal carcinoma cell line over-expressing surface receptors for folic acid. Red = KB cells labeled with folic acid conjugated quantum dots. Adopted from ref. 5 with permission

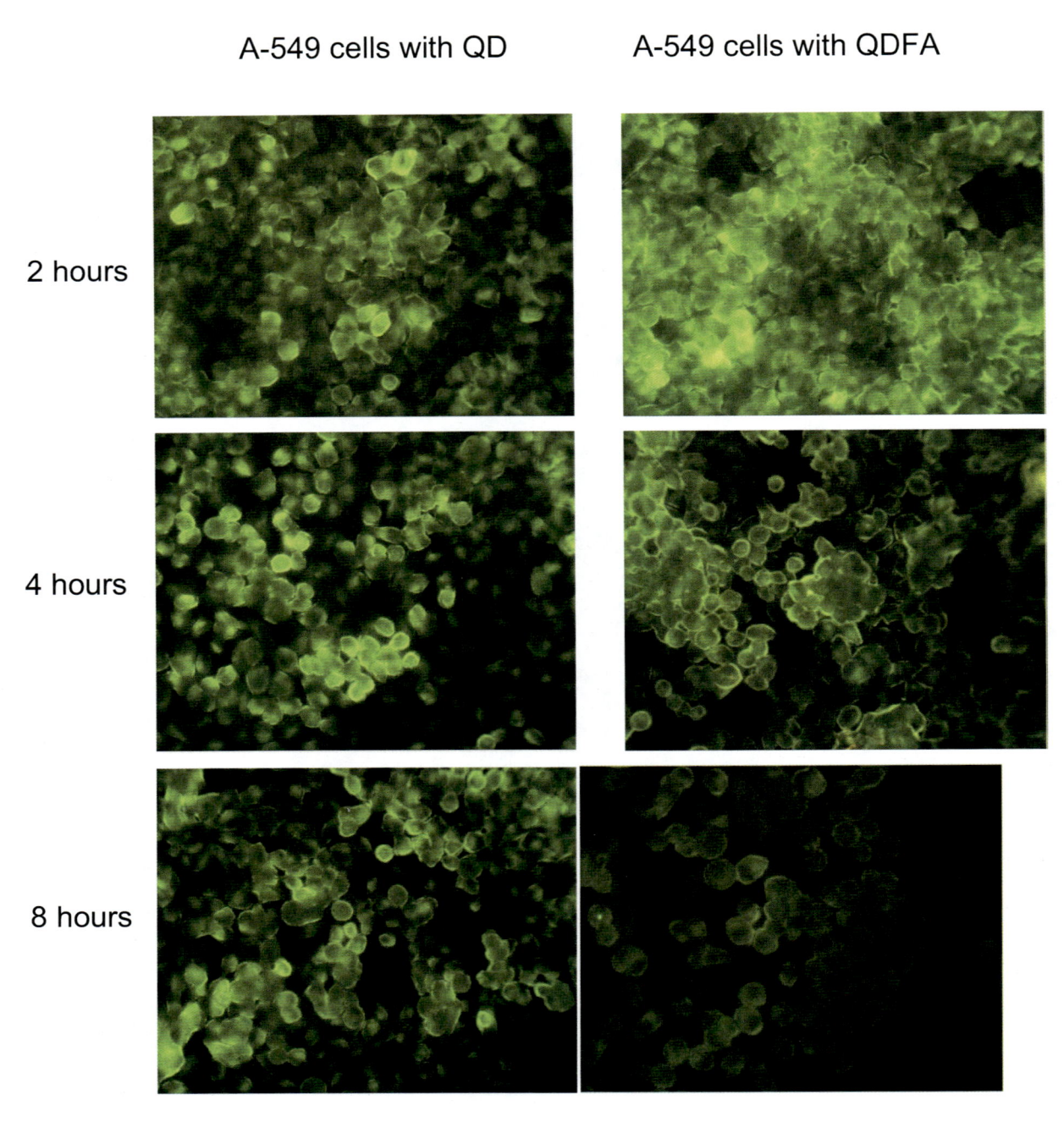

Figure 10-10. Micrographs of A549 cells incubated with QD/QDFA obtained through fluorescence microscopy as observed under the 20X objective. Green = Human lung carcinoma cell line lacking folic acid receptors Adopted from ref. 5 with permission

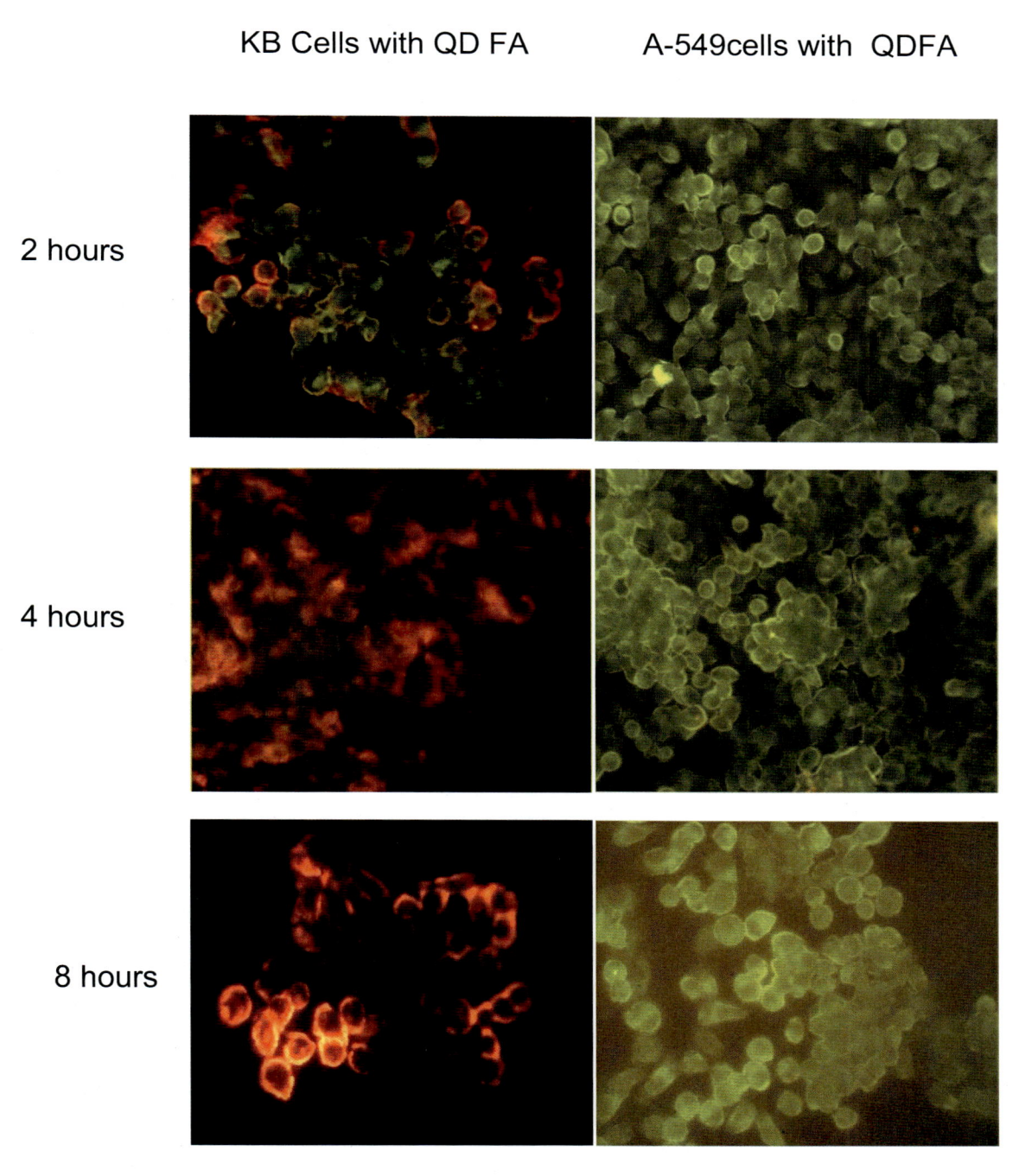

	KB Cells with QD FA	A-549 cells with QDFA
2 hours		
4 hours		
8 hours		

Figure 10-11: Column 1: Represents the ability of the folate receptors to bind to the folic acid coated QDs, thereby labeling the cells. Green= Unlabeled KB cells. Orange/red = KB cells labeled with folic acid coated QD. Column 2: Represents the inability of the A549 cells to bind the folic acid coated QD, due to the lack of folate receptors on their surface. Green (on row 2) = A549 cells
Adopted from ref. 5 with permission

F. Low pH sensitive peptides for tumor targeting

The discovery of low pH sensitive peptides (pHLIPs) is an example illustrating how basic research can lead to translational innovations. In the 1990s, the Engelman lab was investigating transmembrane peptide interactions using a seven-helix membrane-spanning protein, Bacteriorhodopsin. When one helix, isolated from the protein, failed to form a transmembrane helix, the team noted that its transmembrane domain contains two aspartic acid residues, which would bear negative charges near neutral pH. As hoped, when the reaction conditions were made acidic, these residues became protonated and the peptide formed a transmembrane helix. With the realization that the pH at which this transition occurred coincided with the acidity of cancerous tumors, the bacteriorhodopsin C-helix became the basis of what would become an important new tool for targeting such pathologies *in vivo*.

"Wild-type" pHLIP originally derived from the C-helix of bacteriorhodopsin, contains polar ends and a central transmembrane domain, containing two aspartic acid residues, which impart its pH-dependent activity. (Figure 10-12)

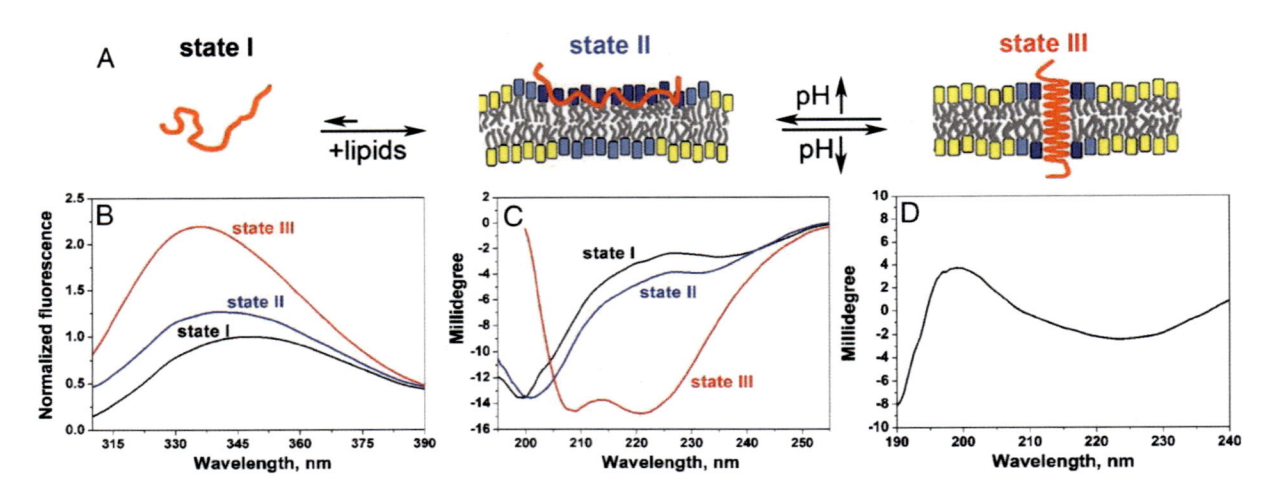

Figure 10-12 A) A schematic representation of pHLIP in solution and interacting with a lipid bilayer at neutral and low pHs is shown. State I refers to the peptide in solution at normal and basic pHs. Upon addition of vesicles at pH 8, the unstructured peptide is adsorbed on the membrane surface (State II). A drop of pH leads to the protonation of Asp residues, increasing peptide hydrophobicity, and resulting in the insertion and formation of a transmembrane α-helix (State II).

Lipids interacting with the peptide directly are marked with blue head groups, lipids influenced by the interaction but not interacting with the peptide directly have cyan head groups, and lipids that are not involved in the interaction with pHLIP have yellow head groups (8). Transitions between states can be monitored by (*B*) changes of fluorescence and (*C*) circular dichroism (CD) spectral signals. The fluorescence and CD spectra of pHLIP at pH8 (*Black Lines*) indicate an unstructured configuration with tryptophan residues fully exposed to solvent. Incubation of pHLIP with liposomes at pH8 (*Blue Lines*) induces the partial burial of tryptophan residues inside the lipid bilayer without helix formation. Decreasing the pH to 4.0 by the addition of HCl (*Red Lines*) induces the insertion of pHLIP and helix formation. (*D*) The transmembrane orientation of the helix has been confirmed by OCD. Adopted from ref. 6 with permission

State I - pHLIPs are largely unstructured as soluble monomers or low-order multimers in aqueous solution

State II - In the presence of membranes, pHLIPs remain largely unstructured at neutral and basic pH and bind reversibly to the outer leaflet of the membrane as monomers

State III - In acidic conditions (below pH ~6) pHLIPs form stable, monomeric transmembrane alpha-helixes, inserting their C-termini into the lumen of liposomes or into the cytosol of cells

pHLIPs Target Acidic Pathologies

At normal physiological pH, ~7.4, pHLIPs exist in States I and II, interacting with the outside surface of cells but exchanging with the aqueous surroundings. A number of pathological conditions produce a more acidic extracellular environment due to the affects of hypoxia, ischemia, or abnormal metabolic processes. A significant example of such acidity is in solid tumors. Due to their heightened metabolic activity, their compromised blood supply, membrane bound carbonic anhydrase activity, and to the Warburg effect, cancerous tumors produce a significantly acidic extracellular environment of around pH 6. In a serendipitous coincidence, this pH is sufficiently low to protonate the aspartic acid residues in pHLIPs' transmembrane domain, causing pHLIPs to insert into cells, where they are relatively stable and thereby accumulate in the cells of acidic tumors. (Figure 10-13)

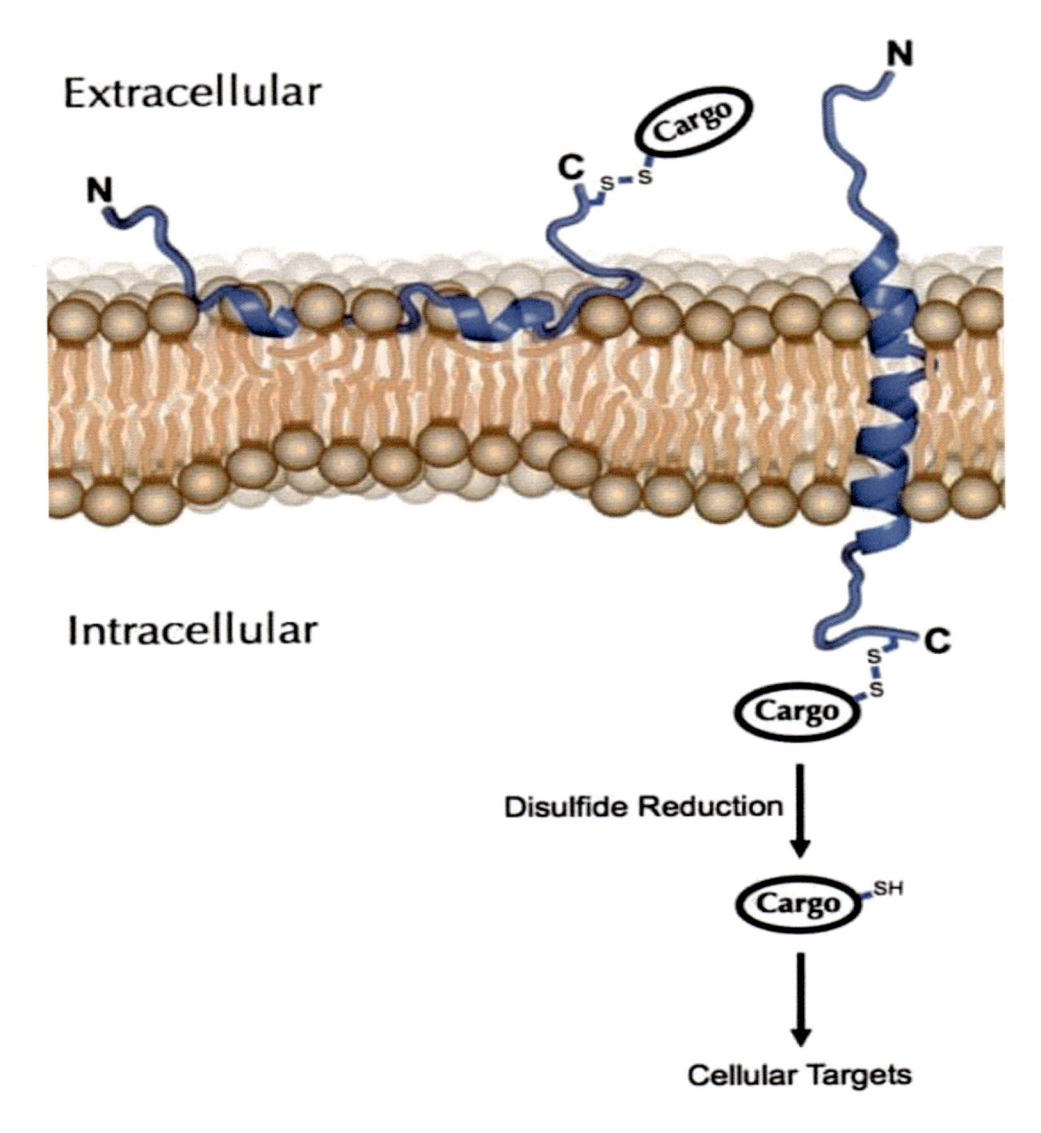

Figure 10-13 Applications of pHLIP Targeting adopted from ref. 7 with permission

pHLIP insertion occurs directionally and with a favorable Gibbs free energy change. Therefore, cargos associated with pHLIPs' N-terminus will be localized to the targeted tissues and upon insertion will decorate the cell surface. Such surface binding has been used to localize imaging agents, such as fluorophores, nanogold particles, and PET or SPECT tracers as well as to deliver liposomes loaded with therapeutic cargos to the extracellular environment of tumors, *in vivo*. (Figure 10-14) The insertion of the C-terminus occurs favorably enough to facilitate the delivery of large molecular cargos bound to the C-termini of pHLIPs. Using biologically labile reversible linkages, such as disulfide bonds between cysteine residues in the pHLIP C-terminus and thiols in the cargo, cytosolic delivery has been achieved for a number of cargoes, including peptides, small molecules, and even large peptide-nucleic acids. These approaches represent a new mode of targeted drug-delivery, directly into the cytosol of the targeted cells without the use of disruptive carriers, such as cell-penetrating peptides (CPPs).

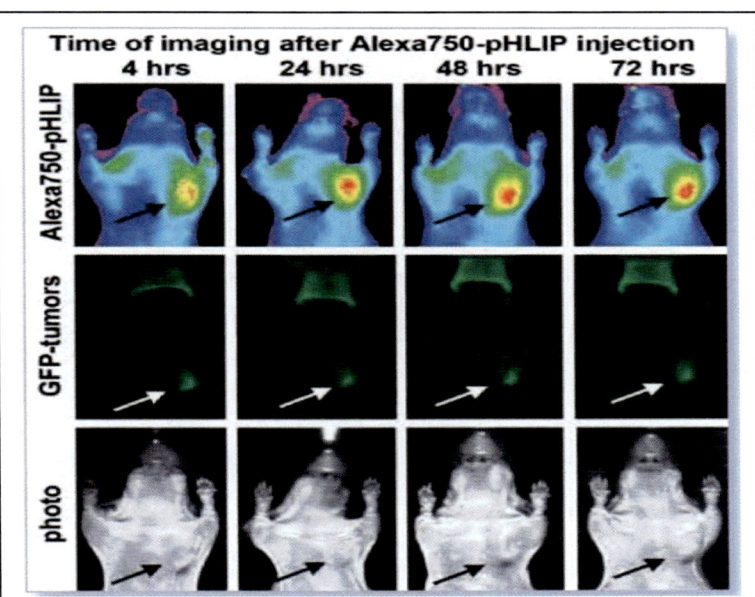

Figure 1-14 Whole-body NIR (Alexa750-pHLIP), GFP fluorescence and light images of mouse bearing tumour are shown. Highly metastatic M4A4 cells derived from the human melanoma cancer cell line, MDA-MB-435, were used to establish tumour. Fluorescently labelled pHLIP (Alexa750 was covalently attached to the Cys residue at the N-terminus of peptide) was given as a single iv injection (0.8 mg/kg). The images were obtained on the FX Kodak in-vivo image station combined with a gas anaesthesia system at 4, 24, 48 and 72 hours post-injection. Tumor indicated by arrows. Tumour targeting was observed already after 4 hours after injection of fluorescent pHLIP, and peptide stays in tumor during several days. Images obtained at various time points presented with maximum contrast between tumor and other tissue. Adopted from ref. 8 with permission

References for this chapter

1. D'Souza GG, Wagle MA, Saxena V, Shah A. Approaches for targeting mitochondria in cancer therapy. Biochim Biophys Acta. 2011 Jun;1807(6):689-96. doi: 10.1016/j.bbabio.2010.08.008. Epub 2010 Aug 21. PMID: 20732297.

2. Smith RA, Porteous CM, Gane AM, Murphy MP. Delivery of bioactive molecules to mitochondria in vivo. Proc Natl Acad Sci U S A. 2003 Apr 29;100(9):5407-12. doi: 10.1073/pnas.0931245100. Epub 2003 Apr 15. PMID: 12697897; PMCID: PMC154358.

3. Singh N, Gupta A, Prasad P, Sah RK, Singh A, Kumar S, Singh S, Gupta S, Sasmal PK. Mitochondria-Targeted Photoactivatable Real-Time Monitoring of a Controlled Drug Delivery Platform. J Med Chem. 2021 Dec 23;64(24):17813-17823. doi: 10.1021/acs.jmedchem.1c00956. Epub 2021 Dec 10. PMID: 34886661.

4. Low PS, Henne WA, Doorneweerd DD. Discovery and development of folic-acid-based receptor targeting for imaging and therapy of cancer and inflammatory diseases. Acc Chem Res. 2008 Jan;41(1):120-9. doi: 10.1021/ar7000815. Epub 2007 Jul 27. PMID: 17655275.

5. Preethi Suriamoorthy, Xing Zhang, Guiyang Hao, Alan G. Joly, Surya Singh, Marius Hossu, Xiankai Sun, and **Wei Chen,** Folic Acid-CdTe Quantum Dot Conjugates and Their Applications for Cancer Cell Targeting, *Cancer Nanotechnology*, 2010, 1(1): 19-28

6. Andreev OA, Karabadzhak AG, Weerakkody D, Andreev GO, Engelman DM, Reshetnyak YK. pH (low) insertion peptide (pHLIP) inserts across a lipid bilayer as a helix and exits by a different path. Proc Natl Acad Sci U S A. 2010 Mar 2;107(9):4081-6. doi: 10.1073/pnas.0914330107. Epub 2010 Feb 16. PMID: 20160113; PMCID: PMC2840156.
https://medicine.yale.edu/lab/engelman/research/phlips/

7. Andreev OA, Dupuy AD, Segala M, Sandugu S, Serra DA, Chichester CO, Engelman DM, Reshetnyak YK. Mechanism and uses of a membrane peptide that targets tumors and other acidic tissues in vivo. Proc Natl Acad Sci U S A. 2007 May 8;104(19):7893-8. doi: 10.1073/pnas.0702439104. Epub 2007 May 1. PMID: 17483464; PMCID: PMC1861852

8. Samana Shrestha, Jing Wu, Bindeshwar Sah, Adam Vanasse, Leon N Cooper, Lun Ma, Gen Li, Huibin Zheng, **Wei Chen** and Michael P. Antosh, X-ray Induced Photodynamic Therapy with pH-Low Insertion Peptide Targeted Copper-Cysteamine Nanoparticles in Mice, *PNAS*, 2019,116(34): 16823–16828

Made in the USA
Columbia, SC
26 April 2024

3364e30f-8aae-45cb-97cf-d4a68a53e499R01